.ibrar

COMPLEMENTARY AND ALTERNATIVE MEDICINE

English edition
First published in 2011 by
Berg
Editorial offices:
49–51 Bedford Square, London WC1B 3DP, UK
175 Fifth Avenue, New York, NY 10010, USA

© Ruth Barcan 2011

Berg is the imprint of Bloomsbury Publishing Plc.

Library of Congress Cataloging-in-Publication Data

Barcan, Ruth.
    Complementary and alternative medicine : bodies, therapies, senses /
Ruth Barcan. — English ed.
        p. ; cm.
    Includes bibliographical references and index.
    ISBN 978-1-84520-742-7 (cloth) — ISBN 978-1-84520-743-4 (pbk.) —
ISBN 978-0-85785-093-5 (e-ISBN (individual))
    1. Alternative medicine. I. Title.
    [DNLM: 1. Complementary Therapies. WB 890]
    R733.B267 2011
    615.5—dc23

                                        2011014898

British Library Cataloguing-in-Publication Data

A catalogue record for this book is available from the British Library.

ISBN   978 1 84520 742 7 (Cloth)
        978 1 84520 743 4 (Paper)
e-ISBN 978 0 85785 093 5 (Individual)

Typeset by JS Typesetting Ltd, Porthcawl, Mid Glamorgan.
Printed in the UK by the MPG Books Group

www.bergpublishers.com

COMPLEMENTARY AND ALTERNATIVE MEDICINE

Bodies, Therapies, Senses

Ruth Barcan

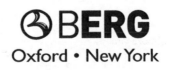

Oxford • New York

CONTENTS

Acknowledgements   vii

1   Introduction: The Body Therapeutic   1

2   The Power of Sight   55

3   Sound: Good Vibrations   111

4   Knowing Touch: Bodywork   141

5   The Sixth Sense: Intuition   185

6   Conclusion   213

Notes   221
References   231
Index   249

ACKNOWLEDGEMENTS

The foundations of this book were laid some twenty years ago, when I did an introductory course in massage at a community college. From that time on my interest in alternative therapies grew steadily.

Research for the book began shortly after I joined the department of Gender Studies (later, Gender and Cultural Studies) at the University of Sydney, and was aided by two grants, for which I am most grateful: one from the School of Philosophical and Historical Inquiry (SOPHI) and the other from the Faculty of Arts FARSS scheme. I offer my sincere thanks to my colleagues in SOPHI and in Gender and Cultural Studies, who provide a warm and insightful climate in which to research and try out new ideas. Indeed, I have been fortunate throughout my academic career to find myself among colleagues who can appreciate the value of thinking waywardly but whose rigour and critical insight have helped keep me on track. And so I warmly thank my colleagues at the University of Sydney and also recall with fondness my former colleagues at the School of Humanities at the University of Western Sydney, in particular Jane Goodall and Fiona Mackie, who helped me find quasi-respectable ways to think the unthinkable.

My thinking has also been enriched by the many CAM practitioners with whom I've come in contact over the years. Thank you for the life-enhancing experiences and the conversations – enlightening, provoking and everything in between. In particular, I thank my interviewees for their time, expertise and generosity of spirit. This book would not have been possible without your input. It is, to recall Maurice Merleau-Ponty, a conversation I did not know myself capable of – indeed, *was* not capable of – until you joined in.

Other participants in this conversation were the colleagues and friends who read drafts of sections of the book. I particularly thank those who read some of the more adventurous sections. I am extremely grateful for the input of Sarah Cefai, Davina Cooper, Shé Mackenzie Hawke, Roz and Bruce Helyard, David Howes, Drew Leder and Jane Simon. Jay Johnston and Anna Gibbs have, in particular, been intellectual companions and critics of the greatest acuity. Many other friends and colleagues have sustained me over the long period in which this book was researched and written, and I thank them all.

David Howes has been a generous reader and supporter of this work, and I am grateful to him for that, and also for his inspiration in his capacity as one of the pioneers of sensory studies and as the series editor of the wonderful *Sensory Formations* books published by Berg. These books brought together in inspiring form a wealth of material from across the disciplines that I have found very useful.

The book's progress was greatly aided by intelligent and efficient research assistance from Scarlet Wilcock, Jane Simon, Jay Johnston and Anna Marie Swanson, and by Kristen Davis's and Lee Wilson's able and cheery transcription of the interviews, along with that of Catherine Forman. It was also greatly assisted by the resources of the Fisher Library at the University of Sydney and its ever-helpful staff.

The staff at Berg Publishers – in particular Hannah Shakespeare, Anna Wright and Emily Medcalf – were unfailingly efficient and cheerful, and I thank them greatly. Copy-editor George Pitcher was meticulous in a way that gladdened my pedantic heart.

A few pages in Chapter 5 draw on earlier published material: R. Barcan (2009), 'Spiritual Boundary Work: How Spiritual Healers and Medical Clairvoyants Negotiate the Sacred', in E.B. Coleman and K. White (eds), *Medicine, Religion and the Body*, Leiden: Brill, pp. 129–46. I thank the publisher for permission to rework this material.

Finally, I want to thank my wonderful family, as ever. I am lucky to have you. To Mark and Sophia, who lived with this book, thanks and love.

1 INTRODUCTION: THE BODY THERAPEUTIC

The other night my bus was late and I had to sprint for the train. Flinging myself down on a seat moments before the train was due to depart, I was out of breath. The exertion and the cold night air had triggered my asthma. I took a couple of puffs of my inhaler and settled back into my seat as the breath came freely. 'That's amazing stuff', said the man next to me. 'The doctor gave it to our fourteen-month-old last night and he was running around like a maniac all evening'. I agreed it was effective. 'My grandfather died of an asthma attack', I told him. 'A couple of puffs of this would have saved his life.' As we travelled on, the man told me about his experience of the Buteyko breathing method, and how it had more or less completely rid him of asthma. 'It's been around for years', he said, 'but it doesn't get much publicity.' Warming to his theme, he continued: 'You know how I know if something's likely to work? I look at who's *not* advocating it. If the drug companies and the surgeons are condemning it, I know it's worth a try.'

For me, this story epitomizes the contradictions, paradoxes and ambivalence that characterize many Westerners' attitudes to, and use of, both orthodox medicine and its alternatives. In one short conversation, my fellow traveller and I indicated both our need and our gratitude for conventional pharmacology and its potentially life-saving benefits, our suspicion of its institutional correlates and our desire for, and knowledge of, alternatives. In miniature, we articulated a politics of medicine and of knowledge, and we switched rapidly from identifying as grateful consumers of the medical mainstream to empowered, savvy selectors of system-beating alternatives. In that, we typified, I think, an ever-growing sector of the modern Western population – those with sufficient economic and social capital to happily move in and out of the various institutions, therapies and belief structures of an increasingly pluralistic medical system.

This book is born out of my enthusiasm for alternative therapies, but it doesn't proceed from hostility to biomedicine, a system of medicine that excels in the management of symptoms, the extension of life and the management of critical incidents. In my view, there is much to celebrate and to be wary of in both orthodox medicine and its alternatives. My fascination, both practical and intellectual, with alternative medicine as a set of often exciting medical or therapeutic techniques and as a significant social phenomenon does not mean an uncritical acceptance, either medically or ideologically. On the contrary, my engagement with alternative therapies has had to struggle with my training in post-structuralist thought, a thought system hostile to many of the types of discourse central to alternative medicine (discourses of holism, nature and spirit), and with my political leanings, which often sit at odds with the undoubtedly individualistic tenor of therapeutic discourse and with the evident material privilege of those able to make full use of therapeutic culture. Through it all, though, I remain compelled by alternative therapies as both medical and conceptual practices, and despite my frequent misgivings about aspects of alternative discourse, I remain committed to the possibility that Cultural and Gender Studies might benefit conceptually from some aspects of the way alternative therapies think about the body.

Certainly, so-called complementary and alternative medicine (CAM) is a significant medical, economic and social phenomenon. Surveys in the US, the UK and other Western nations consistently show that almost half the population uses alternative therapies to treat medical problems and that CAM use is rising steadily. In the US, there are more visits annually to alternative therapists than to orthodox primary carers (Institute of Medicine 2005: 34). In 1997, visits to alternative practitioners represented some $21 billion in the US alone (Ruggie 2004: 43), but almost all users of alternative medicine also seek care from conventional doctors (Goldstein 2004: 927). For an increasing number of (mostly, but not always, affluent) consumers, health care has become a matter of choices made within and between different levels, style and paradigms of care. Much of this process of selection and combination takes place out of the sight of conventional doctors. In the US, most users of CAM (up to 72 per cent) do not disclose their CAM use to their doctor (Eisenberg et al. 2001: 348). This fact has medical implications, with a growing number of medical researchers worried about, for example, unknown and untested combinations of pharmacology and naturopathy. It's also a significant social phenomenon – the rise of a plurality of systems of sometimes interpenetrating health care with patients moving between them in largely unmonitored ways.

But the rise of CAM is more than a medical, economic or even social phenomenon. Alternative therapies are not just purely medical techniques; they are an increasingly popular new form of *cultural practice* bound up in new forms of bodily understanding and perception and new conceptions of selfhood. At once spiritual and bodily, medical and recreational, these practices represent a conceptual challenge to some of the orthodoxies of Western biomedicine. Experientially, they open up rich worlds of corporeal and intercorporeal experience in which the body's senses are opened up, trained and treated as important and legible parts of both the symptom picture and the healing process. The conceptual and experiential world of alternative therapies is one in which bodies know, think, communicate and intersect in radical ways; in which the realm of animals and objects is not utterly distinct from that of humans; and in which bodies are open to intersubjective – indeed intercorporeal – relations of the most far-reaching kind. There is, then, much to be gained from considering the *conceptual* and *paradigmatic* underpinnings of this pluralistic medical economy – this consumer-led sampling of different modalities, this process of lay picking, choosing, combining, sequestering and believing. Since most consumers of alternative therapies are also users of orthodox biomedicine, there is clearly something complicated and interesting going on mentally and psychologically when people adopt multiple, often contradictory, paradigms. What happens when a person moves between, say, the doctor's office, the yoga class and the psychic healer? We can well guess that they are unlikely to tell their doctor that they are 'complementing' antibiotics with spiritual healing, so how do consumers of multiple medical therapies mentally bridge the different body paradigms on which they repose, and negotiate the often stark paradigmatic differences across a variety of institutional contexts? Do they swap mental paradigms, simply ignore or jettison the bits that 'don't fit', or do they find new world-views through which to reconcile often quite starkly opposing views of the body and illness? What are the implications of such strategic silences and private juggling acts?

Such questions are not easily answered, to be sure, but hitherto they have scarcely even been posed. They point to the largely unexamined cultural, phenomenological and philosophical dimensions of alternative medicine. It is a surprise to realize just how rarely these dimensions of therapeutic practice have been studied within my home discipline of Cultural Studies, whose interest in popular and consumer culture and whose focus on embodiment might have made CAM an obvious candidate for detailed study (Barcan and Johnston 2005). Even Gender Studies has not accorded alternative therapies the attention one might have expected given the sheer empirical force of the fact that women predominate both as practitioners and clients and the fact that therapeutic discourses themselves are powerfully gendered, alternative therapies having championed an ethic of care, and having dethroned 'masculine' reason in favour of 'feminine' intuition. While evidence mounts of the medical effectiveness of many alternative therapies, and a secondary sociological and health sciences literature on CAM continues to grow, the new *cultural* terrain opened up by the widespread use of alternative therapies remains largely unexamined. This despite the fact that these therapies are a frequent topic of media interest, a regular part of the daily life of many people, a source of popular concepts of embodiment, and a practice with both medical and philosophical implications. It is this cultural terrain – the meanings, experiences, practices and discourses surrounding alternative therapies – that is the subject of this book.

Alternative therapies are also highly *sensual* practices, and this book uses the senses as a way into thinking about the pleasures of CAM, and the new forms of perception, experience and thinking that regular use of CAM can engender. The sensual nature of many therapies reminds us that they need to be situated within the hedonistic, pleasure-seeking drive of consumer culture – that they are part of what David Howes calls 'the sensual logic of late capitalism' (2005a: 287). Moreover, it points to the fact that many Westerners are seeking spiritual practices based in the *body* – where the senses are not seen as obstacles to spiritual development, as in ascetic religions, but as a pathway to it. Indeed, Constance Classen argued some years ago that the New Age movement (with which alternative medicine is complexly intertwined) indicates a pervasive popular desire for 'a new sensory cosmology' (1998: 159).[1] *Complementary and Alternative Medicine: Bodies, Therapies, Senses* draws on the burgeoning literature in sensory studies in order to highlight the way that different therapies produce different ways of knowing, reading, interpreting and experiencing the body. In reiki (a form of energy healing), the hands 'know' truths about the client's body and emotional life via touch; in aromatherapy, scents have both medical and emotional effects – triggering physical reactions as well as memories; in iridology, the eye is both the method and the object of diagnosis; in medical intuition, the clairvoyant sees the client's body as a multilayered energetic system, in which illnesses may appear as colours, shapes, metaphors or images or may be heard as voices or sensed as smells. By choosing to focus on the senses, this book opens up questions about the relatively unexplored richness of human bodily experience in therapeutic practice and the cultural systems by which bodies are rendered meaningful.

This book starts from the premise that alternative therapies are fascinating and complex. That might sound like a commonplace, but if Cultural Studies has bothered to analyse them at all it has been rather too content to see them as simply complicit with a range of cultural dominants, such as ideologies of the whole self and of nature (Coward 1989), Western appropriation of 'the East' (Stacey 2000), and an individualistic and psychologized relation to the self (Rose 1996, 1999). While such critiques undoubtedly hit the mark, they also risk being one-faceted and missing out on some of the complexities of therapeutic culture, including its positive or resistive potential. Only by seeing alternative therapies as multifaceted and often contradictory – simultaneously conformist responses to the dominant psychological logic of our times and as practices that crack open modernist conceptions of subjectivity – can one begin to gain some sense of their complexity and of what they may have to offer both clients and theorists. Moreover, they need to be not just recognized as part of the modern psychotherapeutic context, but also seen in relation to other histories and trajectories, especially spiritual ones (see Barcan and Johnston 2005, 2011). In this book I argue that despite their complicity with a range of contemporary dominants (consumerism, individualism, neoliberalism, Orientalism), alternative therapies can also offer up rich bodily experiences and, to a Cultural Studies willing to listen and feel, compelling new theoretical models of the body. I am suggesting that alternative therapies are not just worthy as objects of study for Cultural Studies; they might also have something to teach us about the body itself.

Of course, Cultural Studies also has something to teach thinkers and practitioners of CAM. This book is not an uncritical celebration of alternative therapies, but it does take off from a place of engagement and sympathy with them. I have subjected them to a kind of analysis that is rarely found within a more popular literature. I have tried, in short, to bridge the chasm between the usually uncritical rhetoric emanating from popular health discourse and from the New Age and the unremittingly unfavourable attention paid to these practices within Cultural Studies. Doing so means being open to many bodies of knowledge, while trying to remain aware of their points of incommensurability. This book does not just 'apply' Cultural Studies perspectives to alternative therapies as objects of study; rather, it opens a form of dialogue with them. To do so I draw on both my professional training as a Cultural Studies practitioner interested in the body in consumer culture and on my own long-term involvement in the world of alternative therapies, an involvement marked by intellectual and political wrangling, by a seemingly always provisional suspension of disbelief, and by deep bodily participation. I have had many experiences with alternative therapies, both as a paying customer and as an academic observer. I have been fascinated by these therapies for over twenty years. Over the last five years, I have carried out surveys and interviews with regular CAM users, observed and sometimes participated in workshops and training sessions, visited many and varied practitioners as a client, and interviewed just under thirty CAM practitioners, whose voices are threaded through this book.[2] My aim, as I will explore at the end of this Introduction, is not to produce a reconciliation or a synthesis between incompatible belief systems and forms of knowledge, but rather to engage in a kind of intellectual bodywork that I hope others may profit from – not least all those other academics out there who visit masseurs, homeopaths, healers and psychics and wonder how to make it all fit.

In this Introduction, I set the scene in a number of ways: first, by considering the term 'alternative' and its implications; second, by examining alternative medicine's relation to biomedicine; and third, by describing the hybridizing and pluralizing tendencies of alternative therapies. I then give an overview of a number of core principles underlying alternative therapies and put these in a wider social context by considering some of the social factors associated with the rise of CAM. The chapter concludes with a consideration of this book's place in relation to the traditional thematics and politics of Cultural Studies, including a brief consideration of some of the major reservations cultural critics have hitherto had about alternative medicine.

RELATIONS BETWEEN ALTERNATIVE MEDICINE AND BIOMEDICINE
DEFINING ALTERNATIVE MEDICINE

The modern alternative health movement grew out of the countercultural, ecological and alternative food movements of the late 1960s and early 1970s (Sutherland et al. 2003: 320), feminist health activism from the same period (Willard 2005: 121), and a complex intermeshing with the New Age movement. In addition, it overlaps with a range of other social trends, including the rise of what Nikolas Rose (1996: 2) calls the 'psy' disciplines (psychology, psychotherapy, psychoanalysis) and the mainstreaming of therapeutic and self-help culture; the health and fitness boom of the 1980s; the environmental movement; the continued rise of consumer culture; and the globalization of particular healing practices and of the fantasies of nature and authenticity that have accompanied that globalization (Stacey 2000).

Alternative therapies have, in certain kinds of ways, moved from marginal to mainstream (Ruggie 2004), but the question of their relation to a biomedical dominant is neither simple nor politically neutral. It arises right from the outset, even in the question of what they should be called, since almost every name for these therapies proves either conceptually or politically problematic. One historian of alternative medicine, Mike Saks, lists some of the difficulties (2003: 2). 'Traditional' medicine, for example, is shot through with political difficulties,[3] including the implication that non-Western medical practices are static rather than adaptive (Leslie and Young 1992: 5). It also seemingly excludes therapies in which technology plays a major role. (Saks instances biofeedback, and one could also add Kirlian photography, or various high-tech forms of light therapy.) 'Complementary' implies both a paradigmatic harmony and a benign political coexistence between orthodox medicine and its alternatives – neither of which is likely to often be the case. For example, homeopathy, as Saks notes, is based on a diametrically opposed paradigm to orthodox biomedicine (see also Willis and White 2004: 52). Homeopathy's fundamental precept that 'like cures like' (*similia similibus curentur*) could not be more different from contemporary Western medicine's idea of 'combating' disease – evident in its subtle reliance on military metaphors (fighting disease, waging war on cancer, conquering illness. See Stoller 2004: 128).[4] 'Natural therapies', though widely used as a term, is both inaccurate and intellectually weak, calling up a host of fantasies of nature as benign, pure and intrinsically curative. The conception of nature as safe, gentle and non-technological (Coward 1989: 18–19) is, as I will argue below, a very particularized historical view. In any case, what is 'natural' about, for example, mass-produced, synthesized vitamin supplements? 'Holistic' is another problematic term – not only because it buys into the same kinds of intellectual problems encountered with the word 'natural', but also because it is not, as Saks points out, even an accurate descriptor of the ideals of many therapies. (Saks gives the example of osteopathy, which, while it may be practised 'holistically' can also be practised mechanistically (2003: 3).) Saks chooses the term 'alternative', a term that he uses to describe the *political* location of a set of therapeutic practices, rather than a descriptor of some supposedly intrinsic therapeutic 'content' (2). He prefers this relational definition since it allows one to recognize that definitions of orthodoxy and alternatives are historically and culturally variable. An example of such a relational, political definition is that used by medical researcher David Eisenberg and his colleagues, who define alternative medicine as 'medical interventions not taught widely at U.S. medical schools or generally available in U.S. hospitals' (1993: 246). Similarly, an inquiry in 2000 into CAM by a British House of Lords Select Committee categorized CAM modalities in essentially political terms – in relation to their stated aims, their knowledge base and their plausibility in terms of the medical model. On this basis, the report organizes them into three groups: 'Professionally organized disciplines with their own diagnostic approach'; 'therapies which are often used to complement conventional medicine and do not purport to embrace diagnostic skills'; and practices that *do* purport to diagnose but are 'indifferent to the scientific principles of conventional medicine' (qtd in Bensouilah 2005: 139). This last category was itself divided into 'long-established and traditional systems of healthcare' and 'other alternative disciplines which lack any credible evidence base' (qtd in Bensouilah 2005: 139). The precise inclusions and exclusions of normal versus marginalized medicines differ from country to country, even within the West; chiropractic, for example, is quite accepted in the US; homeopathy relatively so in the UK, where it has the endorsement of the royal family. Osteopathy has become a parallel medical system in the US but remains an adjunctive, largely manual, therapy in the UK, Australia and Canada (Baer 2004: xvi). 'Alternative' is a useful term to capture this relational and contingent sense of inclusions and exclusions.

Acupuncture provides a pointed example of the problems of categorization and labelling. When practised in the West, it is usually labelled as an 'alternative' therapy. The fact that it is a major component of the dominant medical system in China, having been practised on millions of people for thousands of years, makes the West's label 'alternative' seem not only graceless but somewhat beside the point, a matter of 'political and cultural judgment' (Lawson 2002: 14). Medical doctor Karen Lawson makes this clear by citing a statement from a Beijing meeting of Traditional Chinese Medicine practitioners in 2001:

> There is sufficient evidence of Western medicine's effectiveness to expand its use into TCM and to encourage further studies of its physiology and clinical value. Western medicine shows promise as adjunctive treatment to TCM. As a stand-alone medicine, however, its efficacy is mainly in the areas of acute and catastrophic care that comprise a relatively minor percentage of total patient complaints (qtd in Lawson 2002: 14).[5]

While I myself am wary of the term 'complementary' because it seems to my feminist sensibility to relegate CAM to the position of a feminized helpmeet, others see it exactly oppositely. Mitchell L. Gaynor, an oncologist who uses sound-based techniques like chanting and Tibetan crystal bowls, considers that 'alternative' downgrades CAM practices, since it may be taken to imply superfluity rather than necessity:

> You'll notice that I refer to these modalities as 'complementary', rather than 'alternative'. I have long since come to accept nontraditional, holistic approaches as necessities, rather than potential options, that must be integrated with the care and treatment of my patients. (1999: 4)

Clearly, the term 'alternative' is by no means unproblematic, but I nonetheless adopt it in this book – not in the wish to champion in romantic fashion some oppressed or marginal medical practices (although I am a fan and user of many alternative therapies), but rather because it points to the paradigmatic, conceptual, stylistic and technical differences between Western biomedicine and the kinds of therapies I explore. Moreover, the term 'alternative' seems to buy into neoliberal notions of the empowered consumer with the ability to *choose* – a discomforting enough notion for me, politically, but in actuality quite an apt one given the current demographics of use, where white, female baby boomers constitute a significant proportion of users (Ruggie 2004: 46). For these reasons I use the term, even while many practitioners do not like the label (one telling me that he hadn't used it since the 1970s) and despite my own interest in the project of a truly *integrative* medicine (see below) as an important medical and political possibility.

The term 'alternative' is also useful because it reminds us that dedicated users of alternative medicine do at times get confronted with real and often painful choices between mutually exclusive options. The Bowen technique, for example, used for structural or muscular problems among other things, claims to effect healing by triggering the brain to correct imbalances, and most practitioners believe that in order not to send conflicting messages to the brain it shouldn't be combined with any other treatment, alternative or conventional (Baker 2001: 52). Another example is some treatments for infertility that require complete detoxifying and staying away from drugs, therefore making them incompatible with IVF. Some women might try them as a last resort, after a failure in IVF; others might try them first, in an effort to avoid IVF. Either way, their mutual exclusivity means they will be tried sequentially and not simultaneously. Given the infamously small window of opportunity in fertility matters, either way it is a difficult choice with potentially serious consequences. This then is the harder side of choice – alternatives not as some superabundance available to indulged Western consumers, but choice as hard paradigmatic decisions whose consequences people must live with. 'We have no choice but to choose', said the sociologist Anthony Giddens (2003: 387) in his classic study of modern identity – a study sparked, initially, by the confronting array of choices offered him when he injured his back. Having over twenty different and often conflicting choices of treatment is, he says, better than having no choices, but it produces 'a complicated mesh of freedom and anxiety', in which choosing a therapist is not only difficult but deeply and troublingly meaningful – not just a question of treating an individual's ailment but, as Giddens found, of 'what it all meant and who I should turn to' (2003: 389).

This sense of hard and mutually exclusive choices is absent from the much favoured term 'complementary therapies', which implies a harmonious interlocking of different paradigms that is unlikely to be true conceptually, medically or institutionally. The term also metaphorically feminizes this form of medicine, it being woman's traditional philosophical fate to 'complement' man. I discuss complementarity in detail in Chapter 5, so for now I will simply signal its place in a gendered dualism that has long underpinned mainstream Western philosophy. As Genevieve Lloyd explains: 'Our ideas and ideals of maleness and femaleness have been formed within structures of dominance – of superiority and inferiority, "norms" and "difference", "positive" and "negative", the "essential" and the "complementary"' (1984: 103).

Orthodox medicine's helpmeets are sometimes construed in more 'masculine' ways. Since the late 1960s,[6] the term 'allied health' has been used in a number of Western countries to name paramedical therapies that are distinct from nursing and medicine, but which are recognized and valued by orthodox medicine. This definition is, again, relational; it is based on exclusion – allied health is that which is not nursing or medicine (Turnbull et al. 2009: 27) – and it is not static – the practices that fall under this label change over time. Examples from the US include occupational therapy, speech therapy, chiropody, ultrasound, dental hygiene, and nutrition and dietetics. While their role is still acknowledged as one of support and supplementation, in the US this category notably excludes the 'natural' or 'complementary' therapies. 'Partners', 'teams' and 'allies' are the masculine lexicon of this paradigm, in which allied health workers are not feminized assistants but 'key players in the multidisciplinary health care team' (Wilde 2006: 2). In Australia, 'allied health' refers primarily to an alliance *between* non-medical disciplines rather than to a relationship between biomedicine and its adjuncts (Turnbull et al. 2009: 27), unlike in the US, where the initial use of the term by the American Medical Association recognized these practitioners as allied with *medicine* itself (Donini-Lenhoff 2008: 47).

Depending on the country, the 'allied' designation has different institutional and economic implications. In Australia, it means that patients can be referred by medical practitioners and that fees can be claimed directly under the national health system (Medicare) rather than having to be paid privately or reimbursed by private health insurance. For this reason, some professions actively seek recognition under this label since it implies a degree of legitimization by both government and the medical mainstream. In Australia, chiropractic has recently (2005) been elevated from the status of a 'complementary and alternative health' practice to an 'allied health' one, a shift that represents an increase in authority (Nudd 2006: 1). That this elevation is a metaphorical masculinization away from the feminized world of nature, natural therapies and 'complementarity' is suggested by the term 'ally', with its militaristic (and more recently managerial) associations, as well as by the criteria for admission to this category, which include an embrace of the dominant evidence-based medical paradigm. As chiropractor Paul Nudd put it in a newsletter to clients:

> Chiropractic has been slower [than medicine] to achieve cultural authority perhaps through a reluctance by some [practitioners] to embrace scientific evidence. Government recognition through the inclusion into *Medicare Plus* [the Australian national health care system] is a significant step towards cultural authority. Modern *evidence based chiropractic* is taking its rightful place beside modern *evidence based medicine* in the partnership of integrated healthcare. (2006: 1, original italics)

Cultural authority is, however, acquired differently in different national contexts. In the US, in the absence of a universal national health care system, the struggle may be less to be recognized as part of allied health than to be recognized as an independent discipline:

> Some professions traditionally considered part of allied health have by and large left that designation behind. Having reached a critical mass of public/ governmental awareness and number of practitioners, they develop more stringent educational/training requirements … and begin to 'brand' themselves as an independent health profession, not an allied health profession, which to some connotes a secondary, subsidiary, and dependent relationship to physicians and medicine. (Donini-Lenhoff 2008: 45)

Perhaps the most common term worldwide, and one with substantial institutional backing,[7] is 'Complementary and Alternative Medicine', or CAM. As its name suggests, the label 'CAM' covers a broad spectrum of alternative healing practices, some of them at least partially compatible with biomedicine, others more remotely connected or indeed diametrically opposed to it. Willis and White note that the term constructs a falsely unified whole out of a range of disparate practices (2004: 52). The term CAM simultaneously smoothes over and points to the split and divisive nature of the alternative-medicine phenomenon, both in its relations to biomedicine and in its own internal diversity and divisions. The term thus accurately renders alternative medicine's complex relations to biomedicine – where non-orthodox techniques can sometimes be an extension of biomedicine, sometimes a supplement and sometimes an active resistance. For that reason, I use the term CAM too – especially when it suits for reasons of brevity, when I want to refer to a self-consciously professionalizing set of practices (and their reliance on scientific evidence), or when I want to point to alternative medicine as a broad *field of practice* rather than particular sets of bodily techniques. But it is not without its own problems. Naturopath Judy Singer points out that the term is 'linguistically efficient' (2008: 20), and that this is a double-edged sword. She cites a number of medical anthropologists and sociologists who have reservations about the term, despite its evident utility (2008: 19–20). Hans Baer (2004: xvi–xvii), for example, agrees with critics like Claire M. Cassidy and Paul Root Wolpe, who both argue that biomedical hegemony is intrinsic to the concept of CAM and that biomedicine has embraced the term as a domestication strategy that privileges Western evidence-based validation.

So what will I be meaning when I use the terms 'alternative therapies' and 'CAM' throughout this book? It is important for me to emphasize that when I am talking about alternative therapies, I am restricting myself to a particular subset of non-orthodox healing practices – those that, while they have often not fully entered the medical mainstream, have certainly penetrated a pop cultural mainstream. At certain points, to be sure, I do describe relatively unknown therapies, where they open up important conceptual points (Psychophonetics in Chapter 3; Zero Balancing in Chapter 4), but in the main, I focus on the point where commodified pop culture meets or overlaps with private therapy culture and state health care. I am thus not considering anything like the full range of non-biomedical healing practices nor the full range of locations and contexts in which they are used – not only because these are so numerous that it would be impossible, but also because I am interested, specifically, in looking at the point where consumption, recreation and medicine blur, and where people turn to a form of medicine not from family or ethnic background or the shared practices of a local community, but through the complex intersections of need, choice, desperation, desire and privilege.

The point about privilege itself needs a little elaboration: when I make passing comments about the privileged nature of the demographic of CAM users I am referring, clearly, to the contexts in which these therapies are currently most commonly available, not to anything inherent in them. On the one hand, the entry of many traditional, often communal, practices into the marketplace means that they become most publicly visible as commodities, and hence accessible seemingly only to those with means. On the other hand, this shouldn't blind us to the fact that non-biomedical healing practices continue to be practised in non-commodified forms in modern Western nations within specific ethnic or other communities (Traditional Chinese Medicine throughout the Chinese diaspora; spiritualism in working-class Britain, and so on), as well as in *new* forms of community, such as the networks of unpaid exchange that spring up around massage and reiki. Moreover, many forms of alternative therapy are practised with particular, often disadvantaged, groups, precisely because public funding is often available for such purposes. Thus, while therapies like reiki, massage and naturopathy are not available for the general public without cost except through informal networks of care, many hospitals and clinics host programmes offering such therapies to particular groups, including refugees, HIV patients, substance abusers, or under the rubric of 'men's health'. Moreover, while the ability to choose between options across the medical landscape undoubtedly increases with social capital, it is important to note that a pragmatic relation between medical systems is not solely the province of the privileged few, as Singer's (2008) study of refugee women's essentially *pragmatic* relation to the various medical systems they encounter makes clear.[8] Indeed, the pragmatic movement across systems characterizes most people outside the First World. In sum, the relations between alternative medicine and biomedicine are institutionally, as well as paradigmatically, intricate.

RELATIONS BETWEEN ALTERNATIVE MEDICINE AND BIOMEDICINE: TOWARDS INTEGRATION?

Any relational definition of alternative medicine also involves deciding what we should call the dominant medical system. Should it be called conventional medicine? Allopathic? Western? Orthodox? Biomedicine? Even 'organized medicine' (Ruggie 2005: 980)? As Saks points out, in the West orthodox medicine currently *is* biomedicine, but the two terms don't mean the same thing and have aligned only in the last two centuries (2003: 2) and only in Westernized nations. Cross-cultural and historical perspectives remind us that despite the potency, pervasiveness and potential persuasiveness of biomedicine as both medical practice and 'curative cosmology' (M. Stacey 1986: 10, n. 2), it is not a truth waiting to be universally acknowledged.

Historically, in Europe, it had to battle to dislodge traditional folk medicines (as naturopaths are fond of pointing out). The spread of scientific medicine outside the West was inextricably bound up in imperialism; Western medicine was 'imposed as an alien form of knowledge and an alien practice' (Cunningham and Andrews 1997: 2–3). Biomedicine construes itself not as 'one medical system among many', but as 'the standard to which all other medical systems should aspire' (1997: 12). Nonetheless, as it gets exported as a globalized paradigm it must still battle to find its place alongside the medical cosmologies it displaces. In the 1960s, the anthropologist Lola Schwartz noted that the people of Manus Island (an island in the Admiralty group north of New Guinea) 'accept biomedicine but take it to be a low-level theory with limited explanatory powers' (M. Stacey 1986: 12), in contrast to their apparent readiness to embrace other aspects of European culture (Schwartz 1969: 201). Schwartz analysed this in terms of a 'hierarchy of [medical] resort' (which systems one turns to, in which order, and for which reasons). This process of sequencing (turning to particular forms of medical practice and then, if they fail, to a series of other systems) is a feature of any culture in which different systems of medicine are to be found, whether through migration, colonization, globalization or consumerism. Indeed, today, almost all countries in the world are medically pluralist.[9] The extent to which the global export of scientific medicine involves the marginalization of traditional medical knowledge and practice varies from country to country. For example, the medical anthropologist Gerard Bodeker considers that in China, biomedicine has resulted in significant losses of traditional medical practice; in India, it has produced hybrid curricula of lower standards; in South Korea, political conflict between traditional and Western medicine has been high (2001: 165). In the West, what we are seeing is not only the use of alternative medicine when the dominant system fails or is seen as unpromising (classically, in the case of cancer patients) but also the emergence of a sector of the population for whom alternative medicine is the medicine of 'first resort' (Goldstein 2004: 940).

While some analysts seem optimistic about the increasing legitimacy of CAM (Mary Ruggie, for example, considers that the change in name from 'alternative medicine' to 'CAM' reflects a shift 'from outsider to partner' (2005: 981)), others are less sanguine, seeing the process of legitimization as one in which difference is progressively lost. Hans Baer, for example, uses the metaphor of 'taming' to describe the professionalization of holistic health into CAM (2004: xiv). Similarly, medical anthropologist Judith Fadlon claims that the gradual legitimization of CAM has been accomplished via a process of 'domestication', in which the paradigmatic differences between CAM and biomedicine have been neutralized. She sees an ultimate medical and scientific hegemony whereby alternative methods are combined with and sanctioned by conventional techniques (2004: 79) and foreign or 'ex-paradigmatic' elements are weakened via the processes of popular dissemination and of professionalization. This integration process reflects both an epistemological shift in biomedicine, on the one hand, and its 'continued hegemony' on the other (70). Importantly, though, she argues that the integrative process is ongoing, and that the future of CAM may involve elements of domestication and/or differentiation (84).

One mechanism of domestication is the imposition of putatively neutral ('scientific') criteria for assessment and legitimization. Some argue that the rise to prominence of alternative medicine means that there can no longer be mainstream and alternative medicine, only, in the oft-quoted words of Angell and Kassirer, 'medicine that has been adequately tested and medicine that has not, medicine that works and medicine that may or may not work' (1998: 841). They argue that 'It is time for the scientific community to stop giving alternative medicine a free ride' (1998: 841); in other words, alternative medicine should be subjected to the same type and degree of tests as orthodox medicine. This is a mixed blessing for CAM. While evidence-based medicine (EBM) may be a workable paradigm for some types of alternative therapies – those underpinned by paradigms at least partially compatible with biomedicine – it is of complex and paradoxical use to those healing or therapeutic techniques that are based on models of the body, modes of knowing or cosmologies so remote from the biomedical model as to be untestable within it. Moreover, alternative medicine's focus on tailoring treatment combinations to individuals and their circumstances means that an emphasis on standardized testing is inappropriate (Willis and White 2004: 56). In any case, evidence-based medicine relies on there being organizations willing to fund the large-scale research on which it is based; it is therefore less likely to be carried out where there is no financial interest at stake for a large company. The call for validation also implies an inaccurate picture of biomedicine, in which all biomedical treatments might be falsely imagined to have been subjected to the rigours of the scientific testing, which they haven't (Institute of Medicine 2005: 17), and in which evidence-based medicine might seem a self-evidently 'objective' analytical tool, whereas it relies on a particular statistical methodology (Bodeker 2000: 4). The primacy of EBM, however, has led many in alternative medicine to seek legitimacy through increasing professionalization and the quest for scientific validation. Meanwhile, other less paradigmatically compatible therapies may repudiate or fail this test, although, paradoxically, one aspect of EBM can work in their favour – an emphasis on *whether* something works rather than *why* it works (Willis and White 2004: 54).

Another component of the professionalization of CAM is a push towards fuller patient disclosure of CAM use to their General Practitioner (GP).[10] The fear of litigation and/or being professionally discredited is driving an increasing number of alternative therapists to urge their patients to discuss their full range of treatments with their doctors. One naturopath told me that a lot of her clients say, 'I can't tell my doctor I'm taking this' and her response is that if they can't then they shouldn't take it. Even a medical clairvoyant told me that she makes her clients sign a form saying that they will disclose to the doctor the fact that they are doing emotional release work because it might affect the dose they should be taking of prescription medicine. It is interesting to wonder whether this simultaneously defensive and 'professionalizing' push from alternative practitioners will produce greater co-operation between systems, or, conversely, more calls from GPs to regulate the alternative industry. Either way, it seems clear to me that the push and pull between systems is far too complex to be considered a process only of 'domestication'.

To some extent, biomedicine and its alternatives co-produce each other, often in relation to the governing regulatory environment. Osteopathy, for example, is practised more esoterically in those European countries where its medical worth is not recognized. The same goes for aromatherapy, which tends more towards the esoteric in countries where essential oils are not classified as health products, such as the US.[11]

The drive towards professionalization and scientific validation has led to splits within many alternative therapies, with practitioners divided as to the extent to 'go anatomical' or 'go crystal', as one of my interviewees so beautifully put it. A particularly politically charged issue is that of training and accreditation. Naturopathic training, for example, is increasingly split between versions in which its traditional holism and vitalism are central, and others that move closer to dominant biochemical understandings of nutrition (Canaway 2007). Commentators point to the divisions and conflicts within and between different CAM modalities over issues as fundamental as the extent to which a traditional knowledge base should be allowed to be (depending on one's perspective) undermined, translated or modernized. In Australia, and no doubt elsewhere, such 'conflict, schisms and fragmentation' (7) have inevitably weakened the political power of CAM advocates to effectively influence government (Jacka, in Canaway 2007: 7).

Domestication may occur in the reverse direction – through the training of GPs themselves in 'natural' therapies, especially ones that have started to find some measure of scientific validation in the West. Acupuncture, for example, now has a Western scientific face in the form of so-called 'medical acupuncture', a form of training open only to physicians. While it is inaccurate to characterize this as a simple appropriation or neutralization, it is nonetheless clear that this represents a process of incorporation rather than an uncontrolled opening out to other paradigms or other experts. The subtitle of the journal *Medical Acupuncture*, for example, is 'A Journal for Physicians by Physicians'. In the promotional literature I have read for courses in medical acupuncture, it certainly looks as though what Fadlon calls 'ex-paradigmatic elements' are weakened, dropped or introduced merely as a kind of 'pre-history'.[12] Such matters have economic and political as well as intellectual force; for example, in Australia acupuncture is covered by the national insurance scheme if it is done by a GP but must be paid for privately if it is done by someone else. As the processes of convergence and overlap make it less and less easy to define alternative practices by their distinctiveness from biomedicine (Fulder 1996: 3), it may be that these other questions – like *who* is practising a particular therapy – become increasingly politically significant.

Despite the evidence of some degree of political and paradigmatic neutralization of alternative therapies, I don't entirely share Fadlon's pessimism. The sense of incommensurability retained in the phrase 'complementary and alternative medicine' is not purely tokenistic. First, there exist a number of techniques, especially the psychic and spiritual techniques discussed in Chapter 5, that remain well outside any biomedical mainstream. Second, the level of paradigmatic and practical accommodation to orthodoxy seems to me to vary enormously not just between the many different types of alternative therapy, but also between practitioners – some of whom actively seek legitimization, and others of whom work happily much more on the margins. Third, some voices, including medical doctors, are calling not for the subjection of alternative therapies to tests devised from within incommensurable paradigms, but for the development of other criteria for validation. Medical doctor Karen Lawson, for example, argues that

> The greatest challenge is to develop good research designs that do not obviate the very processes we seek to maximize, such as the placebo effect, mind-body interactions, self-healing, or the power of intention. Forcing other philosophies of healing to fit into our mechanistic model will decrease the potential of these other approaches. For example, we require proof of a biochemical/mechanical mechanism for energetic systems such as Reiki because we do not know of any other way to measure or understand them (2002: 17)

The fact that most users of CAM keep it private from their doctors points to the continued existence of multiple paradigms whose conflicts, intersections and incommensurabilities are negotiated either privately or socially (among friends) rather than professionally. While this is perhaps not *medically* desirable, *culturally* it points to patients' own perception that what they are doing may be in some measure radical and/or that they don't believe their doctor is qualified to pass an opinion on alternative therapies, and/or that they believe in advance that their doctor will be sceptical or reproving. In other words, patients themselves have a sense of the political contest between paradigms.

The power of orthodox medicine and its advocates is in some measure paradoxical. On the one hand, critics of CAM have for some time seen themselves as custodians of a rationality they see as being under threat. As long ago as 1989, Rosalind Coward, for example, lamented the threat posed by New Age bunkum to orthodox scientific rationality:

> The hard-boiled 'materialists' of the 1960s who scoffed at hippie mysticism see their own systems of thought in pathetic disarray compared with the vigour of their opposites. They perceive themselves as a beleaguered minority in a land peopled with mystics, those, that is, who have not already trained as naturopaths or acupuncturists. (1989: 13)

This theme of the death of reason has, as I have argued elsewhere (Barcan 2009a), gained considerable popular traction, fuelled by the fear of a range of different social and ideological movements, from religious fundamentalism to postmodernism to the New Age. Nonetheless, it is not uncommon for people on *both* sides of the alternative/orthodox 'divide' to see themselves as beleaguered.

After nearly twenty years of personal interest and involvement in alternative therapies, and having watched the huge boom in them as popular practices, I set out on this study assuming that they now had a quite substantial paradigmatic footing. But it is not so simple. On the one hand, alternative therapies are increasingly popular practices, taught in universities and established colleges. On the other hand, they are often *institutionally* far less powerful than biomedicine. During this study I constantly heard stories about biomedicine's political power – for example, of alternative medical programmes being axed from universities after lobbying from the medical establishment, and of attempts to lock out alternative medicine from government funding (Easthope 1993: 289–90). Political resistance to them is often still substantial, and most alternative therapies are still in large measure excluded from national health insurance schemes (where they exist). Despite huge consumer demand, it is, I discovered, often difficult to make a living out of many of the more marginal practices, and many practitioners (even in quite mainstream therapies like naturopathy) feel themselves not to be so much riding a wave of popular acclaim as embattled and always feeling their professionalism and even their existence to be threatened by government, pharmaceutical companies and doctors. To take just one example, the American Medical Association disbanded its Committee on Quackery only in 1990, following a Supreme Court ruling that its practices against chiropractors violated antitrust laws (Ruggie 2005: 981). A number of my interviewees were initially quite wary – scared that a university researcher was inevitably out to debunk them. Stories like this suggest that CAM has not (yet) been safely neutralized into a feminized caring practice rather than a viable, virile alternative; they suggest that there is still a significant degree of political and paradigmatic *battling* actually going on.

In recent years, the rise of a new paradigm – that of integrative medicine – has given advocates of CAM some cause for hope. This term, coined in the early 1990s, describes a medicine that is open to both biomedicine and CAM, and which, rather, like alternative medicine itself, is holistic, patient-centred, and focused on healing rather than disease (Caspi et al. 2003: 61). In stark contrast to all the labels discussed above, the term 'integrative medicine' does not attempt to define by either distinction or exclusion. Opher Caspi et al. warn that integrative medicine should not slip back into 'combination medicine' – that is, it must not be structured as conventional practices 'plus' CAM (2003: 61). This sits somewhat at odds with the rather more cautious and limited definition of integrative medicine given in the preamble to the inaugural issue of the *Journal of Complementary and Integrative Medicine* in 2004, which described integrative medicine as 'incorporat[ing] elements of CAM into [a] comprehensive treatment plan alongside orthodox methods of diagnosis and treatment'. Many commentators see an emphasis on evidence-based science as one of the defining characteristics of integrative medicine (e.g. Sierpina, in Baer 2004: xix), but there is still debate on this among its proponents. The preamble cited above, for example, did recognize that the assessment methods of evidence-based medicine might not be appropriate to all forms of CAM:

> It has been suggested that conventional clinical trials may not be the only source of evidence and other resources, such as good quality case reports, observational studies and traceable traditional references, may have significant contributions to our critical analyses of complementary and alternative therapies.[13]

'Integration', then, isn't necessarily a cover for neutralization, and it isn't wise to assume that all medical practitioners want to keep alternative medicine in its secondary, feminized, 'handmaiden' role. A 2006 editorial in the journal *Integrative Cancer Therapies*, for example, discussed the editor's discomfort with the term 'complementary;' he preferred 'integrative' precisely because it allowed practices like massage or yoga a role that was actually ameliorative rather than simply palliative (although it stopped short of attributing potential curative properties to such therapies) (Block 2006: 3). But to its opponents – and there are many – integrative medicine is deluded and regressive. As Dr Arnold S. Relman, editor in chief of *The New England Journal of Medicine*, put it in a public debate on integrative medicine, 'integrating alternative medicine with mainstream medicine would not be an advance but a return to the past, an interruption of the remarkable progress achieved by science-based medicine over the past century' ('Is Integrative Medicine' 1999: 2122).

Reminders of the unquestionable triumphs of biomedicine always make me uneasy about my fascination for alternative medicine, but I remain intellectually committed to the ongoing project of integrative medicine, despite the evident intellectual, political and practical problems of working across and between different medical paradigms. Over the years of my engagement with CAM therapies, and especially during the research for this book, I have come across many truly gifted practitioners – some who are top-rate specialists in a particular discipline and some whom I would consider multidisciplinary 'cross-over' figures. I met Simon Borg-Olivier, for example, a Sydney-based yoga teacher who is a trained scientist, a physiotherapist[14] and a master yoga teacher. In Chapter 2 I mention the wonderful work of Dr René Mateos, a surgeon turned psychotherapist and hypnotherapist. I have learnt of other cross-over figures through their writing. For example, Fritz Frederick Smith, whose books I cite in Chapter 4, is a medical doctor, osteopath, acupuncturist and bodyworker. As mentioned above, Mitchell Gaynor is an oncologist who uses Tibetan chanting and crystal bowls as an integral part of his practice. Others cross boundaries even more remarkably. Take Mona Lisa Schulz – a medical doctor with a PhD and research career in behavioural neuroscience who practises as a medical intuitive (a medical clairvoyant); or Barbara Brennan – a mechanical engineer who worked as a physicist for NASA, and now as a medical intuitive. Boundary crossing also occurs through collaborations across seemingly incompatible forms of practice. In Chapter 5 I describe the collaboration between medical intuitive Carolyn Myss and medical doctor Norman Shealy. Researching this book, I have found that there exist all sorts of informal or invisible collaborations between people in the medical mainstream and even the most marginalized or esoteric of alternative therapies – for example, General Practitioners who have ongoing but hidden professional relations with medical clairvoyants (see Barcan 2009b).

To critics of alternative medicine, examples like that of a medical intuitive working with GPs prove only that rational people can get caught up in delusions, and that the CAM menace is dangerously contagious. But my intellectual position makes me somewhat wary of biomedicine's universal truth claims even while I marvel at and benefit from the indisputable health and lifestyle benefits that the institutionalization of biomedicine has brought about. I am interested in the cracks and chinks within and between paradigms, and the positive potential of the cross-fertilization of different bodies of knowledge. My embodied experience of alternative therapies also makes me open to the potential *medical* benefits of integrative medicine; I have had not only relaxing and life-enhancing experiences but also deeply curative benefits from some CAM treatments. I remain, therefore, fascinated and energized by alternative medicine and its ongoing relations with the medical mainstream, even while I remain wary about the dangers, both medical and philosophical, of an uncritical acceptance of *any* form of medical intervention. It is possible to remain committed to, and excited by, the possibilities of alternative medicine, including even its more esoteric practices, while simultaneously being aware and wary of practitioners, world-views and practices that are simplistic, naive or ill-founded. In my experience, it comes back time after time to the skills of particular practitioners rather than to generalizable claims about the benefits of particular *practices*. As a good friend reminded me over two decades ago, the New Age is full of charlatans – and to that I would add that it is also full of people who are well-meaning or dogmatic or inexperienced or over-zealous. As a consumer, the game is all about dodging such practitioners – a process of trial, error, experience and maturity that leads, one hopes, to discernment in the selection of modalities and practitioners. But the training of savvy consumers is no fit basis for the social organization and regulation of a health care system. How medical pluralism can be responsibly, safely and economically administered in the bureaucratic, risk-averse, pluralist contexts that characterize modern Western health care systems remains a challenge, to say the least. In this book, I do not address such challenges in detail, though I do periodi- cally discuss questions of professional ethics and accreditation. Rather, I focus on the therapies themselves – as bodily experiences, sensory engagement, and enriched modes of knowing.

ALTERNATIVE THERAPIES
CLASSIFYING, DEFINING AND DESCRIBING ALTERNATIVE THERAPIES

One of the downsides of defining alternative medicine relationally is that in the end such definitions are inevitably unlimited. Defining alternative medicine in- volves categorizing particular practices, but classification is made difficult by the fact that alternative medicine is characterized by a tendency towards eclecticism and proliferation (or, to quote Dr Relman again, alternative medicine is a 'dubious and disparate set of practices' (1999: 2122), a 'hodgepodge' (1999: 2123)). The appendix to a large survey of CAM in the US published by the Institute of Medicine of the National Academies (2005), for example, lists a huge array of practices – from apitherapy (the use of bee products in healing), to juice therapy, pet therapy, biofeedback, chiropractic, prayer and even urine therapy. This eclectic list is prefaced by the rather unvarnished disclaimer: 'The following may or may not be considered a part of CAM, depending on one's accepted definition of CAM' (2005: 283).

Given the vast number and diversity of bodily, mental, emotional and spiritual technologies that can be encompassed within the category, it's tempting to devise internal taxonomies based on particular qualities of alternative practices. Stephen Fulder, for example, divides alternative medicine into eighteen different categories (e.g. mind-body, sense, manipulative, postural), each of which has numerous sub- specialities (1996: xvi–xxiii). The *Hamlyn Encyclopedia of Complementary Health* divides therapies up differently, into Eastern, manipulative, natural, active, therapies involving external powers (into which they also group bodywork, art therapies and diagnostic therapies) (Bradford 1996). Taxonomies such as these, while helpful, have their limits. To begin with, even setting aside the fact that the vast majority of practitioners work across and between a range of modalities, it's hard to think of any one practice as singular in the first place. Within any supposedly singular practice, especially one with a long history, there are often different lineages, traditions and schools. These different styles and traditions evolve, mutate and hybridize, and vary according to cultural context and to the philosophy, interests and style of individual practitioners. The vast majority of alternative practitioners combine and blend therapies, and the therapies themselves multiply and diversify along various lines. The first and most obvious multiplier logic is that of combination. With the exception of the more recognized and more 'scientific' modalities such as chiropractic, combinations seem to be more common than single-modality practitioners. A second process is that of hybridization. Yoga can merge with Pilates, for example, to produce 'Yogalates'; kinesiology breeds with Neuro-Linguistic Programming to produce 'Neuro-Linguistic Kinesiology', and so on. A third logic is that of invention, with many practitioners offering services that appear to be of their own devising: Psychophonetics, Platinum Alchemy Healing, DNA activation. A fourth logic at work is that of specialization. Massage, for example, comes in many forms: relaxation, sports, neuromuscular, deep tissue, lymphatic drainage or trigger point, to name only a few. Such specialization includes the recognition and/or development of niche markets: sports massage, executive massage (fully clothed, in your office chair!), geriatric massage, pregnancy massage or infant massage. Therapies also multiply by analogy. Dr Edward Bach's original forty Flower Essences were made in the UK; now there are Australian versions (Australian Bush Flower essences) and others devised by individual practitioners. A sixth mode by which new therapies emerge in the West is via the finding of healing practices from outside the West, usually of 'traditional' or 'indigenous' origin. This serves consumer culture's need for the proliferation of the new, as well as the West's insatiable appetite for what Jackie Stacey calls 'Easternised nature' (2000: 121). For example, as massage has now moved from marginal to mainstream, more and more forms are imported into Western popular culture: Swedish and remedial massage now vie with, among others, Thai massage, Indian head massage, shiatsu, Hawaiian (kahuna or Lomi Lomi) massage and hot stone massage (advertised by some as an Ancient Chinese practice, by others as a Native American practice).

In this book, I am not concerned with defining alternative medicine per se and in arguing about what should or shouldn't be included under that label. Rather, for the purposes of my *cultural* exploration of alternative medicine, it makes less sense to consider alternative health as a discrete field or even movement than as a set of practices bound up in clusters of overlapping discourses. In other words, their boundaries are not fixed and they look different depending on the discourse through which they are framed. Seen through the lens of medical discourse, alternative therapies are part of the phenomenon of CAM, to be analysed and debated in relation to medical questions (e.g. efficacy, safety or treatment interactions) and professional and institutional questions (e.g. training, professionalization, regulation, funding). Seen as a health (rather than strictly medical) phenomenon, alternative therapies are part of the 'self-health' movement (Stacey 2000: 115), which itself overlaps with the health and fitness boom, which itself shades into beauty and lifestyle practices. Seen through the lens of religion, however, alternative therapies look a little different – they are one manifestation of a changing religious landscape, including the decline of organized Christianity and the advent of a postulated 'spiritual revolution'.[15] These different discursive clusters (medical; health, beauty and fitness; religious/spiritual) are not, of course, distinct, but interpenetrate each other. The same practice may be 'called up' and practised differently within different discursive framings. Yoga, for example, may be carried out as a medical, spiritual, fitness, recreational or therapeutic practice, or, most likely, as some amalgam of the above.

What, then, are some of the lines of coherence among this welter of meanings – the principles or beliefs that bind alternative medicine into a recognizable, if nonetheless disparate, amalgam of practices?

SOME WIDELY SHARED PRINCIPLES OF ALTERNATIVE THERAPIES

Perhaps the most vital principle underlying alternative medicine is the idea of the body's ability to heal itself. This principle in turn usually relies on a belief in a deeper underlying force – the 'life force'. Though conceived of differently in different traditions (Kaptchuk 2001), it is usually understood as essentially a *creative* force that 'acts upon material things, bringing them ever onward and upward to an unknown goal' (Hughes-Gibb 1928: xv). A key corollary of such beliefs is the principle that the healer doesn't heal. The client (a term to which I'll return later in the chapter) is almost universally understood to heal him/herself, with the therapist acting more as a catalyst, supporter, resource, guide or channel for some other healing agent. In Bowen therapy, for example, neither the therapist nor the therapy itself is seen as doing the work; they are both 'merely the helper in the process of assisting nature to do its own amazing work' (Wilde 2006: 24). In the energy healing known as reiki, a sacred or 'higher' energy either heals or catalyses the body's own healing abilities; in hypnotherapy, it is the person's subconscious that does the work; in homeopathy, it is the immune system that is 'kick-started'. No matter whether the healing impetus is understood as coming from within or without, the practitioner is rarely seen as the 'doer'. The relationship between practitioner and client is conceived of as a collaboration or partnership (Williams 1998); clients are, to use Jackie Stacey's term, 'participatory patients' (1997: 3). As reiki practitioner and hypnotherapist Sharron put it:

> [The clients] have all the resources they need. I don't see myself in any capacity, no matter how I'm working, as being the healer. I facilitate. I'm a channel through which the reiki energy comes. The way that I conduct myself can assist to create a space for them to heal. When I'm doing hypnotherapy it is as a facilitator. They're the ones with the knowledge. They're the ones with the inner resources.

The catalytic rather than curative role is a philosophical principle, but it also happily accords with the fact that in most Western countries, claims about diagnosis, treatment or cure have legal implications.[16]

Given this belief in the body's capacity to self-heal, a crucial second principle of alternative medicine is the aim of minimizing certain types of medical interventions – primarily surgical and pharmacological ones – in favour of other, putatively 'natural' and avowedly safe ones. Alternative medicine's 'hesitancy to employ "heroic" measures that often are useless or have disastrous side effects' (Goldstein 2004: 930) has been identified as one of the features that make it attractive. Therapeutic intervention is often aimed less at directly combating the disease so much as at aiding the body to fight the disease, whether by strengthening the immune system, removing root causes of disease, such as emotional blockages, or helping people to break emotional, nutritional or psychological habits. As the naturopath, educator and former Dean of a natural therapies college, Nancy, put it in an interview:

> It's only your own immune system that's going to cure anything. So, they're wellness techniques really, as opposed to disease techniques.

Nancy linked this orientation to the fundamental concept of balance, or homeostasis: 'Natural medicine is always aiming for homeostasis', she said. The word 'balance' appears more frequently in some therapies than in others (in kinesiology, for example, energetic 'balances' form a large part of the treatment regime), but the principle of balance implicitly underlies many therapies. The extent to which holism is foregrounded depends on the therapy in question, but perhaps more significantly on the interests, training and leanings of the practitioner. Many therapies – iridology, chiropractic, massage – can be practised quite technically, even mechanistically, as well as more holistically to include other aspects of the person – emotional, mental, spiritual – in both diagnosis and treatment.

Ideas of self-healing and balance are bound up in a particular idea, or ideology, of nature, linking nature to 'goodness, wholesomeness and virtue' (Coward 1989: 17). In alternative therapies, nature is not the bringer of death, disease, pain or decay;

nor is it the nature of competition (survival of the fittest). Nature is sanitized into the nature of health and renewal rather than that of mess, violence or degeneration. The discourses of natural therapies place much emphasis on process (e.g. the body as dynamic; life as a process of continual change), but they tend to focus on processes of regeneration rather than entropy. This is not to say that alternative therapies see death as a defeat, something to be avoided at all costs. They do not. They usually see death as another part of life's process, to be 'done well' – i.e. peacefully and reflectively. Alternative medicine is often, in fact, less death-denying than mainstream biomedicine, whose approaches tend to focus more on the struggle to maintain life than on its peaceful relinquishment (palliative care being a feminized exception and one in which, moreover, natural therapies are often asked to play a role). Alternative therapies may well even see a 'good death' as itself a form of healing (Barcan and Johnston 2011).

The idealized model of nature is, as sociologist and medical doctor David Armstrong points out, linked to a holistic model of the person: 'The whole-person exists in a natural world, indeed is a part of the natural environment' (1986: 28). Armstrong notes that sociology, with its traditional emphasis on social control, has tended to see a 'pernicious' (31) side to the whole-person paradigm, seeing it as an instrument of the medicalization of everyday life, part of the expansionist tendencies of modern medicine (31–2). This argument was made famous in the 1970s by the sociologist Irving Zola (1972) and later by Ivan Illich (1976), who called for the liberation of an increasingly dependent public from the clutches of a controlling medical establishment. More recently, critiques of medicalization have been influenced by the French philosopher Michel Foucault, and have focused on the ways in which external control has increasingly been internalized as self-surveillance. Nikolas Rose's (1996, 1999) influential critiques of what he calls the 'psy' matrix (psychology, psychiatry, psychotherapy), for example, draw on Foucault to argue that the idea of the whole person is a powerful discursive illusion, 'a fantasy which belongs significantly to this particular historical moment' (Coward 1989: 90). Given the holism of both mainstream medicine and CAM, we can nowadays *all* logically construe ourselves as 'patients' in need of therapy to make us whole again (Armstrong 1995: 397).

Holism is the site of something of an intellectual standoff. In CAM, holism may mean different things,[17] but it usually includes the belief that both illness and healing need to be understood as encompassing physical, mental, emotional, spiritual and social factors. For cultural critics trained in post-structuralism, the very word 'holistic' is likely to trigger an immediate intellectual response of suspicion – perhaps even impatience with the baffling persistence of a self-evidently false notion like the whole person. Meanwhile, the vast majority of practitioners and consumers of alternative medicine remain unaware that this sacred tenet at the core of their practice

– indeed, one of its chief *attractions* – arouses the ire of some cultural critics. For CAM, holism is a form of *recognition* – of the implication of emotions, thoughts and lifestyles in full human (including biological) functioning; for medical sociologists, it is the politically or socially problematic *construal* of an increasing array of aspects of human life as medical problems, which then leads irrevocably down the path of diagnosis and intervention. This great chasm between academic and alternative discourse is unfortunate – both because it means that many alternative practitioners never get the chance to problematize simplistic notions of nature and wholeness, and conversely because it robs cultural critics of their opportunity (and indeed their responsibility) to think more complexly about what wholeness could mean or might be. In that absence, much of the popular CAM literature assumes holism as a more or less unproblematic category whose difficulties are not conceptual but political (i.e. it is something to be fought for in the face of biomedical resistance). A more scientific CAM literature, however, explores intelligently the complexity of biological holism and its relations to non-biomedical models of the body (e.g. Hankey 2005). Indeed, one of the exciting contemporary frontiers of biomedicine itself is psychoneuroimmunology, a field that conceives of itself as demonstrating scientifically 'the fundamental unity of the organism' (Daruna 2004: 1). Psychoneuroimmunology's interest in the interconnection between the brain and the immune system is understood in a fundamentally social way that recognizes from the outset the 'personal and social consequences' of health and illness (2004: 19) and the role of psychosocial factors in biological development. Life circumstances, it is recognized, affect brain activity and hence immune function, and vice versa (2004: 19).

While some fields of biomedicine are moving towards a greater recognition of complex interactions between different aspects of the organism (which is, perhaps, a more biological and potentially less romantic way of thinking about holism), a whole raft of factors still push everyday biomedical *practice* to be segmentist and localizing. While ever this is the case, alternative therapies will continue to attract more and more people because of their typical insistence on the importance of, and interconnection between, the mental, physical, spiritual and emotional. Indeed, philosopher Wouter J. Hanegraaff identifies this feature as one of the core differences between alternative and orthodox medicine and a major source of the former's appeal (1998: 43). As Sharron put it:

> We talk about the mind and the body and the spirit and we have conversations about these aspects of ourselves and it's convenient to be able to articulate those concepts. But you know, they're not living at separate addresses!

Holism continues to be a dominant assumption in alternative therapies not just as a matter of *principle* – i.e. out of alternative medicine's ideological or political commitment to an idea of the whole person – but also as a matter of anatomy or body modelling. Specifically, many alternative therapies are underpinned by the so-called 'subtle' body model, in which the body is understood to be comprised of energy. This concept is foundational to Traditional Chinese Medicine, including acupuncture, where the subtle energy is known as *chi*, as well as to yoga, where the animating life force is known as *prana*. In subtle body models, which are found in various forms in a range of medical cosmologies, the body is imagined as a multiple set of energetic 'sheaths' extending beyond the physical body (Johnston 2008; Johnston and Barcan 2006; Brennan 1988; Dale 2009). Each sheath or body has its own name, and these vary from tradition to tradition, but include the physical body, the mental body, the emotional body and the etheric body. The most well-known lexicon of the subtle body – that of auras and *chakras*[18] – has become central to New Age thought and to many, though not all, alternative therapies. This model, which will be discussed in more detail in Chapter 2, is inherently holistic because it sees these multiple bodies as interpenetrating. An event or intervention on one bodily level (e.g. via physical exercise, meditation or emotional release) will thus inevitably have effects on the others. Moreover, since 'all of reality is *interrelated* and *interdependent*' (Rhodes 1995: 9, original emphasis), reflections, correspondences and resonances occur not just within the boundaries of the body-self, but across the whole 'Divine Oneness' (Trevelyan, qtd in Rhodes 1995: 9) of the universe. But the metaphor of reflection is really an oversimplification of the schema. As yoga teacher Stephen Cope puts it, a better metaphor is that of the hologram, since 'all the aspects of reality exist at the same time and the same place, completely' (1999: 69). This, then, is an *animated* universe – one comprised of an energy that is simultaneously living, material and divine and that unites not only philosophically but *literally* and *materially* all humans, conceived of as 'members of a single holy family, proceeding from the one and only divine substance' (41).

Thus, the subtle body model is holistic not just because it sees the body as an *internally* interwoven multiplicity, but because it sees it as interwoven with the wider world or cosmos. It is comprised of fundamentally the same 'stuff' as the rest of the world (i.e. energy). Acupuncturist Lucy describes it as follows:

> *Chi* is living energy. It makes us alive ... We're standing in an environment of *chi* – there's *chi* coming from the heavens and coming up from the earth. It's moving all the time. That's just the way the world works in this model.

The New Age has accepted this model and typically tries to integrate it with a popularized contemporary scientific explanation of matter. The deep holism of the subtle body model is thus frequently linked to contemporary physics, as in Deepak Chopra's claim that 'At the quantum level *no* part of the body lives apart from the rest' (2001: 14). New Age meditation expert Shakti Gawain likewise uses this pop scientific language: 'Our physical universe is not really composed of any "matter" at all; its basic component is a kind of force or essence which we can call *energy*' (1978: 5, original emphasis). Material differences arise not from ontological distinction but from different densities of energy – the different speeds at which energy vibrates: 'Thought is a relatively fine, light form of energy and therefore very quick and easy to change. Matter is relatively dense, compact energy, and therefore slower to move and change' (6). This monistic principle is mobilized as at once a scientific truth, a philosophical precept and an ethical invitation towards interconnection with others and the collective oneness known to the New Age as 'the universe'.

The energetic model of the body that underpins practices as diverse as yoga, acupuncture and homeopathy is thus an anatomic model bound up in a broader principle of resonance and correspondences, whereby the 'gross physical body that we can see and touch is only the most outward and visible form of a whole layering of energy realities that exist at increasingly refined and less tangible levels' (Cope 1999: 68). Bobby Clennell, summarizing the eighth-century BCE yogic texts the Upanishads, puts it this way: 'Our own being is a miniature universe within which reside the sun, moon, stars and elements. Man is the microcosm of the cosmic being, or the universe' (1997: 14). Thus, as we will see in Chapter 5, the energetic model of the body claims to provide a material explanation for otherwise mysterious phenomena, such as coincidence and intuition. If one takes it seriously, it opens up, as Jay Johnston (2008) has argued in detail, a vista of radical intersubjectivity with profound implications for how one thinks and does ethics.

These core precepts are shared in broad form across many alternative therapies. They involve simultaneously a theory of matter, an esoteric anatomy (that of the subtle body), a principle of microcosm and correspondences, and a dream of a kind of transcendence that does not involve movement away from the physical body, but of unifying the multiple planes of embodied existence, from the gross material plane to the so-called 'bliss' body. Such a project involves the recognition of the elemental oneness of humans. In yoga:

> Though we may appear separate from one another, we are no more separate than the wave is separate from the sea, or than the air in a glass jar is separate from the surrounding air. We are pervaded by and animated by the same spirit, the same nature … (Cope 1999: 41)

In the yogic context, such claims of universal oneness sit within a codified moral framework that includes the *Yama* or universal moral commandments: non-violence, truth, non-stealing, continence and non-coveting (Iyengar 1991: 31). In the New Age context, spirituality is intermeshed within a broader culture of individualism,

and moral prescriptions are usually eschewed in favour of a more floating countercultural idea of moral self-determination. (Indeed, Hanegraaff detects a 'striking
absence' of prescriptive moral injunctions in New Age religion (1998: 280).) The
individual project of self-development and the ethical or political claims on that self
implied by the idea of universal oneness are to some extent in tension in New Age
dogma (see Heelas 1996: 24–5 and Hanegraaff 1998: Ch. 10). Moreover, discussions about social justice are largely absent in popular spiritual discourse (Carrette
and King 2005: x). Given this, and the New Age's notorious individualism, is it
conceivable that alternative therapies could be pushed towards a more *social* (rather
than 'cosmic') vision of interconnectedness, a vision that was perhaps already there
in the countercultural origins of the holistic health movement? If so, this might be
construed as an even fuller holism – one that encompasses not just mind-body-
spirit but mind-body-spirit-society (Baer 2004: xix). The spiritual basis of alternative
medicine did after all ultimately emanate from traditional medicine's role as an essentially sacred and *social* practice (De Rosny 1998: 9), though it has been shaped
within the 'individualization of religious sensibilities' (Carrette and King 2005: 14)
that characterized modernity, and in particular by the individualism of the US metaphysical traditions and later the New Age.

The spiritual character of much alternative medicine is one of its core features,
and a particular point of difference from biomedicine. For, regardless of the beliefs
of individual medical practitioners and patients, and despite a number of well-es-
tablished if relatively minor lines of research concerning the *interrelations* of religion
and health (e.g. into the medical efficacy of prayer (Dossey 1993) or the impact
of religious faith on health),[19] orthodox biomedicine is underpinned by a secular
scientific rationality, and any official discussion of religious or spiritual belief tends
mostly to occur either in relation to (cross)-cultural sensitivity or in medical fields
where it is seemingly more obviously central, such as palliative care.

The spiritual basis of alternative health means that it views illness as deeply
meaningful. First, alternative medicine shares with both psychology and sociology
an awareness of the personal and social impact and functioning of illness. As in the
discipline of medical sociology, where discussions of the sick role (Parsons 1951),
biographical disruption (Bury 1982) and psychosocial factors in illness are prevail-
ing themes, alternative therapists are aware of the impact of illness on a person's
ability to perform his or her social and familial roles, and of the deep impact illness
can have on one's sense of self. Illness is seen as both personally meaningful and
socially significant. A second order of meaning is a psychoanalytical one, since one
of the most fundamental and widely shared of principles underpinning and animating alternative medicine, and reflecting its debt, usually unacknowledged, to Freud,
is a belief in the significance of life events, emotions and thought patterns in causing

illness. Theories of emotional/psychological causation of illness abound in alternative medicine, especially under the influence of New Age thought. Unsurprisingly, they have been the object of fierce critique from mainstream medicine and within cultural commentary; Susan Sontag's (1977) seminal denunciation of the metaphorical understanding of tuberculosis and cancer is the most well known. When queried on this issue, almost all alternative practitioners will ultimately say that there may well be causes other than emotional ones (environmental, perhaps genetic), but one gets the impression that this often functions as a kind of conceptual residue used to explain failure of emotion-based treatment (i.e. an idea of organic illness arrived at as a final retreat) and/or as a kind of quasi-legal disclaimer. For example, a book about intuition by Mona Lisa Schulz (the remarkable figure mentioned above, who is simultaneously a physician, a neuroscientist and a medical clairvoyant) focuses on the emotional meaning of illness. In the inside cover, however, there is a legal disclaimer that includes the following:

> Human vulnerability to disease cannot be reduced to a single physical or emotional cause. Many genetic, nutritional, environmental, emotional, and other unknown reasons contribute to the development of illness and disease. Although many studies will be cited in this book that discuss specific emotional factors that contribute to illness, no study is perfect. There are limitations to any scientific inquiry. Patients should work with their health care practitioners to examine for themselves which problems, relationships, habits, and situations in their lives contribute to health or disease. (1998: n.p.)

That this multifactorial account of illness occurs in a disclaimer in the inside cover rather than constituting the body of the argument suggests the role of 'other' (i.e. non-emotional/spiritual) causes of illness as a kind of supplement. This is internally logical since, as we have seen, the subtle body model makes no fundamental ontological distinction between spirit and matter (Johnston 2008: 2).

Metaphysical accounts of illness have had a significant place in the US religious landscape well before they were codified into something known 'officially' as the New Age. Catherine Albanese's history of American metaphysical thought contends that metaphysical thought was 'a *major* player' in the evolution of US religiosity in the nineteenth century (2007: 4, original emphasis), alongside evangelicalism and mainstream Christian denominational practice (2007: 5). Metaphysical thought has diffused into a broader popular culture, of which the New Age is the most visible exemplum. Perhaps the most famous New Age proponent of metaphysical concepts of illness, Louise L. Hay (to whom I will return in a moment), developed her theories within the Church of Religious Science, founded by Ernest Holmes in the early decades of the twentieth century.[20] Holmes had read Freud, as well as texts from Eastern mysticism, such as the Bhagavad Gita, and Western hermeticism

(Albanese 2007: 426–7). This type of formation helps explain why contemporary alternative/New Age thought not only embraces a Freudian-influenced idea that repressed emotions might account for *some* symptoms or illnesses, but often extends this into a universal metaphysical theory of illness.[21] In esoteric anatomy derived from Eastern religions, illness is generally understood as emanating in the more 'subtle' bodies before eventually manifesting in the denser, physical layer (Brennan 1988: 7). In the New Age, this trickle-down model, in which illness is a 'distortion' transmitted gradually through all seven auric bodies before finally manifesting in the physical body (141ff), is often rendered in a kind of shorthand as a stark dualism: illness starts in the mind and manifests in the body. This haziness is again traceable to the synthesizing work of thinkers like Holmes, who understood spirit as 'both the Universal Mind (God) and the subjective, or unconscious, mind of humans' (Albanese 2007: 426). Albanese characterizes Holmes's conception of divine action as having a 'mechanical quality', since the Universal Mind produced a form in the physical world to match each idea (426).

These influences and this mechanism are visible in the writing of Louise L. Hay, one of the best-selling New Age self-help writers of all (Oppenheimer 2008).[22] Hay's enormously influential books invite you to 'look up the mental cause' for your physical problem (1987: 149). In its most strenuous form, this intersection of a psychologized culture with a spiritualized anatomy can result in fundamentalist prescriptions, such as Hay's unequivocal statement that 'Every cell within your body responds to every single thought you think and every word you speak' (127). In such a view, emotion is not part of a multifactorial account of illness; it is a universal root cause able to be decoded for its metaphysical 'meaning'. Her book *You Can Heal Your Life* (1987) contains not only a general emotional anatomy (e.g. the back represents our support system (132); the colon our ability to let go (139); the skin our individuality (140)), but also a minutely detailed dictionary of symptoms and illnesses, where you can 'look up' the 'meaning' of your illness. A fuller version of this schema was published separately as *Heal Your Body* (1988), where the metaphysical 'meanings' of bodily symptoms are matched with corrective affirmations. In Hay's schema (and there are a number of similar ones), rheumatism means feeling victimized (1988: 60); ringworm means allowing others to get under your skin (60); insomnia is fear, lack of trust, or guilt (44); and flatulence 'Gripping. Fear. Undigested ideas' (36). Not all the practitioners I interviewed shared Hay's belief in universal, prescriptive always-emotional meanings of disease. In my experience, belief in metaphysical causation seems more practitioner-dependent than modality-dependent, but Hay's ideas are nonetheless very influential. There is, moreover, a shared precept even beyond New Age accounts that many modern illnesses are 'diseases of meaning' (Jobst el al. 1999).

The metaphysical view of illness means that illness can be 'read' and translated as an index of one's psychological or spiritual wellbeing. Your body is, to quote the title of Annette Noontil's book (1994), 'the barometer of your soul'. Often, this takes the form of a pedagogic discourse, where illness is seen, especially by New Age practitioners, as a spiritual 'lesson':

> It is essential that we deal with the deeper meaning of our illnesses. We need to ask, what does this illness mean to me? What can I learn from this illness? Illness can be seen as simply a message from your body to you that says, *Wait a minute; something is wrong. You are not listening to your whole self; you are ignoring something very important to you. What is it?* (Brennan 1988: 7, original emphasis)

So it is that illness can paradoxically be conceived as 'good for you' – as suggested by titles like Dethlefsen and Dahlke's *The Healing Power of Illness* (1992) and Harrison's *Love Your Disease* (1984).[23] Illness is a tap on the shoulder from 'the universe', a 'lesson you have given yourself to help you remember who you are' (Brennan 1988: 131), 'a key to the education of the soul' (145). It is more than an affliction or punishment to be borne stoically or heroically; it is viewed more optimistically – as a 'manifestation of health' (Jobst et al. 1999: 495), a healthy sign that the body is striving to regain equilibrium (495). New Age versions of this idea of illness as an opportunity for growth and self-improvement bear the trace of the pragmatism of some of the nineteenth-century US spiritual movements that informed the New Age, like Emerson's Transcendentalism (Melton 1988: 36–9).

The pedagogic discourse is one means of reconciling the sense of illness as both punishment (in this case, for 'bad' thoughts) and blessing. It also reconciles the idea of a fundamentally beneficent universe with the existence of suffering, since the universe brings 'lessons' that become increasingly unsubtle to those who refuse them or do not know how to listen. Thus illness and suffering can be 'useful' but ultimately needless: 'Suffering is not good for the soul, unless it teaches you how to stop suffering' ('Seth' qtd in Hanegraaff 1998: 280).[24] This pedagogic concept of illness, in which there is no place for accident, luck or chance, sits quite happily in consumer culture, since it involves both comfort and control. It is also one of the ways in which the New Age influence on alternative medicine is most at odds with conventional medicine. For any alternative therapy (or practitioner) strongly influenced by New Age thought there are no accidents – only signs, lessons, meanings. As can be imagined, it is this facet of alternative/New Age thought that has attracted the most ire of all, both from mainstream medical practitioners and from cultural analysts.

THE RISE OF ALTERNATIVE THERAPIES: SOCIAL FACTORS

As I noted at the start of this chapter, CAM is one of the fastest growing areas of health care (Ruggie 2004: 43), with up to half the population of many Western nations making use of some form of alternative therapy. This is economically very significant: in Australia in 2000, for example, people spent nearly four times as much money on complementary medicine as on prescription drugs (MacLennan et al. 2002: 170). Why is CAM so attractive? Mary Ruggie suggests three main reasons: a disenchantment with conventional medicine; a search for self-control; and an increasing match between the values, beliefs and philosophies embodied in CAM and the world-views of CAM users (2004: 45). This philosophical dimension is highlighted by medical doctor Karen Lawson. She sees CAM as reflecting a number of philosophical trends she (somewhat oddly) calls postmodern: 'a movement to-wards holism, a renewed desire for spiritual meaning, an increasing belief in intuitive knowledge, and the recognition of the power of intention for healing' (2002: 16).

In the chapters that follow, I aim to connect these philosophical trends to a larger sociocultural picture, as well as to matters of embodiment and sensory experience. What new forms of bodily imagining and bodily life does alternative medicine open up, and why might these be both plausible and attractive in the contemporary moment? To address such big questions, I move between three registers of analysis: the *cultural* (questions to do with the meanings, mechanisms and models of the body bound up with these therapies); the *social* (in which the therapies' popularity is linked to social questions – such as gender, consumerism and changing relations to the self); and the *experiential* (i.e. what new forms of bodily experience these therapies open up). In order to set the stage for the next chapters, which focus on the senses in order to explore the embodied experiences made possible in alterna-tive medicine, I will survey a selection of sociocultural factors implicated in the rise of CAM: 1) dissatisfaction with orthodox biomedicine; 2) the rise of the New Age movement; 3) the rise of consumerism; 4) neoliberalism; and 5) the body as a project.

DISSATISFACTION WITH ORTHODOX BIOMEDICINE

In an essay on the relations between alternative and conventional medicine, medical anthropologist Judith Fadlon (2004) discusses the question of modern dissatisfac-tion with orthodox biomedicine. She identifies a prevalent argument about the attractiveness of alternative therapies – that the popularity of CAM represents a rejection of biomedicine (2004: 70–1). Modern Westerners, it is commonly argued, have become increasingly unhappy at the technological interventionism and negative side-effects of much biomedicine, and alienated by its construction of the patient as a passive recipient of treatment rather than as an empowered individual with many dimensions (physical, emotional and spiritual). For an increasing number of patients, CAM is the medicine of 'first resort' (Goldstein 2004). This reading, says Fadlon, tends to situate the rise of alternative therapies in the larger countercultural movements.

It is true that orthodox medicine has particular (perceived) shortcomings. Frequently cited limitations include its perceived reductionism and secularism (Rhodes 1995: 13); its mechanism (seeing the body as an object to be repaired) (Scott 1998: 22); its dualism; its paternalism, especially towards female patients (Birke 1999); its 'communicative and psychological shortcomings' (Willard 2005: 115); its doctor-centredness (Goldner 2004); its highly interventionist practices (e.g. surgery and pharmacology); and the consequent potential for side-effects or medically induced illness, known as iatrogenesis. Two specific limitations frequently cited are the treatment of emotional, psychological and psychiatric conditions including depression, anxiety and stress, and the treatment (rather than 'management') of chronic conditions like back pain, sinus and asthma. These two broad categories of biomedical weakness suggest that the rise of CAM is linked not only to changes in the nature of medicine, but also to changes in the nature of illness itself. The rise of chronic and degenerative illnesses, for example, is a paradoxical result of biomedicine's success in promoting longevity (Turner 1992: 155). Moreover, medical success has raised our expectations about what constitutes a healthy body.

The CAM literature on dissatisfaction with biomedicine contains a second sub-theme – that the rise of CAM is not a result of blanket dissatisfaction with orthodox medicine, as much as of its specific failures (Fadlon 2004). According to this argument, CAM users are socially quite diverse, and CAM is not perceived as 'an esoteric choice' (Fadlon 2004: 71) nor is it part of a wholesale rejection of orthodox medicine. Rather, this view sees CAM use as a 'practical choice' (71) in the choice-rich environment offered by postmodern consumer cultures. Its use, then, is an indication of pluralism rather than resistance. This is the view taken by Mary Ruggie, who, it was noted earlier, saw dissatisfaction with biomedicine as a major contributor to the rise of CAM, but who was quick to note that disenchantment is not the same thing as rejection (2004: 47). Patients recognize the spectacular successes of biomedicine in emergency medicine, public health,[25] pharmacology (e.g. antibiotics); short-term pain relief (e.g. epidurals in childbirth) and so on. Not even the most ardent fan of 'natural' methods would be likely to reject an anaesthetic during a tooth extraction, let alone during surgery! Most people do not totally reject biomedicine but pick and choose what they want.

What is it, then, that people seem to want? The 'pull factors' *towards* CAM are widely reported, and include: the minimization of technological and pharmaceutical intervention; the foregrounding of an ethic of care; the treatment of the patient as an individual; holism, especially an emphasis on psychological and emotional factors; connection to larger philosophies of life, including to spirituality; personal attention and time devoted to clients; and a close, ongoing relationship with a practitioner, often involving a kind of intimacy, whether physical (e.g. massage) or emotional (e.g. counselling). The naturopath Nancy pointed to an increasing lack of personal connection with the GP: 'I think another thing that's gone is the concept of the GP who knew people for a long time. I mean, you might never see the same doctor twice nowadays.' While reports of the death of the family GP are, to invoke Mark Twain, greatly exaggerated, it is certainly true that leisurely consultations and a personal, ongoing relation with a family doctor are under threat, a fact that has medical implications, but also social ones, as people increasingly desire a sense of having been recognized and acknowledged in the medical encounter. This was made clear to me on one occasion as I arranged to interview a home-based alternative therapist. She wanted me to know that hers wasn't a large practice, lest I be disappointed. 'We're a small practice,' she said. 'We don't have many clients come through. But every one of them is cherished.' This kind of personal attention stands in clear contrast to the standardized, time-limited exchanges that all too often characterize a visit to the local GP. If I were feeling stressed I could chat to a GP about it for my allotted fifteen minutes, or I could have a massage (an intimate, sensual experience lasting up to an hour and a half). Moreover, I could also join up with others in a similar situation. For not all alternative treatments take place as commodified exchanges where a client purchases a service from an expert; rather, there exists a vast and largely invisible network of informal amateur social exchanges where friends, often women, swap treatments like reiki, massage or Touch for Health in their homes in informally organized networks of care.

As a response to late modernity, then, alternative medicine must not be understood only 'negatively' – as a response to the limitations of biomedicine and a challenge to its authority – but also positively. Its regular users create for themselves networks of care – not only the often intimate commodified relations between clients and practitioners, but also more informal, democratic, social networks operating outside of the market.

THE RISE OF THE NEW AGE MOVEMENT

The appetite for both commodities and community is part and parcel of the New Age spirituality with which alternative medicine is so deeply intertwined. For despite the individualistic *philosophy* of the New Age, as a cultural *practice* it nonetheless shares the emphasis on life-changing emotional experience and communal testifying that characterized American revivalism (Albanese 2007: 5). And although as a movement it is dispersed and resistant to organization, to the extent where many question the validity of the term 'movement' to describe it (Hanegraaff 1998: 1), the formation of groups and networks is nonetheless an important part of popular spiritual practice.

Over the last two decades, the New Age has escaped its boundaries as a specific spiritual movement of the counterculture and pervaded a broader popular culture (Sutcliffe 2006: 160) in the form of more free-floating 'methodologies' amenable to the market (Melton 1988: 42). It has attracted those unsatisfied by the rationality of atheism, wary of religious dogma, or unwilling to trade in the pleasures of consumerism for those of asceticism. As such, it is part of the broader 'subjective turn' of modern culture (Heelas et al. 2005: 2). This 'subjective' (rather than alienated) modernity is characterized by a movement away from a role- and duty-based understanding of selfhood towards one in which aspects of *inner* experience become primary: 'states of consciousness, states of mind, memories, emotions, passions, sensations, bodily experiences, dreams, feelings, inner conscience, and sentiments – including moral sentiments like compassion' (3). In this version of modern culture, the 'good life' consists, as Heelas et al. describe, 'in living one's life in full awareness of one's states of being; in enriching one's experiences; in finding ways of handling negative emotions; in becoming sensitive enough to find out where and how the quality of one's life – alone or in relation – may be improved' (2005: 4). The New Age has provided a vehicle in which these modern values can have a spiritual dimension. Insofar as alternative medicine interpenetrates with the New Age (which it does significantly, though the two are not coterminous),[26] it appeals to those seeking a spirituality not based on a denial of materialism, the body, sexuality, pleasure or the senses. New Age spiritual practices are often based in the body, and the senses are not seen as obstacles to spiritual development but as a pathway to it.

THE RISE OF CONSUMERISM

Spirituality-in-the-body also chimes with a consumer culture in which inner states are increasingly bound up with commodities. The rise of CAM is undoubtedly a consumer-led phenomenon (Bodeker 2001: 164). Although the alternative health movement dates from the counterculture of the 1960s and 1970s, where it had at least some connection to back-to-nature ideologies and an ethic of simplicity, the therapeutic practices that constitute contemporary alternative medicine are now firmly embedded in the pleasure-seeking, individualist, body-focused drive of consumer culture. In particular, they are bound up in the aestheticization of every-day life and the appeal to the senses increasingly offered by the market.

In his essay 'Hyperesthesia, or, the Sensual Logic of Late Capitalism', David Howes (2005a) argues that Marx's focus on production made him more aware of the sensory *losses* imposed by industrial capitalism than of the new forms of sensory experience it engendered. Marx vividly described the 'stripping of the senses' effected by capitalism (Howes 2005a: 282) – the alienation of the senses caused by poverty and by the deafening and dulling conditions of factory life. He argued that even among the bourgeoisie the senses were dulled – through their fixation on only one object, capital (283). He paid little attention to the appeal to the senses offered to the bourgeoisie by the developing commercial and visual culture. This appeal to the senses – what Howes calls 'the sensual logic of late capitalism' (287) – has become ever more pervasive, culminating in the 'hypersensuality of the contemporary mar-ketplace' (290).

Alternative therapies can certainly be understood as part and parcel of this (hy-per)aestheticization of everyday life. For those with economic means, they offer rich bodily experiences of touch, smell and sound, which set them apart from the every-day. For regular users they form part of a (privileged) art of living – where the purely medical function of biomedicine is replaced, supplemented or enriched via practices based in an ethic of self-care, of bodily sensuality and, sometimes, of reciprocity, and where sensual self-care becomes a reward for the (perceived) hardships of everyday life. Often offered by the self to the self as a reward for the pressures of everyday life (motherhood, family responsibilities, longer working hours, stress), they are spaces of sensuality, experimentation and relaxation. In short, they offer 'time out' from modernity understood as rational, secular and controlling. In this sense, alternative therapies are part of an emerging art of living in which the medical, the sensual, the spiritual and the recreational may coalesce. Alternative medicine may well be an extension of the medicalization of everyday life as its critics contend, but it's also part of the aestheticization of that life. (Note how the term 'client', the standard term used in alternative medicine, recognizes the commodity relations involved, and paradoxically *de*-medicalizes the therapeutic encounter.) Indeed, one of alterna-tive medicine's chief features is the re-aestheticization (and the re-sacralization) of medicine itself. The sensuality of massage, the aromas of essential oils or the warmth of touch are precisely the kinds of bodily experiences the market hopes to capture, evoke and sell.

The contemporary quest for sensual experience is thus both a backlash against some aspects of late modernity and an expression of other core aspects of it. As the neoliberal economy brings less job security, longer working hours and incessant demands to increase our 'productivity', some people fall through the cracks, while others fall into the willing arms of a consumer culture promising us solace, reward and escape.

NEOLIBERALISM

I stated earlier that most clients of CAM use it in combination with orthodox medicine, picking and choosing what they want to use. This is especially true of the demographic that most typifies CAM use – discerning, educated consumers with a sense of entitlement, money to spend, and a belief in consumer choice. Alternative therapies may have spiritual origins and a countercultural history, but they have a neoliberal present. In a funding context in which the economic burden of health care grows at an exponential rate (thanks to the combined effects of an ageing population, an increasingly technologically sophisticated medicine, and a diminishing tax base), there has been a paradigmatic shift towards a model of an empowered health consumer taking responsibility for his/her own health, making informed choices from a variety of different modalities, and being prepared to pay out of pocket. Citizenship 'is increasingly being defined in terms of consumer identities' (McDonald et al. 2007: 432) and making good health choices becomes a responsibility of citizenship (432). This model brings the two cornerstones of neoliberalism – choice and responsibility – into the marketplace, and also into modern psychology, via a discourse of 'empowerment'. Critics see this discourse as a 'subtle mechanism for shifting responsibility from the state to the patient' and a mechanism for surveillance and social punishment of those who make 'bad' health choices (434). In neoliberalism, 'personal responsibility for risk avoidance is structured as a model of citizenship' (Dovey 2000: 79). It goes hand in hand with a decline in authority of the GP resulting from biomedical specialization (Pringle 1998: 156–7) and from the growth in the idea of lay expertise, a democratic sentiment fuelled, in part, by the Internet (see Ziebland et al. 2004). This can certainly be empowering, but mainly for those with considerable intellectual or social capital. It is also a double-edged sword. Doctors and critics lament the rise of a cohort of the so-called 'worried well', and GPs report that the phenomenon of Internet-fuelled lay expertise results in more informed, more demanding and more anxious patients (Ramachandran 2007: 12). Moreover, consumer pressure cuts two ways: doctors may feel the pressure to train in a CAM therapy, or at least to familiarize themselves with the range of options available, especially as in some countries the question is arising as to whether doctors' legal requirement to discuss a full range of treatment options with their patients might increasingly be taken to include CAM options (Weir 2003: 297).[27] Thus, to give an accurate sense of the picture, any analysis that focuses on patients being required to take responsibility needs also to note the complexity of forces and counter-forces at work, such as increasing patient litigation against doctors, which relates in quite complicated ways to the idea of responsibility.

The theme of responsibility can easily morph into a discourse of control, and indeed the desire for control was one of the factors cited by Mary Ruggie above as one of the attractions of CAM. Jackie Stacey characterizes contemporary health cultures – both biomedical and alternative – as bringing together 'care, control, will-power and surveillance' (1997: 179). The idea that health is a reward for self-control is becoming increasingly self-evident (Crawford 1985). In this, the New Age is a powerful ally of neoliberalism. Indeed, Jackie Stacey considers the idea that one should take responsibility for one's own health to be 'perhaps the most glaring overlap' between alternative health and 'the Thatcherite legacy of the cult of the individual' (1997: 3). New Age thought builds a traditional US ethic of self-reliance into a fully developed theory of personal responsibility. In her bestseller *You Can Heal Your Life*, Louise L. Hay proclaims:

> I believe that everyone, myself included, is 100% responsible for everything in our lives, the best and the worst ... No person, no place, and no thing has any power over us, for ... we create our experiences, our reality and everyone in it. (1987: 7)

Paul Heelas connects this New Age axiom to the importance placed by the New Age on an 'internalized locus of authority' (1996: 25), and in turn to 'one of the absolutely cardinal New Age values', freedom (26). The New Age typically understands freedom as a personal rather than a social value. The idea that 'we have the freedom to choose every step of the way the manner in which we are going to respond to and deal with [oppressive social] forces' (Scott Peck, qtd in Rimke 2000: 64–5) is another of the New Age doctrines that has infuriated cultural analysts (e.g. Coward 1989: 92).

Control isn't, of course, a New Age invention; it was a feature of some of the ascetic traditions taken up in alternative medicine. The theme of control of the body recurs in yoga and also in Ayurvedic medicine, at least as popularized by the physician and 'poet-prophet of alternative medicine' Deepak Chopra.[28] I do not know how accurately Chopra's writings reflect traditional Ayurvedic thought, but his metaphors of control, choice and perfection certainly resonate with the broader Western culture in which his writing has found such favour. Chopra's exegesis of Ayurvedic medicine certainly reverberates with what Stacey calls 'the recognizable metaphors of Western individualism (control, autonomy and personal output ...' (2000: 116) as well as with the core modern (US/New Age) values of freedom and choice: 'The first secret you should know about perfect health is that you have to choose it' (Chopra 2001: 10). Or: 'The purpose of Ayurveda is to tell us how our lives can be influenced, shaped, extended, *and ultimately controlled* without interference from sickness or old age' (11, my emphasis). It also resonates with the preservationist tendencies of consumer culture, for ageing is, in fact, 'a mistake' (2001: 213). 'The ancient sages', Chopra writes, 'ascribed aging to a "mistake of the intellect" (called *pragya aparadh* in Sanskrit) ... Seeing yourself as free from aging, you will in fact be' (214).[29]

Jackie Stacey sees this obsessive 'desire for mastery' as typifying contemporary health culture, whether alternative *or* biomedical (1997: 238). This is undoubtedly true, but the pedagogic concept of illness can in some cases work to destabilize the idea of control. Jobst et al., for example, argue that 'Disease is not necessarily to be avoided, blocked, or suppressed. Rather, it should be understood to be a process of transformation' (1999: 495). Of course, neither biomedicine nor alternative medicine is animated by a single desire. In the case of alternative therapies, a range of cultural dominants converge and coalesce, sometimes contradicting each other. The desire for control meets the search for pleasure but it may also rub up against the concept of the spiritual journey with its unknown goal; the frisson associated with resistance to medical orthodoxy often sits alongside a sense of consumer entitlement. The user of CAM can be simultaneously a good citizen, a privileged consumer and a spiritual journeyer.

Although the idea of spiritual journeying often relies on the relinquishment of control, it is certainly true that the rhetoric of control is never far out of view, even among those committed to the unpredictability of healing rather than the certainty of cure. Take the following, quite complex example, from a medical clairvoyant I interviewed:

> I'm a great believer that you should take control and responsibility for your life. Then if you are diagnosed with a terminal illness or an illness, take control of it. Find out what emotions, thoughts and actions created it; you can let all those go. Well then if you die at least you've done the best you can; there's nothing else you can do. But if you get rid of all that, well you're still in control of it, aren't you?

Here, the idea the idea of control is absolutely central, but it is not equated only with medical 'success'. As I have argued elsewhere (Barcan and Johnston 2011), alternative medicine, especially in its more spiritual guises, is animated by contradictory impulses – the desire for control and mastery, certainly, but also by the more open-ended idea of 'healing', which is usually construed as a letting go rather than the taking of action, and which may or may not be equated with physical recovery, and may encompass a broader range of transformations, including mental and emotional ones. Interestingly, though, the medical intuitive quoted above uses the term 'control' to cover all eventualities, equating it with the taking of conscious action, regardless of the outcome.

The idea of responsibility for one's health sits at the intersection between a paradigmatic dominant (neoliberalism), a socio-economic phenomenon (consumer culture), a spiritual axiom and a particular demographic – the wave of ageing baby boomers with a rebellious past, high expectations for their health and the habit of buying solutions for problems. As I have already observed, well-off baby boomers constitute a significant proportion of CAM users. Mary Ruggie reports that in the US, alternative medicine is used more by people who have more education; people who have higher income; whites; women; people aged thirty-five to fifty-five; and (in the US) people who live in the Western states (2004: 46). This was echoed in my interview with the naturopath Nancy, who considers that 'a small group of usually affluent-ish women, usually in the twenty-five to forty-five group, probably make up the bulk of the people I see'. But the picture is more complex, since the demographics of use also include people who are in poorer health and people who suffer from chronic illness (Ruggie 2004: 46). Users thus include people for whom it is a last resort (the terminally or chronically ill, the desperate seekers of solutions) as well as the more visible contingent for whom it is a lifestyle choice, an ongoing body management regime, perhaps a first resort (Goldstein 2004), or a luxury indulgence (the corporate weekly massage). Thus Nancy's clientele also include a 'smattering of strange men' and a group she terms scrapheap patients, who may or may not be affluent. In particular, she sees women wanting to have a baby who have run out of standard medical options, having typically had a number of unsuccessful IVF attempts:

> For a lot of my women I'm their last resort because I work with endometriosis and fertility. They've all been tossed on the scrap heap. They've been ruined by drugs, the poor things – but you can do heaps! Get them believing that things can change and they do!

The desperate and the chronically ill, then, can come from across the social scale, and may or may not feel 'empowered'. One can be a 'chooser' consumer (Gabriel and Lang 1995: 27–46) but still be desperate, especially when ill. In her capacity as an educator and media expert as well as a naturopath in private practice, Nancy saw it as an important component of her role to 'convince people of the power of taking back responsibility for their own life and their own health'. 'You make them so happy', she says. 'It's often a concept they hadn't thought of.' I was surprised to hear this, since we hear so much of the rise of concepts of personal responsibility and empowerment that I think of them as a cultural dominant. When I put this to Nancy, she accepted that there was a small group of people for whom this was the case but that in general this was not so:

I think the dominant idea is I am *not* in charge, I am *not* in power. I am powerless. I am a puppet moved by the whims of government, people, this, that and the other. People feel powerless, they don't feel empowered.

Critics of neoliberalism would perhaps agree – citizens are increasingly interpellated as empowered, but they may not *feel* empowered.

THE BODY AS A PROJECT

As we have seen, neoliberalism works in tandem with the market; in the case of responsibility for one's own health, it works with consumer imperatives like the cult of beauty, the refusal of ageing, and competitive performance. The late-modern relation to the self is characterized by a welter of body techniques structured into everyday life that aim to monitor, discipline, develop, preserve or enhance the self – from gym work to cholesterol tests; low GI diets to facials; 10,000-step walking programmes to regular pap smears; jogging, yoga or bikini waxes. Such daily activities blur the realms of medicine, recreation and aesthetics. The body becomes an ongoing project, simultaneously a citizenly responsibility, a reflection of one's moral character, a site of pleasure and leisure and a source of anxiety.

Thus, although alternative therapies are part of what Turner (1996) calls the 'hedonistic' tenor of modernity, this does not mean that they are purely frivolous or pleasure-seeking. The body-as-project is a site of anxiety as well as freedom; it conjoins the two in what Nikolas Rose acerbically terms 'the obligation to be free' (1999: 258). An emerging psychological literature on the burdens of so-called 'hyperchoice' (Mick et al. 2004) tells us what an increasing number of modern citizens already know – that choice is not a simple moral good and that, once a certain level of affluence has been achieved (a crucial point), there is no automatic correlation between increased choice and happiness (B. Schwartz 2004). Although some social critics may have little truck with what might be construed as the burdens of the privileged (the so-called 'choiceoisie' (Savan, qtd in Probyn 1990: 152)), it is nonetheless true that in the neoliberal consumer economy, choice is a responsibility of citizenship, and 'bad' choices can be punished.

Nor does these therapies' place in hedonism mean that they are necessarily resistive, my frequent use of the term 'alternative' notwithstanding. Rather, as Turner points out, one of the 'peculiar features' of the new hedonism is that 'it is also compatible with asceticism' (1996: 124). Hedonistic fascination with the body exists, claims Turner, 'to enhance competitive performance': 'We jog, slim and sleep not for their intrinsic enjoyment, but to improve our chances at sex, work and longevity' (1996: 124). One of the contradictions of alternative therapies, then, is that they can be imagined as self-indulgent time-out from or reward for a stressful job, but their pleasure-enhancing capacities may be ultimately recuperable as a form of 'productivity':

> The new asceticism of competitive social relations exists to create desire – desire which is subordinated to the rationalization of the body as the final triumph of capitalist development. (Turner 1996: 124)

Read this way, alternative therapies start to sound very much like disciplinary techniques in the Foucauldian sense, techniques aimed at disciplining of the body, 'the optimization of its capabilities, the extortion of its forces, the parallel increase of its usefulness and its docility, its integration into systems of efficient and economic controls ...' (Foucault 1979: 139). In this critical tradition, in which forms of medicine are interrogated for their role in securing and managing populations, it is possible, then, to see alternative therapies as not very 'alternative' at all – indeed, as an *extension* rather than a repudiation of the surveillance functions of biomedicine (Armstrong 1995). I have discussed both the benefits and limitations of such arguments in detail elsewhere (Barcan 2008). Here, I want to focus on some of the other major lines of critique from within Cultural Studies.

CRITIQUES OF ALTERNATIVE THERAPIES AND OF NEW AGE CULTURE

In his introduction to the 1988 collection *Not Necessarily the New Age*, Robert Basil claimed that although millions of people had experimented with non-traditional spirituality and with alternative therapies, and although hundreds of books had been written on New Age thinking, there was not one 'intelligent tour' of the New Age movement and very few sceptical studies (9). Twenty years on, a substantial social and medical literature on CAM and CAM science now exists, but intelligent *cultural* studies either of the New Age or of alternative therapies have not proliferated at the same rate. Cultural and Gender Sciences, in particular, have had relatively little to say about alternative therapies. I have addressed this lacuna in detail elsewhere (Barcan and Johnston 2005) so I will treat it only briefly here. But it is worth restating the oddness of what seems to me a glaring gap, given the fact that millions of people worldwide engage with these therapies, that they constitute significant consumer practices and that many of their core ideas are 'diffused through the general culture' (Sutcliffe 2006: 15).

Such cultural analyses as do exist are likely to treat alternative therapies with almost unremitting negativity, in sharp contrast to the populism that has characterized much Cultural Studies since the 1980s. To take just a few examples from the smattering of cultural studies of either alternative therapies, the New Age or the self-help genre: for Heidi Maria Rimke, the public sphere and public responsibility 'are negated by a life of self-help' (2000: 73); for Rosalind Coward, the emphasis on personal responsibility 'rarely generates political empowerment' (1989: 204); for Deborah Root, 'much of the New Age seems almost deliberately to leave itself open to ridicule' (1996: 87); for Nikolas Rose, the psychological disciplines produce governable selves 'obliged' to be free (1999: 258); for Jackie Stacey, self-health culture is based on a desire for mastery (1997: 238); for Andrew Ross, the New Age's emphasis on either individual or universal goals means that it of necessity forsakes the goals of social growth (1991: 74). In short, most Cultural Studies approaches to alternative therapies have been examples of what Eve Sedgwick calls a great 'unveiling' (2003: 141). Nature is unmasked as culture; intuition is unmasked as social rules; liberation and empowerment as still more subtle forms of enslavement or narcissism.

Given my stated predilection for alternative therapies, it is important that I stress from the outset how important these critiques are. I share many of the political and philosophical cautions of these writers, in particular a frustration with the naive concepts of nature so often wielded in popular alternative and New Age discourse (though less so in the professional CAM literature). Part of the bridging work of this Introduction, then, is to give a brief overview of some of the critiques of alternative therapies that come from the cultural disciplines and which are divided from much of the popular alternative rhetoric by something of a conceptual and ideological chasm.[30]

The inevitable starting point in the Humanities for thinking critically about alternative therapies is Susan Sontag's (1977) critique of metaphysical views of illness in *Illness as Metaphor*. Sontag attacks metaphysical and psychological views of illness, seeing them a 'powerful means of placing the blame on the ill' (1977: 61). Although she does not address alternative therapies specifically, the centrality these therapies accord to theories of psychological causation and their tendency to metaphorize illness make Sontag's book an important contribution to the debate about alternative medicine. Sontag condemns the use of cancer as a metaphor for something else, whether it be a plague, a curse, an ill society or a psychological disorder, and compares it with the historical metaphorization of tuberculosis. She argues that 'the most truthful way of regarding illness – and the healthiest way of being ill – is one most purified of, most resistant to, metaphoric thinking' (7). That this idea of 'purification' is itself metaphorical, and that, indeed, Sontag's own book begins with an extended metaphor – 'Illness is the night-side of life, a more onerous citizenship' (7) – is an irony that was not lost on critics, who noted the impossibility of non-metaphorical thought. Sontag herself subsequently explained her opening metaphor as a deliberate and ironic rhetorical flourish (1988: 93), and muted her original manifesto into a call for vigilance about the use of metaphor, a call that resonates in my head whenever I hear alternative therapists' confident reduction of illness to a single causality.

Another early text is Rosalind Coward's *The Whole Truth* (1989), a thorough critique of the concepts of nature and wholeness that underpin alternative health practices. Coward's key intellectual targets are the essentialism, romanticism and ahistoricism of the alternative health paradigm. As mentioned earlier, she rightly condemns it for its romantic vision of nature as virtuous, non-technological and benign. These intellectual reservations are bound up in political ones. For Coward, holism is a religious fantasy inextricably bound up in the moral imperative to live 'wholesomely' and in conceptions of illness as sin: 'At the very moment traditional religious and moralistic views of the personality began to lose a hold intellectually, they have regrouped around health' (92–3). This, in turn, is connected to the neo-liberal questions of personal responsibility and illness explored above, and to the potential to blame people for illness identified by Sontag.

Jackie Stacey, as noted above, is another powerful critic of the conjunction of neoliberalism with contemporary alternative medicine, as well as of the transnational politics of the contemporary appetite for all things 'Eastern'. She connects the obsession with holism to a 'new fantasy of a panhumanity' (2000: 125), in which the West avidly consumes, appropriates and commodifies selected non-Western beliefs and practices, in the process purging them of their histories and politics. The West, she argues, seeks cultural authentication and redemption in nature, which it not only romanticizes but also 'Easternises' (122). For Stacey, the desire for 'interconnectedness' celebrated in alternative therapies is yet one more instance of the West's consumption not just of global products and ideas, but of globalization *itself* as an idea: 'The global gets inside us, not just because we consume it (eat it, drink it, rub it on our bodies, feel it on skins), but also as we imagine we embody it through our integration within the universal energy systems that characterise its power' (127). In other words, she continues, it is not only that we ingest the global commodity but also that we believe we embody and unify a new globalism.

These philosophical and political critiques are important, especially as they appear to have made no real dent in dominant therapeutic discourses. It is vital that they be made, and re-made, but it is also time, given the paucity of interesting cultural studies of alternative therapies, for these therapies to be explored from other angles, even if that means temporarily downplaying some of their problems. For such critiques themselves run the risk of becoming programmatic, especially when they are not based in a deep bodily engagement with alternative therapies. (Stacey's work is an exception in this regard.) Sympathetic to many of the critiques of alternative medicine, I would nonetheless like this current book to be more about *looking at* than *seeing through*.

APPROACH AND OUTLINE

So it is that I depart from the mainstream Cultural Studies response in five main ways. First, I want to avoid the intellectual problems associated with big-picture critiques of ideas like 'holism' or 'intuition' that aren't based in an empirical study of them as ideas operationalized within particular subcultures. I therefore apply to alternative therapies, even fringe ones, a social analysis that is empirically based. In the case of clairvoyant intuition, for example, which I explore in depth in Chapter 5, I apply an ethnographic mindset, asking, in the words of Alexander Massey (1998), "What's going on here? How does this work? How do people do this?' I have found that taking a genuinely curious approach to culturally marginal practices like clairvoyance (in which one aims not to prove them true or false but to look at how they work) allows one to cut through some of the intellectual deadlocks – the refusal to even *open up* a dialogue – and to see whether any of this deadlock is based on assumptions that remain invisible because they are seemingly too obvious to investigate. It is up to the reader to decide whether this curious rather than hostile approach has produced something more useful than the mutual disregard that mostly characterizes New Age/Cultural Studies (non)interaction. A second, related, departure from most cultural studies of alternative therapies is that the book derives from, and focuses on, bodily experiences themselves, which are so often omitted in favour of sweeping sociological readings or cultural interpretations narrowly focused on a disembodied concept of identity. Thirdly, the book is not structured as a one-way traffic between Cultural Studies and alternative medicine, in which the latter serves only as an object of analysis rather than a potential source of insight, which so often means that Cultural Studies is missing out on opportunities to learn *from* alternative therapies and to borrow concepts of the body from them. I have made it clear when I find a particular alternative idea about the body exciting or useful. Fourth, as part of this two-way process, I have drawn on substantial interviews with practitioners themselves, as well as on my own experiences as an amateur practitioner of reiki. This bridging process has given me the opportunity not only to compare different schools of thought but also to put criticisms, cautions and doubts drawn from my academic training to the very people who are so often the objects of this critique. In the process I have been able to listen to and learn from their responses and, occasionally, to incite them too to further thought. My fifth point of difference is that I am prepared to be uncool – indeed, to expose elements of my own investment that a more cautious guarding of the academic persona might warn against. For I suspect that on occasion Cultural Studies' intellectual reservations about these therapies can also mask (and/or be intertwined with) the maintenance of the authority and cultural capital of intellectuals themselves. I detect a certain squeamishness when it comes to the multiple sins of these therapies: they are mainstream and middlebrow rather than subculturally 'cool'; (seemingly) mundane rather than spectacular; they talk about happiness rather than resistance; and they are founded on a combination of discourses unpalatable to Cultural Studies – combining psychological, humanist and spiritual discourses.[31]

In fact, such has been the squeamishness around the middlebrow and the spiritual that it is actually truer to say that alternative therapies have been less the object of wholesale critique within Cultural Studies than that they have been largely ignored. They have slipped under its radar – or, perhaps more accurately, they have been met with an embarrassed silence, whether as medical, bodily or spiritual technologies. I have explored this special distrust in detail elsewhere (Barcan and Johnston 2005), but two reasons behind it are worth reiterating here. The first reason for the almost exclusively negative stance taken towards therapeutic culture is Cultural Studies' taken-for-granted scepticism about the discipline of psychology, especially in the wake of the significant intellectual uptake of Foucault. The second reason is the almost total exclusion of questions of religion and spirituality from Cultural Studies for a long time, where religion was not so much critiqued as sidestepped, either for reasons of cultural sensitivity, or because its falsity is taken as self-evident. In short, religion is, in the words of John Frow (who nonetheless argues for its absolute centrality to Cultural Studies), 'an embarrassment to us' (1998: 207). This despite the increasingly glaring fact that, as Arjun Appadurai presciently noted well before September 2001, 'religion is not only not dead [as surmised by modernization theorists over a number of decades] but … it may be more consequential than ever in today's highly mobile and interconnected global politics' (1996: 7). As Frow notes, Cultural Studies, despite its core interests in identity, belief and power, has failed 'to come to terms with, to theorize in any adequate way, what is perhaps the most important set of popular cultural systems in the contemporary world, religion in both its organized and disorganized forms' (1998: 207). There are signs, though, that the global climate, among other things, is forcing Cultural Studies to expand its horizons.

Despite my reservations about the way Cultural Studies has treated alternative medicine so far, the rich and nuanced approaches that generally characterize the discipline provide the essential starting point and the critical repertoire for this study. So too, the new feminist work that contests conventional feminist rejection of the biological sciences is of great inspiration in opening up new ways of thinking about the body. I am following the lead of feminists like Lynda Birke (1999),

Elizabeth A. Wilson (2004), Anna Gibbs (2002) and Elspeth Probyn (2000), who critique or resist the non- or anti-biologism that often underpins even nuanced cultural approaches. Wilson, in particular, has been a vehement critic of feminist anti-biologism, arguing not only that biology offers an as yet untapped resource for feminists, but that anti-biologism actively undercuts even the most subtle of cultural readings of the body:

> [P]roblematically, much of the feminist work on embodiment seems to gesture towards a flat organic realm elsewhere as a way of securing a more valuable or dynamic account of the body closer to home. The organic – conceptually dull and politically dangerous – lurks at the periphery of these texts, underwriting the claims about embodiment that are made. (2004: 78)

Feminist work on the body has been extraordinarily successful in helping us recognize the subtle, intricate work of social factors, including ideology, in concretizing particular truths about the body. But an almost inevitable side-effect has been aversion to or distrust of biology as a field of knowledge. But in the words of Eve Sedgwick and Adam Frank, if we *automatically* and *uncritically* discard biology we lose access to a whole conceptual realm (1995: 15). Indeed, it is interesting to note that the feminist health movement that was one of the progenitors of the alternative health movement was, in fact, one of the few places that continued to insist on the importance of biology to feminism during the high era of feminist anti-biologism (Birke 1999: 1). Nowadays, it is increasingly common for academic feminism to take an interest in the biological body beyond that of repudiating patriarchal or biomedical control over it or deconstructing the gender politics of seemingly neutral scientific writing, vital though both of those projects continue to be. Many contemporary feminists want to engage with the body more corporeally, even *viscerally*. For my own part, I have found myself conjoining a traditionally feminist recognition of the importance of experience with a form of ethnographic practice that has been able to learn from what David Howes has called the 'experiential turn' in anthropological theory and practice (2009: 31). This process of finding my way has been driven by my own ongoing curiosity about alternative therapies. I am animated by a curiosity about what the body can do in different circumstances. I genuinely want to know what effects Tibetan crystal bowls may or may not have on the body, or what it means to live in a body you imagine as multiple, or whether clairvoyants see in colour. And, as a post-structuralist, I also want to know what role beliefs, expectations and ideologies have in producing such bodily experiences, and what sociocultural factors make them plausible to different audiences.[32]

My approach, then, is to interweave different forms of analysis (the social, the cultural, the experiential) and in so doing to try to bridge the chasm between the usually uncritical rhetoric about alternative medicine emanating from the New Age and the unremittingly unfavourable attention paid to it within Cultural Studies. In this book, then, I am proposing not just that alternative therapies are plausible and even important as objects of study – they are, after all, practised by millions of people around the globe and are highly significant even just as consumer practices. More, I'm suggesting that alternative therapies have the potential to enrich and invigorate – even to radicalize – Cultural Studies' own theorizations of corporeality, affect and intersubjectivity. Taking up Alan McKee's (2002) useful provocation to consider some elements of popular culture as forms of theory, I do not just 'apply' Cultural Studies perspectives to alternative therapies as objects of study; rather, I open a form of dialogue with them. After all, if one is serious about rethinking the body in non-dualist ways, why not start by examining, *and learning from*, bodily practices that claim not to be based in dualisms? In Chapter 2, for example, I examine the concept of the subtle body – in which the human body is imagined as comprised of multiple layers or sheaths of energy vibrating at different densities, suggesting, following Jay Johnston (2008), that Cultural Studies might be interested in this model and the radical intercorporeality it implies. In Chapter 4, I consider the concept of an embodied unconscious (cellular memory; the fascia as a kind of unconscious, located not in the brain but dispersed throughout the body), seeing in it real possibilities for an anti-dualist philosophy (and practice) of the body. The book aims, then, to explore and describe new forms of bodily experience opened up by alternative therapies, and it also hopes to suggest particular bodily concepts that could help enrich Cultural Studies' own theorizations of corporeality. As such it is both a cultural mapping and a modest theoretical intervention.

In being open to dialogue, I do not, however, suppose that all aspects of alternative therapies will be amenable to Cultural Studies and vice versa. I know their incommensurability all too well, since my autobiography and my intellectual biography (Skeggs 1995: 194) have so thoroughly, and often so painfully, intertwined them. Let me illustrate this intertwining of contradictions with two stories, both dating from the beginnings of my interest in alternative therapies, which coincided almost exactly with the beginning of my postgraduate training. These stories serve both to clarify what my own speaking position in this book will be, and to situate my personal dilemmas within a larger politics of knowledge.

I recall in my first week of postgraduate study a fellow student asking me about my personal interests. When I mentioned alternative therapies he replied bluntly that it was OK to study New Age beliefs so long as I didn't actually *believe* in them. But *did* I believe in them? I hardly knew. At that point, the rupture between belief and practice seemed insurmountable. I would attend a weekly class in post-structural theory, after which I would jump in my car and drive to a reiki group. I left the space of 'there are no universals' and drove to one where healing was understood as the channelling of 'universal energy'. Both experiences seemed (and still seem to me) to be 'true', but in completely different ways. One was a convincing intellectual schema; the other a powerful bodily experience. This struggle – almost embarrassingly banal in its embodiment of a split between mind and body – continued for many years. For a while, I learnt to live with it by convincing myself that alternative practices themselves were much richer than the discourses in which they were popularly explained. There is no doubt some truth in that, but it is also rather too convenient, and once again a veiled reiteration of a mind-body split, separating out explanations from practice.

Travelling along these parallel, or perhaps opposing, tracks was very destabilizing, and for a while I sought a theory that would allow them to be compatible. Today, my aims are more modest, and more realistic, in that I no longer seek synthesis. Some elements of these paradigms *are*, ultimately, incompatible, and many more are incommensurable – but that doesn't mean alternative medicine and cultural theory don't have interesting things to say to each other. My suspicion of New Age discourse has, by and large, increased over the years, but my regard for alternative therapies remains strong. I still haven't entirely decided what I do and don't 'believe' in alternative medical discourse. But I've learnt to operate, both conceptually and practically, across disparate fields of thought and practice, and have met many people whose work brings them into intersection and co-operation rather than opposition.

Moreover, twenty years on, I can now take some distance and see that my struggles were part of broader politics of knowledge in which gender plays a significant role. That clients and practitioners of alternative therapies are overwhelmingly female, and that the discourses and values underpinning the practices are deeply and explicitly gendered, is no mere sidenote to the sense of confusion and shame I felt. The secrecy and the shame surrounding some types of alternative medical practice are part and parcel of the feminization of alternative medicine, for both practitioners and clients. At the beginning of this Introduction, I noted that most users of CAM do not disclose it to their doctors. Even some *practitioners* are guarded about their work, as I discovered when I explored how CAM practitioners working in the more feminized-stigmatized areas like spiritual healing negotiate their professional identity (Barcan 2009b). This is especially true for more esoteric, traditional or non-Western practices. Hans Baer has noted the role of the class and race of both practitioners and clients in establishing how a particular therapy is ranked and valued (2004: xvii–xviii). Similarly, Alex Hankey (2005) has pointed out the cultural bias inherent in the report to the House of Lords Select Committee on CAM mentioned earlier, which ranked non-orthodox techniques according to their plausibility. Traditional systems of medicine, such as Traditional Chinese Medicine and Ayurveda, were relegated to the lowest level. Hankey points out that their knowledge base was unknown to the British committee and their theoretical texts written in languages other than English (2005: 5–6), and he notes the resultant protests from the governments of their countries of origin. Such systems of knowledge and the practices that arise from them are prime examples of what Bob Hodge (1995) terms 'monstrous knowledge' – forms of knowledge that are 'annulled' and dismissed as 'quaint', 'naive', 'outrageous', or 'unthinkable' within any dominant epistemology (1995: 8). I am no champion of the stigmatized and the devalued simply for their own sake, but if this current book is in part a process of personal reconciliation (at least letting post-structuralism and reiki speak to each other over the dinner table, even if they don't get on that well), it is also, it seems, a process of coming out.

The burgeoning field of sensory studies has provided me with a way through, if not out of, this impasse. Pioneered by scholars such as Constance Classen, David Howes and Anthony Synnott, it draws on a longer anthropological tradition (including the work of Walter Ong) and has attracted historians, sociologists, geographers and literary scholars (Howes 2006: 114). David Howes conceives of sensory studies as a corrective to the textualism and visualism of the 'overliterate world of academia' (2005b), an attempt to recover a full-bodied understanding of culture and experience' (1). Its focus on embodiment, its recognition of the historically and culturally variable nature of perception, and above all, its curiosity and openness have provided both a conceptual repertoire and an appropriate *disposition* through which to approach my topic. For one of the appeals of sensory studies is its unabashed *relish* of the body. There is something very alive in its openness to the world and to all shades of bodily experience, and in its invitation to us to more fully participate – both in scholarship and in living – in the richness, both delighting and disgusting, of the senses. The senses are also particularly pertinent to any gendered analysis since women have traditionally been associated with the senses, especially the 'lower' senses: 'Women are the forbidden taste, the mysterious smell, the dangerous touch' (Classen 1998: 1).

The major tenets underpinning contemporary cultural approaches to the senses are the historical separation and hierarchization of the senses; the phenomenological interdependence of the senses; the variation and cultural specificity of sensory understanding, valuation and experience; and the connection between the senses and social values, including the gender, class and racial meanings associated with different sensory orders. These precepts are appropriate to an analysis that hopes to highlight why alternative therapies are both attractive and plausible to so many Westerners, what implications this has for bodily understanding and experience, and how particular sensory practices are implicated in the market. The senses are also a useful lens through which to consider how in alternative medicine bodily experiences are linked not only to pleasure, but also to information. For not only do alternative therapies offer up particular forms of experience that aren't available in biomedicine (such as lying down being caressed by waves of sound made by crystal bowls; or the sensuous touch and smells of aromatherapy massage), these are also linked to the offering of information or new ways of knowing the body. In alternative therapies, then, the senses act as diagnostic tools, as therapeutic modes, and as different modes of knowing the body.

Each chapter in this book focuses on a particular sense. Chapter 2 is a study of a number of diagnostic and therapeutic practices, through the lens of vision. It focuses on one theme in particular – the power relations involved in looking, and the construction of therapeutic authority. Who has the ability and the right to read the body? What are the relations between visualization practices and the desire for control? Can therapeutic visual exercises escape the politics of capture and mastery? Chapter 3 begins with a survey of the traditional connections between sound, sociality and harmony, before focusing on a relatively obscure therapy, Psychophonetics. Derived from the philosophy of Rudolf Steiner, this therapy is interesting because it uses sound not as an adjunct (like the relaxing music played during a massage, for example) but directly as a tool in healing. Chapter 4 deals with touch, via a study of a number of bodywork practices. It concludes with my attempt to make sense of my own years of amateur reiki practice and to submit it to the same kind of ethical scrutiny used for the visual techniques explored in Chapter 2, while also holding out hope for an expanded idea of what kinds of knowledge bodies might be able to bring into being through interaction. This theme of an expanded reason is the bridge into the final chapter, on the 'sixth' sense, or intuition. This chapter draws on interviews with medical clairvoyants and spiritual healers, in which I explore what they see, hear, smell or feel. It shows how intuition functions in alternative medicine as an overarching category that makes use of particular senses but ultimately transcends any particular form of sensory perception, and whose intersensoriality might, indeed, be seen as a model for sensory perception more generally. The decision to begin with vision and end with intuition is deliberate. For as well as providing a series of separate case studies, the book charts a path from the most familiar starting point (vision, viewed cautiously as a tool of power, as in so much cultural analysis) to the most esoteric. This arc from the familiar to the esoteric describes the shape if not of a bridge, then of a jumping off into the unknown.

Inevitably, I have had to focus in on just a few of the senses, even within the 'now-standard five-fold arrangement of the sensorium' that characterizes the modern West (Howes 2009: 3). For reasons of space, a chapter on smell and aromatherapy could not be included. It is worth noting here, though, how the gendered tension between esoteric and scientific versions of aromatherapy makes it an interesting case for those interested in the professionalization of alternative therapies into CAM, and how aromatherapy also demonstrates the enmeshment of CAM in the marketplace, since one cannot practise it without buying essential oils, which are luxury products produced around the globe.

I have also not written a chapter on taste. It is a curious thing that taste has dropped out of the repertoire of biomedical diagnostic techniques; the physician no longer tastes the patient's various secretions and excretions as he may have done in Galenic medicine or the Renaissance clinic![33] Nor does taste appear very centrally in the more visibly commodified forms of CAM. Despite the central role accorded to taste in the contemporary sensorium, and especially in the modern marketplace, and despite the role of ingestion (of vitamins, nutritious food, etc.) in therapies like naturopathy, taste per se has little diagnostic or therapeutic value in the CAM therapies that have become most well known in contemporary Australian popular culture. In the West, we encounter taste in relation to pleasure not cure, belief in its more literal therapeutic effects having long waned. Indeed, Judith Farquhar argues that the English language does not have a lexicon that could recognize this potential (2002: 66),[34] though consumer culture and pop psychology are doing their best to provide us with one ('chocolate therapy' being one example). This absence is in contrast to the traditions in which taste does play a central role, such as Traditional Chinese Medicine (TCM) and Ayurvedic medicine. Each of these systems of healing centralizes and uses taxonomies that include taste: TCM's Five Elements[35] and the herbal medicine of Ayurveda.[36] In the end, I decided that I was insufficiently versed in either of these traditions to do them justice. The absence of a detailed consideration of both TCM and Ayurveda is a considerable omission, especially in those Western countries in which they are moving out from a diasporic community practice to a pop cultural mainstream, and one I hope to rectify in future work.

This book is intended as a gentle provocation to both 'sides' of an increasingly blurred and fractured health care environment – an environment, indeed, in which the idea of 'sides' is increasingly irrelevant as practices spread, blur, hybridize and integrate. I seek to prod CAM therapists with the suggestion that their field could well benefit from a fuller engagement with the political awareness that characterizes critical theory. Chapters 4 and 5, on the other hand, aim to provoke Cultural Studies to consider the limitation of conceptions of the body that do not engage fully with the body's expressive, memorializing and communicative potential – its ability to hold memory and experience to the subtlest degree, its capacity to know, and 'its' ability to articulate and/or act on that knowledge. These chapters also aim to demonstrate the richness of the body-self's radical extensivity through space and time. Chapters 2 and 4 raise cautions about power relations in CAM. Well-trained, experienced, mature and ethical practitioners are highly aware of the ethics and interpersonal subtleties of therapeutic encounters, but, as in all medical practices, there are elements in the discourses of alternative health and the New Age that can unhelpfully feed the do-gooders, the ill-trained, the power-hungry, and the naively exuberant.

This book, then, describes a struggle, an intellectual wrestle. But it also describes a journey towards some form of co-habitation of differences. I am happy to call this co-habitation an integration, if by integration we do not mean either a false synthesis or a fixed resolution. But if by integration we can mean a mutual provocation between different bodies of knowledge, the valuing and mobilizing of different modes of knowing, a comfortable passageway between public and private identities, an engagement of mind and body, and a celebration of all the senses, then I am happy to say that this book charts a journey towards integration.

2 THE POWER OF SIGHT

Ours is a visual age, the art historian Ernst Gombrich famously observed (1972: 82), and indeed it has become a commonplace of cultural criticism to point out the special place reserved for sight in the modern hierarchy of the senses. Western modernity is, it is frequently claimed, 'ocularcentric'. There exists a venerable tradition in which vision has been understood as the truth-bearing sense, inextricably intertwined with reason. Freud understood the pre-eminence of sight as a sign of civilization itself, bound up in humans' evolution away from the 'lower' senses like smell towards an upright posture and a correspondingly visual perceptual order (1973: 36). In the nineteenth century, sight was elevated to the 'pre-eminent esthetic sense' (Smith 2007: 24); in contrast to the proximate senses like touch it was seen as 'safe, distanced, and true' (24). Vision is seen as crucial to the development of a sense of self: 'Our language conflates the I with the eye', as Martin Jay so neatly puts it (1993: 284).

But the so-called 'great divide theory' (Smith 2007: 21) – which relegates the non-visual senses largely to pre-modernity and posits 'the victory of the rational eye under modernity' (21) – should not be overstated. For modernization also involved ambivalence about vision and visual culture. The elevation of sight did not do away with long-standing traditions in which both the objects of sight and sight itself were variously understood much more negatively. From Plato, for example, the West inherited a tradition in which the knowledge provided by images is to be mistrusted as ephemeral, insubstantial and deceptive, and its delights condemned as dangerous seductions or mere mirages. Even in the Enlightenment, where vision was apt to be understood as a tool of reason (Vasseleu 1998: 4), the equation between seeing and believing was countervailed by a long tradition in which vision is believed to set 'decoys and traps' (Stafford 1991: 8). This epistemological suspicion took a political turn in twentieth-century European philosophy, whose famously 'antivisual' (Jay 1993: 14) strands critiqued sight as a tool of power, emphasizing its ability to capture, sanitize or make safe. 'Radically antiocular critiques' (Smith 2007: 14) were a particular feature of French philosophical and cultural theory. The philosopher Jean-Paul Sartre, for example, understood the gaze as a tool of objectification. The feminist conception of this objectifying gaze as 'masculine' was an extremely influential idea in the latter decades of last century.

The 'venerable contempt and mistrust of phantasmagoric pictures' (Stafford 1991: 9) also found new objects in the twentieth century with the development of technologies of mass entertainment, which was greeted by fears expressed in predominantly feminine metaphors (Huyssen 1986). Cinema and later television were instruments of 'mass deception' – technologies seducing the unwary masses into dangerous fantasy worlds (Adorno and Horkheimer 1979 [1947]). Contemporary accounts of visual culture sometimes still make use of these gendered tropes, as in the dramatic opening sentence of Fredric Jameson's *Signatures of the Visible*: 'The visual is *essentially* pornographic, which is to say that it has as its end in rapt, mindless fascination' (1990: 1, original emphasis). *All* films are like pornography, argues Jameson, since they 'ask us to stare at the world as though it were a naked body' (1).

Yet alongside such suspicion of a visual culture designed to lure us into a deceptive and eroticized fantasyland, ideas like the light of reason and light as divine emanation continue to flourish. Metaphors of illumination and enlightenment are deep-seated in both religious and secular discourse. Light is 'the founding metaphor of metaphysics' (Vasseleu 1996: 130), pointing, in subtle and changing ways, to that which lies beyond material reality (Blumenberg 1993: 31). From Plato on, metaphors of light naturalize the connection between Being and truth (1993: 32). Plato conceived of light as 'an invisible medium that opens up a knowable world' (Vasseleu 1998: 3) – 'the "letting-appear" that does not itself appear' (Blumenberg 1993: 31). After the Enlightenment, argues Hans Blumenberg, illumination (allowing something to become visible) transmuted into 'lighting' (directing light at something), and light was imaginable as a kind of tool – a 'directed beam' (1993: 31) that allows one to examine phenomena in the world (Vasseleu 1998: 4). In the Western metaphysical tradition, then, light is a recurring, but continually changing, metaphor for truth. In Blumenberg's masterful summary, light can be 'a directed beam', 'a guiding beacon in the dark', 'an advancing dethronement of darkness', 'a dazzling superabundance', or the condition of visibility of other things (1993: 31). Light and darkness can be absolute metaphysical opposites, or light can be the force that conquers darkness (1993: 31). For my purposes here, suffice to say that in our cultural unconscious, the artificial lights of film and photography continue to do metaphoric battle with the pure light of reason, or the divine light. Vision as dangerous capture and light as benevolent healing force both endure as metaphors, and deep ambivalence around vision persists.

This chapter takes ambivalence about vision and the visible as a useful lens through which to consider some alternative therapies in which sight plays a central role. It is divided into two broad sections: diagnostic and therapeutic uses of vision.

In the therapies described in the first part of the chapter – iridology, bodywork and medical clairvoyance – the practitioner does the looking. The second part uses the meditative practice of creative visualization as its key example, in order to explore whether issues of power look a little different when an individual decides to develop his/her *own* power of inner sight. Is the shift in power away from an external therapist a welcome democratization, a burdensome shift in responsibility, a fanciful hope, or a complex mixture of all these things? Before turning to the therapies, I will sketch out a few themes from the sociocultural literature on sight that are important as they provide a critical lineage useful for considering the relations between vision and power.

When it comes to philosophical reflection on the pre-eminence of sight, it is commonplace to begin with Aristotle, whose *Metaphysics* opened with the claim that humans prize sight above all other senses for both practical and pleasurable purposes (1960 [350 BCE]: 3). Sight is superior at bringing knowledge because it is intrinsically analytical; it 'best discerns the many differences among things' (3). Sight, for him, was both trustworthy *and* pleasurable, both truth-revealing and sensuous.

The connection between seeing and analytical knowing has frequently been understood as reaching its epitome in the eighteenth-century Enlightenment, which has traditionally been read as the era of the rise of 'visualism', in which the other senses were supposedly eclipsed (Classen 1993: 28). Enlightenment thought is widely characterized as marked by an 'ocular obsession' (1993: 28) and as having naturalized the association between sight and insight, particularly rational knowledge. With the Enlightenment, or so the dominant narrative goes, sight became 'the pre-eminent means and metaphor for discovery and knowledge, the sense *par excellence* of science' (Classen et al. 1994: 84). This is both in material terms – via the development of visual technologies like the telescope and the microscope – and in more abstract terms, via the subtle visual metaphors that connect seeing and knowing. ('I see', as commentators frequently point out, means 'I understand'.) According to Mark Smith, both the Protestant Reformation and the scientific revolution helped strengthen the association between seeing and believing (Smith 2007: 24–5) and both Protestantism and science 'ended up agreeing on the supremacy of vision' (25), though of course Protestantism remained suspicious about the seductive power of images. A powerful and sustained feminist argument, made over many decades, has been that the naturalization of the connection between sight and knowledge involved the naturalization of particular modes of conceiving of gender. Classen et al., for example, claim that from the Enlightenment onwards sight 'increasingly became associated with men, who – as explorers, scientists, politicians or industrialists – were perceived as discovering and dominating the world through their keen gaze' (1994: 84).

As this argument suggests, feminists have been acutely aware of the power of vision and visual technologies to objectify, fix or master the object of the gaze and of the falsity of the modern idea of vision as disembodied, coming from 'nowhere'. They have insisted that analyses of vision and visual culture are not adequate unless they take into account the gendered dynamics of looking. Laura Mulvey's (1975) highly influential analysis of the male gaze, for example, was a crucial moment in the feminist articulation of looking as a mode of gendered domination. Her famous analysis of the gendered nature of spectatorship in classic Hollywood cinema contributed a specifically feminist perspective to the more general psychoanalytical reading of cinema as 'an instrument of totalizing social control' (Cartwright 1995: 8), and was taken up, somewhat problematically, in a large variety of projects and disciplines, well beyond the cinema studies readership for whom it was originally intended.

The link between vision, power and control is a recurring theme in philosophy. The story of the power of the gaze to rob us of our freedom is, as Stephen Melville says, 'a deeply familiar one in contemporary theory' (1996: 104). It figures prominently, for example, in the philosophy of Jean-Paul Sartre, who developed a phenomenology of ocular capture in which, as Melville puts it, 'He who looks is free; and he [or she ...] who is looked upon falls into nature, mere being, shame and mortification ...' (1996: 104, my brackets). In this conception, the eye fixes and captures: 'More than any other sense, the eye objectifies and it masters', as the feminist philosopher Luce Irigaray put it (qtd in Vasseleu 1996: 129). This isn't, of course, the end of the story, and there is an alternative, more positive, strand of the phenomenology of vision. For example, Sartre's contemporary, the phenomenologist Maurice Merleau-Ponty, complicated Sartre's analysis of ocular capture by emphasizing the interpenetration of self and other, self and world, and the interconnectedness of the senses. Perception was, for him, neither the passive recording of external stimuli, nor a creation of consciousness, nor a brute capture of the world, but rather, a 'communion' (1962: 213) between the world and an embodied subject. In his last, unfinished, work, he describes vision in even more tactile terms, as a 'palpation with the look' (1968: 134). This more optimistic, embodied and indeed *tactile* conception of vision is implicit in some of the bodywork therapies discussed in this chapter, and again in Chapter 4.

This, surely, is where the philosophical debates about sight will eventually need to travel. Kelly Oliver, for one, suggests that accounts of the denigration of vision, such as Martin Jay's (1993), need to recognize that what is at stake is the denigration of 'a very particular notion of vision' (2001: 57). In place of a view of vision that reposes on an idea of space as 'essentially empty' (Oliver 2001: 57) and which understands people to be separated by a physical and/or ontological gap, she proposes a model of vision that doesn't rely on a model of space as a 'void or abyss' (59). Drawing on and extending the work of Merleau-Ponty and Irigaray, Oliver argues that space is, rather, *filled* with the 'density of air' (67). Vision, she argues, is actually part of a 'vision-touch system' (70), and the look can be a caress as well as a capture (70).

Sight, then, need not be conceived of as inherently predatory, despite the dominant antivisual tradition of modern Western philosophy. So it is that over the last decade, classic critical accounts of vision, including feminist accounts of 'the gaze', have themselves been critiqued – accused of abstraction, generalization, ahistoricism and a paradoxical lack of attentiveness to the body. Many branches of inquiry, including feminist theory itself, now routinely call into question overly simple tales of the unqualified dominance of perspectivalism and Cartesian space since the Renaissance, or of vision as inevitably bound up in dynamics of domination and capture, in favour of historically and culturally specific accounts of particular 'scopic regimes' (Metz 1982: 61) (which Mulvey's essay was, it should be noted, always intended to be). Contemporary studies of visual culture are now likely to be marked by an acknowledgement of the historical specificity of visual cultures, the complexity of power relations, and an increasing recognition of the multiplicity of ways of looking – an interest not just in some putatively male or modern gaze, but also in glances, glimpses and looking back (Brennan and Jay 1996) and in the situated and embodied nature of all vision. Such approaches do not consider vision to be monolithic, but instead show an interest in the training of specific forms of visual perception, and their relation to dominant technologies. The rise of sensory studies has also complicated the tale of the ascendance of vision and has opened up the 'other' senses for analysis. As Mark Smith argues, historians should not overstate the tale of the 'hegemony of the eye' (2007: 15) in modernity, and nor should they understate the important role of vision in pre-modernity (18).

Nonetheless, the intense academic attention paid to vision over many decades has bequeathed us a number of insights useful to a study of alternative therapies. The first general point is the long-standing ambivalence about vision. Modern Western philosophy is not completely antivisual, but it is marked by a suspicion of the visual. This chapter is itself an example of that. I am cautious about the use of vision in alternative therapies to capture supposed truths about another person, and likewise wary of techniques that promise that the individual has the ability to create truths for him/herself, for example by using visualization techniques to 'manifest' a desired reality. And yet I recognize the value of, and have benefited from, therapies that celebrate and activate connections between image-making, creativity and freedom, or that focus on the therapeutic power of images, image-making and indeed light itself. After all, if vision is the principal medium of the unconscious (as its role in dreams might suggest), it might well follow that it can have a special role in healing.

In the second half of this chapter, then, I consider the meditative practice of creative visualization as an instance of the potentially therapeutic power of vision, noting, though, that the purpose and experience of visualization depend very much on the particular meditative tradition in which it is framed and the sociocultural context in which it is practised.

A second point is that the deep-seated equation between seeing and knowing means that medical and therapeutic techniques involving vision are understood to be providing hidden information. We will see that this is true of the diagnostic techniques examined in the first part of the chapter, and of some forms of meditation and visualization.

A third point is the insight that vision is not a natural given but a set of trainings or 'techniques of the observer' (Crary 1990). If even the most fundamentally 'human' of ways of using the eyes – the imperceptible flickering that characterizes the way we look at faces – is learnt (Ings 2007: 147), then there must certainly be a host of much more obviously cultural visual practices. Vision is neither singular nor universal, but rather a set of naturalized practices embedded in particular contexts, ideologies and practices, which John Berger (1972) famously called 'ways of seeing'. The visible can thus be thought of as a form of practice rather than 'the natural result of human sight' (Alcoff 2006: 180). It therefore follows that there is no single visual mechanism, 'only highly specific visual possibilities' (Haraway 1991: 190), whether organic or technological, each of which is an 'active perceptual syste[m]' (190) that allows its own form of access to the world. Each of the therapies examined in this chapter, for example, represents a particular mode or training of vision, whether on the part of the practitioner or on that of the patient. This is so whether the vision occurs through technological means (as in iridology), through the naked eye (as in bodywork), or through a putative sixth sense, as in medical clairvoyance.

Medical perception – what the practitioner looks for or sees – is therefore not a neutral capture of visible things but the interaction of perception, semiotics and systems of belief and knowledge. Particular medical or therapeutic paradigms or practices imply and produce their own sets of bodily signs or symptoms. What counts as a plausible, legible and meaningful sign in one practice might be impossible, invisible or insignificant in another. The brown spots or white rings in the iris that iridologists read as signs of constitution, predisposition or history are irrelevant to a GP or even an optometrist; the dark colours in the aura that the clairvoyant claims to see are invisible to ordinary perception and a biomedical nonsense. Medical perception and interpretation are thus subtly and deeply intertwined. Moreover, visual signs are connected to visuality at an even more abstract level – the fundamental model of the body on which any system of medicine is based. It is this, more subtle, level of visuality to which I turn next.

BODY MODELS, MEDICAL GAZES: THE CRITICAL TRADITION

For many critics interested in the visual cultures of modern medicine, Michel Foucault's *The Birth of the Clinic* has provided a decisive starting point in considering both the subtle visual metaphors that underpin medical knowledge and the power relations embedded in specifically modern medical ways of seeing. In his account of the transition in early nineteenth-century France away from a medicine based on the classification of disease towards one focused on the body of the patient, Foucault prefigured his general reading of modernity as characterized by particular forms of visual and surveillance technologies, focusing on the pivotal role played by vision in modern clinical medicine.

According to Foucault, the modernization of medicine involved the centralization of visibility as biomedicine's grounding metaphor and the rise of the 'perceptual act' (2003: 133) as the chief mode of interaction between clinician and patient. He charts the development of the new 'spatial and visual metaphors' (Stacey 1997: 58) that, he argues, underpinned this evolving medicine and of a new, specifically modern, 'medical gaze' (the 'anatomo-clinical gaze' (2003: 179)), which involved diagnostic techniques centred on the body of the patient. While pre-Enlightenment medicine was, he argues, 'classificatory' in nature (that is, its 'fundamental act of medical knowledge was the drawing up of a map' (2003: 33)), post-revolutionary French medicine turned increasingly towards the observation of an individual body. Instead of disease being primarily configured in abstract space – the tables and charts of seventeenth- and eighteenth-century classification systems, which treated disease like a botanical species (2) – it was now to be found 'in the secret volume of the body' (1). Illness was now to be found not in textbooks but 'in the space in which bodies and eyes meet' (xi). Moreover, the medical gaze would not content itself with peering at surfaces, but would strive to 'confront this embodiment by finding ways of penetrating into the deepest recesses of the body' (Philo 2000: 13). The physician's task was now to attempt to chart and know the patient's body, to render even its interiors knowable, in the face of symptoms which 'may quite easily remain silent' (Foucault 2003: 196).

The medical science *par excellence* of the new clinical medicine was anatomy.[1] Unlike the traditional clinician's gaze, which analysed pathological events as they unfolded, the newly developed gaze of the anatomo-clinician sought to 'bring to the surface what was given only in deep layers' (2003: 200). Anatomy literally embodied the Enlightenment project of 'dissect[ing] in search of a deeply lodged, dark or luminous, truth' (Stafford 1991: 7). Bringing the invisible to light thus became the base metaphor for a form of medicine that nonetheless involved all the senses. Foucault argues that the medical gaze is 'a plurisensorial structure' – 'a gaze that touches, hears, and, moreover, not by essence or necessity, sees' (2003: 202). But vision provides the base metaphor for a form of medicine in which the body is imagined as ever more knowable. Foucault's own metaphor for this metaphor is (perhaps unconsciously) gendered. He depicts clinical medicine as a kind of metaphorical striptease – the lifting of a never-ending series of veils:

> The structure, at once perceptual and epistemological, that commands clinical anatomy, and all medicine that derives from it, is that of *invisible visibility*. Truth, which, by right of nature, is made for the eye, is taken from her, but at once surreptitiously revealed by that which tries to evade it. Knowledge *develops* in accordance with a whole interplay of *envelopes*; the hidden element takes on the form and rhythm of the hidden content, which means that, like a *veil*, it is *transparent* ... (2003: 204, original emphases)

The naked body exposed to a powerful gaze is, metaphorically, a feminized body. Medical knowledge thus becomes a particular form of (gendered) quest underpinned by a desire for revelation. Barbara Stafford's characterization of this period accords with Foucault's, insofar as she characterizes Enlightenment medicine (and fine arts) as marked by a desire to grasp the ineffable: 'the wish to know intimately the unseizable other' (1991: 1).

Much of contemporary medicine is still bound up in this quest and its attendant metaphors; it is 'an era from which we have not yet emerged' (Foucault 2003: x). The 'compulsive search for truth through the power of vision' (Stacey 1997: 155) continues through an expanding array of biomedical diagnostic technologies that give us access to new ways of seeing, mapping, imagining and 'knowing' our bodily interiors. The body has become 'transparent' (Van Dijk 2005). As medical imaging technologies proliferate, it is no longer only the doctor who has the privileged knowledge of bodily interiors. Patients themselves are increasingly given access to this view from/of the inside, with a concomitant shift not just in medical authority, but also in our self-perception, fears, anxieties and hopes, as the body's new-found 'transparency' becomes part of the lived experience of embodiment.[2] The metaphorical nakedness of this new transparent body seems to guarantee its ability to tell us the truth of itself. The body stripped bare right down to the DNA is a body out of which all metaphoricity has seemingly been emptied. The medical gaze that knows this body seems on the surface to be equally neutral: it is an 'unprejudiced gaze' characterized by 'purity' (Foucault 2003: 241). Despite these appearances, fantastical elements and hidden metaphors still characterize the medical gaze. After all, nakedness is not a pure, uncontaminated truth but a *metaphor* for truth – indeed, a metaphor for the lack of metaphor (Barcan 2004).

To its critics, the dream of perfect visualizability is not just illusory but politically dangerous. The fantasy of the inner body as a world to be explored arose, not uncoincidentally, at a time of unprecedented global exploration and the birth of colonialism. Feminists have noted that the parallel developments of medical imaging techniques like the X-ray and new visual entertainment media like cinema helped reinforce the idea of the female body as a spectacle awaiting discovery (Cartwright 1995). They have been especially wary about the gender politics of 'the intensification of the *visualisability* of the body's interior' (Stacey 1997: 157, original emphasis), especially with regard to reproductive technologies, and have typically treated these new technologies with a mixture of caution and wary engagement. Either that, or they have sought to give women themselves the power to see into their own interiors, most famously exemplified in the 'radical challenge to medical power' when the feminist health groups of the 1960s and 1970s encouraged women to look inside their own vaginas with mirrors and specula (Birke 1999: 9).

Imaging technologies undoubtedly give both doctors and patients information about the body that can be medically very useful indeed. And dynamic techniques like ultrasound, molecular, biodynamic or bioelectric imaging investigate the body as an active, moving system, not just an inert and passive corpse awaiting opening up. Nor do they just extend the practitioner's gaze; they can also create new vantage points, hitherto unimaginable vistas and perspectives (Crary 1990).[3] In so doing they make possible new connections between seeing, knowing and feeling. These new ways of imagining the body have an impact on our experiences of our own bodies and on our expectations of doctors or therapists. The more we develop surgical, digital and optical modes of making visible the interior of the body, the more credence we place in what we (think we) see. It is easy to forget that not everything in the body, nor every disease, is necessarily 'visualisable' (Van Dijk 2005: 7), and that reading X-rays and ultrasounds is not just a matter of looking, but rather a way of seeing requiring training and interpretation. As visual technologies continue to develop, the fantasy that we might 'ultimately be able to "map" each individual body' (Van Dijck 2005: 7) is fed by, and feeds into, 'the idea that seeing is curing' (7).

The idea that knowing more about the body is tantamount to cure makes sense in the 'informational cultures' (Stacey 1997: 231) in which modern consumers live, since the production and exchange of information has become central to our way of life and our ways of being and thinking:

> The expansion of information technologies and communication systems, which have increasingly come to replace the manufacturing industries of Western countries, have laid the foundations for the formation and validation of different forms of knowledge and new ways of seeing the body and the self. (158)

People who live in such cultures have, Stacey argues, become more curious, more entitled, more needy about knowing our psychological and bodily 'interiors':

> [T]hose of us who have been influenced by the information cultures of the last twenty years are more susceptible to the desire to know and to the fantasies of knowledge as power. We are encouraged to seek out information about ourselves with an obsessive curiosity. (2–4)

This curiosity can lead to new forms of identity based on quite detailed knowledge of one's own biological or medical condition, especially in the case of injury or stigma.

The need to know slips easily into the requirement or responsibility to know, and thus meshes with the neoliberal conception of health as one's personal responsibility and citizenly duty. This new 'biological citizenship' (Rose 2007: 131) is double-edged; it gives us new responsibilities but it can also allow individuals and collectives to claim *rights* as a citizen. Like Stacey, Nikolas Rose sees the ready availability of detailed medical knowledge as having a major impact on the contemporary sense of self, coining a new term, 'informational biocitizenship' (2007: 135), to draw attention to the way in which contemporary information culture intersects with neoliberalism to promote new forms of self-knowledge. As noted in Chapter 1, Jackie Stacey connects these new relations to information and to the body with fantasies of control, which she sees as applying equally to modern science and to 'the self-health culture of the 1990s', which are, she argues, united by

> the desire for mastery. It is the desire to see, to know and to control. It is the desire to fix meaning and to make outcomes predictable. It is the desire to prove that one has power over disease, the body and the emotions. (1997: 238)

While I think Stacey overstates the case somewhat,[4] her claim that both orthodox and alternative medicine are united by the desire for mastery usefully reminds us that even disparate medical paradigms can be connected along other cultural lines.

ALTERNATIVE VISIONS? THE VISIBLE AND THE INVISIBLE IN ALTERNATIVE MEDICINE

A number of the practices discussed in this chapter represent a challenge to biomedicine's tacit (or alleged) claim to provide the best modes of seeing and knowing the body currently available. Nonetheless, some of the ways alternative medicine configures relations between the visible and the invisible are not so distant from biomedical ones. As with biomedicine, they often construe the body as truth-telling, and structure the search for medical truth as a kind of metaphorical stripping away towards an always-receding state of nakedness. They differ, though, in their particularity: each therapy perceives different visual signs as diagnostically significant; requires different visual training or modes of vision of the practitioner; and is based on different models of the body.

Alternative medicine provides a set of body models that both compete with a classic anatomical picture and yet are also in a broad sense congruent with some contemporary shifts in the biomedical imaginary. The energetic conception of the body construes it less as a fixed entity than as a *set* of unbounded bodies, most of which are invisible to ordinary perception. While this seems far-fetched to those who have not encountered or adopted it, biomedicine itself is working less and less with a classic anatomical body than with conceptions of the body that emphasize systems and networks (Stacey 1997), and which construe the body as an *information* system (Stacey 2000: 129). Moreover, an increasing number of medical technologies convert bodily experience not just into the numbers, graphs and charts of classic modern medicine but also into digital signals, *in vivo* images and live flows of information. This new body's clues lie not only on the skin or even in the interiors opened up by anatomy, but are more deeply and invisibly encoded – encrypted in the DNA – and more dynamically tracked in the ebbs and flows of the body's ceaseless processes. It is a 'de-materialised' (Fadlon 2004) and 'informational' (Stacey 2000: 129) model of the body. In this context, it is hard to know if the energetic body that so typifies alternative medicine represents a point of difference from biomedicine or a convergence.

For some, the existing traction *within* biomedical science of the concept of information is a key part of its future value as an integrative paradigm. Beverly Rubik, a biophysicist who was Director of the Center for Frontier Sciences at Temple University, Philadelphia, considers that the concept of information is so fundamental to the biological sciences as to be a 'unifying concept' within them – so palatable conceptually and metaphorically as to constitute a viable 'bridge from alternative to mainstream medicine' (1995: 37). Writing in 1995, Rubik, a specialist in the science of energy medicine (a broad term that encompasses, among other things, homeopathy, reiki, spiritual healing and electromagnetic therapies), considered that an expanded concept of information – one that goes beyond the molecular level – is 'a fundamental feature in bioregulation' (37) and as such is the basis for a new paradigm for biology and medicine (34). This new informational paradigm would, she argued, allow us to recognize the myriad of connections, both internal and external, that comprise and sustain biological life. It enables a new holism based on the scientific principle that the human being is sustained by 'a web of relationships at many levels of order' (37) and that health is maintained and recovered via 'a wealth of information exchange, or "conversation", between and within the elements of these levels of order' (37).

The new informational paradigm, then, is not strictly speaking a 'de-materialisation' as posited by Fadlon (2004). Rather, it is a 'new' form of understanding materiality itself. Though the model of the subtle body – with its mostly invisible 'layers' of interpenetrating bodies – may seem to be a less material body than that focused on the solidity of bones, organs and tissues, in actuality, it reconstrues both materiality and information themselves, seeing no intrinsic ontological difference between thought and matter (Johnston 2008: 2).

What of the power relations attached to this rising paradigm of information that is so deep-seated and pervasive as to be able to provide a bridge between biomedicine's ability to provide us with 'data' about formerly inaccessible bodily recesses and inconceivable registers of bodily life and something as paradigmatically remote as medical clairvoyance? If they both speak to the same dream of perfect knowledge, hoping to reveal invisible truths, are they both part of the same vast web of surveillance technologies? Certainly, this is how it looks to those schooled in the 'social control' (Armstrong 1986: 30) traditions of social theory.

Judith Fadlon suggests that the paradigm of the energetic body is at least as ripe for the exercise of power as the biomedical paradigm, since 'the notion of energy offers innumerable opportunities for diagnosis, treatment, and ultimately, control' (2004: 76). She cites a homeopath whose claim to render the invisible (indeed, the *unformed*) visible will read to some as a reassuring and benevolent gaze reducing the body's exposure to risk and to others as a chilling pathologization of the normal:

> Even when a person does not have any disease, and he assumes that he is healthy, he has no way of knowing what is seeping through his body ... According to the method in which I work, it is possible to diagnose the weak points in the body, understand what might develop, and treat it before great distress develops (Maariv qtd in Fadlon 2004: 76).

One can never, it seems, be too vigilant.

In this, as critics like Stacey (1997) have noted, biomedicine and alternative medicine are not poles apart, but are part of a broader culture of so-called 'surveillance medicine' (Armstrong 1995). The Foucauldian tradition provides a strong tool to understand this rise of a culture of constant bodily surveillance by both self and other, and its role in helping to produce a cohort of people who may feel both entitled and anxious. Writing in this tradition, Nikolas Rose (1996, 1999, 2007) and others have demonstrated the connection between hypervigilance and neoliberalism, understood as both an economic policy regime and a lived experience of the self. Such critical approaches recognize the dual potential of medical diagnosis: as a useful tool and as an instrument of subjection. Seeing-as-curing and seeing-as-domination are not necessarily diametrically opposed. Surveillance medicine is both medically and morally ambiguous: it extends the terrain of medical power by opening the body up to a scrutiny that becomes almost impossible to evade in some form or another, but it simultaneously enables the detection of risk, and the possible enhancement of life. While Foucault himself treated such 'optimization' with a degree of suspicion, despite its evident 'utility', others may find the fantasy of the body's ultimate know-ability appealing, or reassuring, or at least regard it with ambivalence, as the price we pay for contemporary medicine's evident capacities. Many of us have reason to be grateful for the mammogram that spotted the tumour, the X-ray that showed that our lungs were clear, or the blood test that explained our fatigue.

Beverly Rubik, for one, is hopeful about the human and ethical possibilities of this new science and its medicine. She argues that the new paradigm of information requires scientists to continue to think beyond the molecular, and that its emphasis on systems, interactions and communication implies and pushes us towards 'an extended science' (1995: 38) that has to take account of the kind of phenomena described and mobilized within alternative medicine: the exchange of information as something more than a mere 'transaction' of data but as inevitably implicating all parties and involving 'communion' and 'meaning' (38); the ability of information to be distributed and exchanged 'nonlocally' (both within the body and between bodies) and in response to intention (38); and the necessary recognition of the human implication in science. For Rubik, information is something far more, and far more significant, than the 'pile of numbers' we call 'data' (38). In her view, the new medicine will have to be underpinned not by a mechanistic science, but by one able to 'address life in its fullest capacity' (38).

Despite Rubik's optimism, my aim in this chapter is not to argue that when alternative therapies open up new forms of seeing that they necessarily create new and friendlier power relations than those biomedical technologies of seeing that have been so repeatedly denounced as important components of surveillance medicine. On the contrary, some of the instances I will examine in this chapter look very similar to the types of optic capture mistrusted within Sartrean philosophy, feminist theory and critiques of biomedical technologies. But it is equally important to be open to the possibility that a new science might be able to be more than just a repeat of the old – for visual technologies, and the model of a particular form of optical capture that has underscored them, to be able to take us somewhere else. This, as I see it, is the ongoing and vital role for critical theory at its strongest – to help us see when the new is simply the old re-made and to help push us towards more ethical and socially just forms of science and medicine. But to do this, critical theory itself must be able to see things anew rather than just capturing the same old images.

Each of the practices described in this chapter not only makes medical or thera-peutic claims but also opens up rich ways of seeing the body. Perhaps some of the visual experiences encountered in alternative medicine can form part of a rethinking and revaluing of the visual, not as a disembodied view from nowhere as in the classic modernist/masculinist formulation, or as a process of capture, but as fully embodied, as suggested by Kelly Oliver (2001). Feminist philosopher Donna Haraway likewise argues that feminism should strive to reclaim the visual, via a recognition of the inevitably situated and embodied nature of all visual perception (1991: 188). Her highly situated and embodied account of vision emphasizes the myriad of different visual systems, whether organic or technological, human or non-human. Vision is never vision from nowhere: the fly, the dog, the meditator, the satellite, the X-ray and the webcam all have their own 'wonderfully detailed, active, partial way of organizing worlds' (190). I close the chapter with an account of a practitioner whose ability to work with the visual is remarkable, and demonstrates that caution about the use of sight to capture, fix or master its objects shouldn't blind us to the possibility for experiences of the visual that are nourishing, eye-opening and even liberating.

DIAGNOSTIC USES OF VISION: MANIFESTING THE INVISIBLE IN IRIDOLOGY, BODYWORK AND MEDICAL CLAIRVOYANCE

The purpose of 'diagnostic disciplines', writes Barbara Stafford, is to 'discover and exhibit the inarticulable relationship of interior to exterior, idea to form, private pathos to public pattern' (1991: 2). All medical practice involves a dialectic between the visible and the invisible, but different medical practices or systems involve their own particular repertoire of visible signs and hidden truths. Thus, what counts as a detectable and meaningful sign in alternative medicine may be invisible, unrecognizable, implausible or meaningless within biomedicine, though of course there are also points of overlap. Many alternative health practices are predicated on models of mind-body-spirit in which the vast majority of the body is understood to be invisible to the untrained, unaided or unendowed eye. Symptoms may be buried deep within the body, or be in some other way beyond the reach of normal perception or even of linear temporality, having perhaps not yet manifested in visible form in the physical body, as in the case of the homeopathic beliefs quoted above. In these cases, diagnosis involves bringing something to light that may belong to the distant past, a foreshadowed future, or even another plane of existence.

Diagnosis, as its etymology implies, is a form of discernment, one that implies a degree of translation whereby symptoms are converted into numbers, or images into words, words into explanations, sounds into meanings, feelings into categories, or the present into possible futures. Making a sign, symptom or illness manifest involves explanation and interpretation, and so it resides almost inevitably in the realm of narrative, judgement and prescription. Diagnosis, whether in biomedicine or its alternatives, is thus a good place to go looking for political, ethical and personal ambiguities about the pleasures, uses and dangers of being 'seen through'. What actually counts as something that can be seen or that is worth seeing? What forms of visual training, technology and literacy are needed to see knowingly? Who has the power, authority and ability to name an illness and who can tell its stories? The historical ambivalence about the power of sight returns as an important theme. On the one hand, there is the evident utility of vision as clear-seeing: vision, the provider of useful knowledge and insight. On the other, there is the spectre of vision as capture, oppression, domination and control.

The three diagnostic practices examined in this section – iridology, bodywork and medical clairvoyance – all involve the activation of a specialist external gaze. In iridology, the practitioner looks the patient in the eye, either directly or through a special machine. In bodywork, a trained gaze is brought to bear on the body. In medical clairvoyance, a special, contestable, mode of sight is used to tell the client the truth of him- or herself. With each therapy, I examine the relation between seeing and knowing, looking at how each practice enables particular truths of the body and soul to be told, and exploring the seductiveness – indeed, almost the romance – of the dream of being known perfectly by another.

LOOK INTO MY EYES: IRIDOLOGY AND THE WINDOWS OF THE SOUL

Iridology is a diagnostic technique that involves the close study and analysis of the coloured part of the eye, the iris (pl. 'irides'). Developed in the nineteenth century by the Hungarian doctor Ignatz von Peczely and, independently, the Swedish clergyman Nils Liljequist, it found favour in Germany, and reached the US in the early twentieth century (Jensen and Bodeen 1992: 8–10). Iridologists look at the colour, structure and markings of the iris to analyse the patient's underlying constitution and state of health. Each person's irides are different, 'the genetically determined evidence of your uniqueness' (Jackson-Main 2004: 8). This is why they are potentially so useful in security identification systems, where they are claimed to offer 'approximately ten times greater security of identification than your fingerprints' (8). In iridology, the iris is examined with an iris torch and a magnifying lens or through ophthalmological devices like slit-lamps, which provide greater magnification. Since iridology is diagnostic rather than therapeutic, most iridologists are trained in a range of therapies, and iridology is rarely found as a stand-alone practice.

I have called iridology a 'diagnostic' process, but in fact, according to its practitioners, iridology offers a way of understanding the body that both falls short of and exceeds medical diagnosis:

> It gives you a read-out of your constitution, your essential makeup. Your constitution defines your health predispositions, not as predictions written in stone, but as guidelines to your body's innate mode of response. Iridology also may provide you with clues as to how your constitution has been affected by the choices and conditions of your life. (Jackson-Main 2004: 10)

One of the foremost twentieth-century practitioners and proponents of iridology, medical doctor Bernard Jensen, stressed that iridology was both a science and an art (Jensen and Bodeen 1992: 6). In the account just cited, taken from a popular handbook, the idea of interpretation as a human art (Jensen and Bodeen 1992: 27) has given way somewhat to a language of choice and empowerment that is deliberately counterpoised to a critique of the medical experience of prognosis, in which we are (allegedly)

> ... entirely in the hands of the experts and we usually have no choice but to believe what they tell us, which may not be what we want to hear. What power do we have to influence or change that prediction? (Jackson-Main 2004: 10)

Here, medical science is critiqued as 'prediction'. It is, paradoxically, *insufficiently* empirical, too abstract, failing to take into account the individuality – indeed the desires – of the patient, in contrast to iridology's alleged ability to give a nuanced account of both individual constitutional predisposition and the impact of current lifestyle choices. In a way entirely congruent with the neoliberal discourses described in the previous chapter, iridology is framed as empowering and illness is construed as rationally controllable via the provision of accurate information and the making of informed choices:

> [It] makes crucial information available to you – your strengths, weaknesses, opportunities, and threats. With this information you can make effective decisions about your health. (Jackson-Main 2004: 10)

This neoliberal construal of the medical encounter as an empowering communication of information enabling positive action belies of course the complexity of such encounters in the flesh. What of the power relations and the emotional complexities inevitably involved in such communications? Can communication ever feel like revelation, the practitioner less a collaborator or facilitator than an all-seeing expert, revealing to you the secrets of both your genetic inheritance and your life course? If so, is it really so different from the biomedical technologies against which it is here contrasted? Jensen himself deplored such practices, declaring that the iridologist 'truly cannot name any disease by merely observing the iris' (Jensen and Bodeen 1992: 18). He noted that practitioners may succumb to the sense of power and satisfaction associated with naming a disease, but also that patients unknowingly put pressure on iridologists, through their unstated expectation that every malady should have a name (18).

Certainly, there are those who would use iridology as an opportunity for self-aggrandizement, sometimes via a 'party trick' approach. There is no shortage of anecdotal material about alternative practitioners of many kinds, not just iridologists, who delight in making precise medical pronouncements before hearing any case history, based on visual examination of the tongue, the eye or posture. Judith Fadlon (2004) illustrates how diagnostic techniques from Traditional Chinese Medicine, for example, can be used in spectacular fashion, describing an introductory lecture given at an Israeli CAM college at which the dean asked the students to stick out their tongues as he moved around the lecture hall inspecting them and making quasi-diagnostic comments, including announcing to one woman that she had her period. According to Fadlon, he moved on without awaiting a response and the woman turned to those near her and excitedly confirmed the reading (78–9). We will see in the next section that some bodyworkers cannot resist similar temptations. The workshop mode that typifies the New Age end of the alternative health spectrum, and which is especially popular in the US, is a pedagogical mode that enables public displays of the power to declare the truth of another, as when bodyworkers call for volunteers and then proceed to 'read off' elements of personality and emotional make-up from their body. Such manifestations of visual power, whether in the public space of the alternative health workshop or the privacy of the therapeutic clinic, can be seductive and pleasurable. The pleasure and relief in being seen right (through) can resemble the excitement of first love: at last someone sees me as I really am; at last, someone understands me, and knows I am not making up my malady. Viewed critically, that is the insidious nature of spectacular diagnostics – they play on the all too human need for recognition, on the dream of the perfect legibility of the self, and sometimes on a pressing medical need, offering the hope of cure-through-recognition.

If, as a critic, one has no belief that the information such techniques provide is likely in any way to be true, then this story of power would be the whole ghastly truth of these practices – that they prey on the needs and yearnings of vulnerable people and aggrandize the authority of people who are at best naive and at worst cruel charlatans. But what if techniques like iridology *can* give detailed, useful, individualized information about the health state of a person, including information about illnesses that have not yet developed? How, then, could one frame the ethics of such diagnostic encounters?

I write as someone who remains open to the possibility that this is the case. I haven't had many experiences of iridology, but my fundamental belief in the complexity of the body, coupled with the frequency with which I have heard people tell tales of extraordinary diagnostic accuracy (not only with iridology, but also with other non-biomedical diagnostic practices, such as Ayurvedic ones), leaves me at least agnostic on the question. So, as someone who believes that iridology may well have useful truths to offer (some) patients in (some) situations – truths that may not always be accessible via biomedical diagnostics – I am drawn into the complex terrain that lies between the naive neoliberal belief in the 'empowering' nature of 'offering' people 'information' and the reactive critical mode in which iridology is yet another manifestation of the cruelty and dangerousness of a naively wielded and spurious medical authority. This, then, was the terrain I explored with two iridologists I interviewed.

From the outset, it must be said both my interviewees were acutely aware of the problem of the iridologist's power, which threatens to go contrary to alternative medicine's fundamental commitment to healing as a collaboration rather than a course of treatment imposed from above (Williams 1998). They were both evidently genuinely committed to a principle of diagnostic caution not only for legal reasons (alternative practitioners in Australia are not allowed to 'diagnose') but also as a fundamental human courtesy: 'you've got no right to frighten and alarm people', as the naturopath Nancy (who uses iridology as one of her tools) straightforwardly put it. Nancy was particularly aware of the power of language to alarm, instancing the potential of a word commonly used in naturopathy – 'toxins' – to seriously concern people to whom it was unfamiliar. Similarly, Geoff was aware that mention of, say, the heart could 'scare the daylights out of someone'. Accordingly, he said, 'rather than coming out and saying it and being the all authority, it's best as a therapist to encourage them to tell *you* what's going on'. To a Foucauldian, this is an example precisely of the 'humane-ness' of contemporary therapeutic authority – not the abolition of power, but its reconfiguration in seemingly more democratic, 'productive', forms. But such critiques, while they provide an important contribution to understanding contemporary forms of power, sidestep the question of whether the information provided, in this case by iridology, is medically accurate or useful. If, as I do, you want to take these practices seriously both as medical techniques and as sociocultural phenomena, then their medical value is not a peripheral issue.

The caution of the two iridologists I interviewed concerned professional ethics rather than reflecting scepticism about the ability of iridology to provide accurate information about the inherited constitution, the history and the current state of the patient's health. Professional confidence and ethical caution can be a complex mixture:

It's not a magic device – which a lot of people seem to think it is – where you look in people's eyes and you can say all sorts of things about them. Although if you've got a lot of experience like I have, you probably could, but it's not something that I would use as a party trick, and I don't like to see it used in that way. (Nancy)

As we saw, Geoff's professional ethics mean that he prefers the patient to lead discussion of some of his/her problems, but this is not always possible, since some people really *want* to be read by a culturally licensed authority, as Jensen noted. Geoff says:

It's funny, because people sort of – if they know you're an iridologist they say, 'What do you see in my eyes?' And of course I'm never drawn into that, because eye-to-eye – just on a one-to-one – you can't really see very much, whereas under the iriscope ...

Clearly, the idea that someone might be able to speak the truth of them delights some clients: 'People really do like it and I think that in a way people tie iridology in with the concept that the eyes are the window of the soul' (Nancy). Nancy was aware of the cultural power of the eyes, which are widely seen as central to the perennial human drama of honesty and deception. When she says that the eyes 'do give away an enormous amount', she is signalling iridology's place within a broader set of interpretive practices, including everyday empathic ones. When a practitioner scrutinizes your eyes at close range it is impossible to repel the tradition of the eyes as windows of the soul. In the popular imagination, the iridologist sits somewhere between scientist, charlatan and clairvoyant – hence, perhaps, the perceived need in the handbook quoted above to turn the tables and accuse biomedicine of 'prediction'. Rather like many clients of clairvoyants, some iridology clients are reluctant to give away too much in the case history part of the consultation – because they want to test iridology out and/or be delighted by its abilities:

When you do a consultation to begin with some people are a little bit reluctant to tell you too much then anyway – for fear of giving you information prior to the iridology. So they want you to do the iridology and tell them what's wrong with them, rather than them telling you in the first place. (Geoff)

Of course, this may also be nervousness, since iridology's putative ability to see hidden truths also frightens many:

I find that you have to approach people quite cautiously. You mustn't just get into their face – you've got to [proceed] very cautiously. I always put my hand on their face. I come closer in stages so that I don't intimidate, because I can see the hesitation, especially with men, for some reason. They are sure that all their dirty secrets are going to be revealed. And in a way there are secrets than *can* be revealed if you know what you're doing; you can see ways of people operating. (Nancy)

Some people find the prospect 'terrifying and affronting' (Nancy). Others reject it completely: 'When someone can look me in the eye and tell me the state of my hemorrhoids, then I will believe it', harrumphed one Australian newspaper letter writer, angry at a proposal that an iridologist be considered a 'registered health professional' (Doyle 2006: 10). In fact, in popular discourse about the illegitimacy of alternative medicine generally, iridology seems to surface quite frequently as an exemplary instance.

As the reference to haemorrhoids perhaps suggests, both the threat of the revelation of inner truths and the clinical process itself are in their own way quite intimate, like so many medical and therapeutic encounters. After the detailed taking of a case history, the practitioner examines your iris at close range. Some prefer to use an iris torch rather than a slit lamp. While this may give less intense magnification, it allows the practitioner's other senses to be more fully involved in the diagnostic process:

> I think if you do it a lot you develop all sorts of other senses within yourself whereby there's all sorts of visible and non-visible cues that you do pick up things about – and I think you're better off with that contact. I don't think we should over-medicalize too many things, and I think our basic premise has always got to be, that we're the facilitators – we're there to guide someone or point out the pathway back to health. We're not there to over-complicate matters. Most things are simple, they really are. (Nancy)

Equally, but differently, intense is the experience of sitting at the slit lamp, which resembles the experience of being examined by an optometrist. Seated so close to the practitioner, it is impossible to be anything other than acutely aware that someone is looking into your eyes not for physical anomalies as at the optometrist, but for clues about your character, constitution, physical weaknesses, strengths, diet, medical history, emotional makeup and potential future. Some scrutiny indeed!

I interviewed both iridologists in the same week. Each offered me a brief 'consultation' at the conclusion of the interview, and both saw the same physical signs and interpreted them in the same way. Despite my long conversations with both practitioners about how iridology didn't reveal simple truths but was a useful indicator, and despite both practitioners' evident self-reflexivity and ethical intentions, I still succumbed to the power of iridology's professed ability to reveal the unseen. To put not too fine a point on it, I was thrown into a mild panic. Of course, a quick, unplanned 'go' at the end of a research interview is not the same thing as a planned, carefully structured and usually ongoing therapeutic encounter. And my analytical focus on just the diagnostic force of iridology – extracting the diagnostic technique from the broader naturopathic context in which it is always found – is somewhat distorting, since iridology is intended to work hand in hand with other therapeutic systems, especially nutrition (Jensen and Bodeen 1992: 2). Nonetheless, I was struck by how powerful this dual 'diagnosis' had been and by the bodily reaction it produced in me.

As Nancy herself said: 'In the right hands it's good, in the wrong hands it's quite dangerous'. 'Look into my eyes', is, after all, both the lover's invitation and the hypnotist's ploy.

READING THE BODY: BODY TYPING AS AN ELEMENT OF BODYWORK PRACTICE

I turn now to a group of manual therapies in which the practice of 'reading' the body often plays a role. In alternative parlance, these physical therapies are known as 'somatic therapies' or 'bodywork', which are loose terms that encompass a range of distinct and yet frequently overlapping or combined techniques (many of which also have their own internal schools and traditions), including massage, myofascial release, Rolfing, Feldenkrais and osteopathy. No specialized visual technology is used except, perhaps, in an initial consultation, in which more biomedically trained practitioners may require an X-ray. Instead, the practitioner's expert perception, itself a commingling of vision and touch, becomes a specialized 'technology', in which trained vision and touch act in concert to encourage, allow or force the body to release tension in the muscles, nerves, fascia or ligaments. To re-tool an apt phrase from Barbara Stafford, bodywork therapies combine 'sensory detection and a tactile craft' (1991: xvii). What can be seen and known by a skilled and experienced bodyworker? What truths, histories or stories can a body reveal, and what are the professional ethics of 'reading' the body of another? Is the practitioner a meddler, or a magician who reveals hidden histories, layered muscular tension, stored emotions, bodily memories? Or is s/he something more like a supportive catalyst, interested less in revealing the body's truths than in triggering the body to do its own work?

I enter the osteopathic consulting room for my regular appointment. The osteopath has already seen the hidden architecture of my body through spinal X-rays, and he knows some of its history and its habits – what injuries it has suffered, how and where it is constricted, where it is happy to move, how comfortable it is with the process of unwinding. Perhaps too he knows more than that – like what kind of person makes a body like that. Now that I have been coming for quite a few sessions, we have a workable trusting relation. He, perhaps, has nothing to prove and I, perhaps, have no obligation to make my body perform. My body is used to the touch of his hands and so is willing to sink into receptivity – or perhaps even to lead the way.

He asks where I believe he should begin today. I say that deep in my nose and cheek-bones there is no room to move and that I would love to breathe easy. Well yes, he replies. Your mandibles are compressed, so it is no wonder you have trouble breathing through your nose. Your face, cheeks and jaws are held tight. And so he begins, the procedure uncomfortably intimate as his gloved fingers find the right spot high inside my mouth, and as we both wait, over many minutes, to see if and how the body might respond.

The intimacy and occasional awkwardness of therapeutic touch, the process of waiting for the body to respond rather than forcing it to release, and the interweaving of touch and sight are themes to which I will return in Chapter 4. Here, though, what fascinates me is the way a highly trained and experienced eye is capable of reading me – of knowing my body better than I do, in certain ways. I am intrigued by the professional restraint involved in *not* speaking these truths, over many weeks, until the questions or desires arise from me, as the practitioner and I play a careful and subtle game of revelation and silence, in which authority – the power to name and describe my body, its habits and its history – is batted silently between us. Again, a Foucauldian response to this game would be to note the depth and subtlety of therapeutic power – its ability not just to confer authority on the practitioner but also to imbue me with new ways of sensing, describing and problematizing myself. This is, in the Foucauldian use of the term, the 'productive' nature of power: it 'establishes the individual in his irreducible quality' (2003: xv). This power, which simultaneously makes us, enables us and constrains us, is not, in this instance, something I resent. After all, why would I resent a form of physical engagement that has loosened my frame, relieved my posture, given me more energy and taken me out of two years of near-constant back pain – and which is, after all, a substitute not for 'liberty' but for some other form of power – dependency on pharmaceutical companies or surgical intervention being the two most likely contenders in my case? No, I resent it only when it is clumsily, ineffectually, moralistically or normatively wielded. As with so much in alternative medicine – as indeed, with *all* forms of medicine – this depends as much on the practitioner as on the modality of practice.

Any good bodyworker, just like more mainstream physical therapists, combines biomedical knowledge of anatomy and physiology with highly developed powers of visual observation, including the power to detect patterns of movement, holding, structure and behaviour.[5] A masseur told me that this type of perception becomes naturalized, and is hard to switch off, even when at the cinema:

> In looking at a person, what I tend to perceive, and therapists do this, is how does the person hold themselves? How do they walk? They start doing postural analysis. Is one shoulder sitting higher than another? Are they tending to slouch to one side? This sort of thing.

Visual acuity involves not only attention to the now, but also the development of a particular form of visual imagination and memory, for practitioners need also to compare their clients over time, sometimes over a number of years. My osteopath can casually note that my facial muscles are less taut than usual; my Pilates teacher can look around a busy class and note that someone's left hip is moving more freely than the previous week, or that a person's thoracic area is tighter than usual. Bodywork uses visual acuity as one of its important tools, to be complemented with sensitive, sometimes interpretive, touch and with a form of intuitive knowing that claims to use but also to transcend ordinary senses. The eyes may be open, but they are not always looking in the same way. The cranial osteopathy of Hugh Milne, for example, involves not only acute professionally trained vision but also two forms of more intuitive vision: one with the eyes open, 'but in a deeper, more penetrating way than ordinary seeing', and the other, which uses 'the same apparatus' but works 'through a different channel' – keeping the eyes shut and using inner sight (1995a: 78). The bodyworker's 'gaze' is thus, to recall Foucault's phrase, 'a plurisensorial structure' in which vision plays an important but not isolated role. Moreover, it is not just that vision is 'supplemented' by other senses; it is, rather, that there are many different modes of vision itself. Sight's infamous power to 'distinguish, separate, [and] judge distances' (Serres 2008 [1985]: 67) is just one of the many things sight can do.

One of the interesting dimensions of the emerging science of neuroplasticity, which emphasizes the brain's ability to forge new neural connections throughout life, is the finding that neural 'firing' can be triggered not just by obvious actions in the world, but also by *imagining* such actions and by observing *others* performing them (Doidge 2008), a finding that would seem to confirm the importance of imitation and visualization in practices like yoga and meditation respectively. This type of sympathetic looking undoubtedly has ethical import; no doubt it also has therapeutic potential. Perhaps, indeed, we can consider it to be a core ingredient of many existing therapeutic practices. For some forms of professional seeing, such as the bodyworker's gaze, may move between distanced judgement and something far more entangled, such as that described by the drawing teacher Kimon Nicolaides as 'an observation that utilizes as many of the five senses as can reach through the eye at one time' (1941: 5). Margaret Mayhew calls this form of vision 'seeing with feeling'.[6] As the masseur quoted above put it, 'What I teach [my students] is that you see not with your eyes but your hands.' And his technical vision is not merely some form of optic capture; it is inseparable from the hands that touch and from practices of care. When he sees a body, even on the cinema screen, he is not just seizing an object of sight but also being seized by a desire – to reach out and to soothe. The bodyworker's gaze, while it cannot be disentangled from interpretive processes, is thus no simple objectification, but a complex form of seeing that is at once technical and empathic, visual and tactile, one which runs counter to the high-modern 'dissociation of touch from sight' (Crary 1990: 19).[7]

There is a certain irony, then, in the fact that in order to start my exploration of alternative medicine and the senses in familiar ground, I risk replicating this separation of touch from sight. For in this chapter I focus on the visual elements of diagnosis and on the interpretive practices of some bodyworkers, reserving my exploration of the tactile elements of both diagnosis and treatment till Chapter 4. My focus on the visual dimensions of bodywork is somewhat distorting, but I start here since the questions it raises about power are commonly levelled against alternative medicine, and I want to begin my bridging project at a place where Cultural Studies has already recognized the stakes as being high. As will be seen, the later chapters move to more tactile forms of knowing and to forms of body practice less commonly discussed in Cultural Studies. In this way I hope to bring some much needed critical interrogation to alternative medicine, but also to open possible avenues where Cultural Studies' conception of embodiment might be enriched through openness to some aspects of alternative thought and practice.

For example, I welcome the expanded concept of the body with which most alternative practitioners work. In a skilled and experienced bodyworker, precise, informed seeing turns into something much more, for bodyworkers typically work far more holistically than their biomedical counterparts and may well draw a range of inferences from the patterns they see – about the client's history, lifestyle, personality and emotional patterning. Like many other alternative therapists, they see the body as fundamentally *expressive*, and their holistic paradigm opens up greater potential for narrativization, interpretation and philosophical reflection than does a more mechanistic view of the body.

This interpretive potential of bodywork is both a strength and a danger. Conventional physical therapies tend to restrict themselves to more or less functional attitudes to the body, reserving, perhaps, some minor role for emotional patterning in the construction of body habits and shapes. Aside from a rather vague notion of 'stress', most mainstream physical therapists do not centralize questions of emotion. For some bodyworkers, however, anatomy can be understood *only* as inherently emotional: 'Human anatomy is ... more than a biochemical configuration; it is an emotional morphology' (Keleman 1985: 58). The body is understood as holding and embodying emotional experience and thus, eventually, being patterned by it. In that sense, the body remains the harbourer of dark secrets. For some practitioners, these secrets are understood as discrete and potentially retrievable; for others they are understood more processually, as part of the 'complex emotional configurations' that have shaped us (149).

The view of the body as storing experiences and emotions and having an innate propensity towards expressivity is not only inimical to the more mechanistic forms of biomedicine, but has also, as I have said, been the object of a number of trenchant philosophical and sociocultural critiques. But since my aim is to put such critiques into proximity with potentially more sympathetic perspectives from the 'inside' of alternative practices, I won't repeat them here, preferring first to build a thicker sense of the field of practice. Bodywork is quite internally diverse in its understanding of how the body processes and holds emotions and how significant a role emotions should play in therapy. In some practitioners' world-view, emotional experiences are held whole and complete like tiny time capsules deep in the body's inner space; for others, they have patterned the body and made it what it is; for others, they are significant but difficult to disentangle from all the other things that have got us in the shape we're in – habits, lifestyles, accidents, genetics. Practitioners vary greatly in how much weight they give to interpretation in the therapeutic process, as well as in the rigidity of their interpretive frameworks, and how openly their interpretations are expressed. Some agree with Freud that bringing the repressed into cognition is an essential component of 'cure' (Reich 1969: 11); others think the analytical mind is best left out of the process. These kinds of differences are linked to the practitioner's training, his/her relation to both metaphysics and biomedicine, his/her understanding of professional ethics, and the strength of his/her desire to articulate to mainstream medicine.

In some modes of practice interpretation ('reading' the body) is central; in others, it is treated with intellectual, professional or ethical caution. Fritz Frederick Smith, for example, calls the bodywork practice he developed, known as Zero Balancing, 'non-diagnostic' (2005: 2), but this does not mean that metaphysical, psychological or spiritual interpretation plays no part in it. The question of interpretation is usually as much a matter of practitioner as of modality. Among those practitioners who do 'read' the body, there is considerable variance around the role accorded to emotions, ranging from the bodyworkers who see the body as always, only or ultimately expressing truths about emotions, thoughts and feelings, to those who offer up multifactorial explanations that take into account other things, like genetics, accidents or life habits (factors that in a fully fledged New Age account would *themselves* be understood as having arisen from emotional states). A further spectrum of differences involves the corollary question of how the practitioner chooses to *articulate* these readings. Whose job is it, if anyone's, to reveal the body's truths? Is revelation always necessary, helpful or ethical? At one end of the scale are dogmatic practitioners who will naively or doggedly insist on their 'meaning' of a bodily event and for whom clients' potential resistance is merely a form of psychological defence or denial. (For an account an experience interpreted that way, see Stacey 1997: 37–9.)

Other practitioners may wait for patients to bring up questions of interpretation. Still others may believe that the practice of interpretation is either impossible, unnecessary, unethical, or a distraction from the real work of the body. In practice, the waters are muddy: though there are plenty of dogmatic practitioners, there are also many whose views are professed or operationalized differently in different contexts, including in response to the different views, interests and desires of their clients. This variability demands an informed, discerning and assertive patient-consumer.

Perhaps the most absolute, and certainly the most well-known, exponent of a psycho-spiritual theory of illness, in which all illness, indeed, all discord, ultimately derives from one cause – emotional dis-ease – is the New Age writer Louise L. Hay, whose work I described in Chapter 1. Though Hay is not a bodyworker, her metaphysical theories have enjoyed enormous popularity and have taken on the force of received New Age wisdom, such that many bodyworkers (and their clients) have been influenced by them. Hay is unequivocal about the place of emotion in illness:

> When people come to me with a problem, I don't care what it is – poor health, lack of money, unfulfilling relationships, or stifled creativity – there is only one thing I ever work on, and that is LOVING THE SELF. (1987: 14, original emphasis)

Hay's *Heal Your Body* (1988), described in Chapter 1, is a dictionary of illnesses, symptoms and body parts, alongside their metaphysical 'meaning' and a corrective thought pattern or affirmation. Her metaphysical schema sheds light on the mysteries of illness and invites readers to use this light to re-order their own dark psyches and hence correct their bodies. This exercise in decoding and re-coding blends spiritual views of illness with modern psychology. It is also an intriguingly modern take on the kind of classificatory medicine described by Foucault (2003) as typifying (French) pre-modernity, in which diseases are understood as a form of botanical species abstracted from the individual (and indeed from each other).

The abstraction and universalism of such metaphysical schemas sits somewhat at odds with modern individualism and especially with the psychologized tenor of therapeutic culture. Some practitioners may indeed be torn between the seductiveness of universal metaphysical templates and the individualist tenor of contemporary psychotherapeutic practice, in which every person is understood as a complex interiority in need of its own individual narrative. The relation to Freudian psychoanalysis, with its rather more universalist tendencies, also complicates the picture. Despite many alternative practitioners' lack of awareness of the influence of Freud on their world-view,[8] Freudian thought is, as Jackie Stacey notes, a deep influence on the contemporary alternative view of the body as holding and ultimately reflecting emotional or psychological patterning. Stacey points to a number of similarities between Freud and Breuer's theory connecting hysteria to emotional repression and contemporary alternative approaches to illnesses such as cancer, including a 'belief in the damaging nature of unexpressed emotions', the importance placed on early trauma and its possible link to adult illness, and the 'pathogenic qualities' ascribed to ideas and feelings (1997: 119). These psychological and alternative beliefs share what she calls a 'hydraulic model of repressed feelings' (119), in which emotions are understood as a bodily force requiring expression. She is, however, keen to point out differences between early psychoanalytic theories and modern alternative accounts.[9]

The view that (many) bodily symptoms are the result of the repression or conversion of mental or emotional events, states or habits is, as Stacey explains, a reversal of earlier theories in which the body was understood as affecting the soul, rather than the other way around (1997: 125).[10] With Freud, this 'redirection of the causation' of illness became 'pronounced':

> Thus, although the mind and the body have been seen to affect each other since ancient Western thought, the typical direction of this influence before Freud was from the body to the mind ... To put it crudely, popular beliefs today are more likely to attribute physical symptoms to depression than they are melancholia to too much 'black bile'. (126)

True enough, but the advent of the so-called 'Decade of the Brain'[11] – in which experiences like depression or anxiety are increasingly understood as neurochemical disorders as much as (if not more than) psychological ones – is starting to constitute a new orthodoxy, and one that puts blunter forms of alternative medicine, with their theories of emotional causation, starkly back at odds with the mainstream.

Bodywork construes mind-body relations in quite complex ways. For most bodyworkers 'it goes both ways: if the state of one's body directly affects one's mind, then the reverse also holds' (Hanna 1977: n.p.). The Freudian lineage remains strong in somatic therapy, through its elaboration in the work of Wilhelm Reich,[12] whose work is at the roots of much somatic psychotherapy today. Reich worked as a psychoanalyst under the tutelage of Freud. Medically trained, including in neuropsychiatry, he believed in the importance of the body to psychoanalysis and saw the aim of psychoanalysis as essentially ameliorative: detecting then releasing the muscular 'armouring' that is the human's main defence mechanism. Reich agreed with Freud that neuroses arose from the conflict between instinctual demands, especially sexual ones, and the ego that represses them (1969: 3). But he 'saw repression not as a psychic activity but as a somatic event' (Hanna 1977: n.p.), with the muscular system being the 'site of repression' (Hanna 1977: n.p.):

> The psychic structure is at the same time a biophysiological structure ... The muscular attitude is identical with what we call 'body expression'. (Reich 1969: 300–01)

Reich believed in the preventable and ameliorable nature of human suffering. The task of psychoanalysis as he saw it was to unlock blocked body/character structures, thereby releasing a stream of primordial energy, which he characterized as inherently sexual, into the organism. Reich combined this bodily vision with a political one (he was a Marxist), seeing neurosis not merely in individual terms but as the result of particular forms of education and socialization (1969: xx). His utopian impulse, his radical social consciousness and his emphasis on sexuality and the body made him controversial (he was imprisoned and died in gaol), but also made him the psychoanalyst of choice in the US counterculture.

A contemporary practitioner whose work was influenced by the Reichian lineage (among other traditions) is the US somatic psychologist Stanley Keleman. Trained in chiropractic, and later in humanistic psychology, he brought the Reichian tradition to the US West Coast (Hanna 1977), where he has directed the Center for Energetic Studies in Berkeley since 1971. He is the author of a number of vibrant books, including *Emotional Anatomy* (1985) and *Your Body Speaks its Mind* (1981). Keleman's view of anatomy is highly dynamic, bearing little relation to the exposure of inert matter for which anatomy is so often used as a metaphor. He is insistent that abstract anatomical knowledge needs to be turned into active, embodied knowledge. 'Life makes shapes', he declares in the opening line of *Emotional Anatomy* (1985: xi), and the human body is a multilayered, dynamic result of the innate urge towards organization and form. Anatomy, therefore, makes sense only when it is holistically and processually conceived:

> Anatomy is destiny as long as it is a somatic process. We must learn to re-envision anatomy more than as a static materialism, more than pictures of the dead, abstractions in the form of physiological formulas, ideas about nature rather than nature itself. Anatomy is really about a dynamic living process, a mystery, an initiation, the shape of experience which gives rise to feeling, thought, and action. It is about ourselves as feeling forms. It is about genetic, embryological, and personal history. (1985: 160)

To bodyworkers like Keleman, the body cannot help but speak the truth:

> The body cannot lie. It is incapable of lying. Only what comes out of the mouth can lie; the body never lies. (1981: 66)

Though in Keleman's model the body is the repository of truth, it does not hold that truth like an apricot holds a kernel. Rather, it embodies and manifests truths that are multilayered, complex and often inarticulable by other means. So is it bodywork's task to make this mystery manifest – to *reveal* these different forms of history – or merely to work productively with them?

Although some bodyworkers are very engaged in reading signs, and making legible the body's invisible stories and histories, Keleman clearly does not imagine this process as anything remotely so blunt as the revelation of a hidden universal truth, in the way that Hay's metaphysical schema does; if life makes shapes, then different lives make different shapes. His bodywork involves less the revelation of a universal truth than a process of *working with* particular embodied truths. Nonetheless, Keleman's debt to the Reichian tradition is evident, at least in his earlier books, in that he accords some degree of generalizability to these truths, insofar as different emotions are understood as producing different types of bodily response: stiffening, collapsing, slumping, rigidity or swelling. His book *Emotional Anatomy* (1985) includes numerous diagrams of typical holding postures accompanied by an explanation of the emotional states they are understood to embody.[13]

The invitation to read and interpret the body is especially hard to resist in public contexts like the workshops and demonstrations so common in the New Age circuit. In the Californian tradition especially, where the taste for spectacle and public catharsis is reputedly quite strong, there is likely to be an element of showmanship at work, and recipients of bodywork may well respond with visible emotion or bodily reactions. Having participated in a goodly number of such workshops in Australia myself over the years, I understand how easy it is for the practitioner's diagnostic or therapeutic skill to slip into showmanship, and the patient's release into performance. I have now learnt to understand such catharses as neither genuine nor faked in any simple sense, but as somatic responses to the expectations generated by the context, including the national context. An Australian myofascial release trainer, 'Barbara', who has worked with a number of prominent US bodyworkers, told me that the bodily unwindings[14] produced in North American workshops tend to be much more visibly cathartic than those in Australia or the UK, 'and I think that goes with the nation'. We will see throughout this book that the need to feel something happening – the need, at times, to *perform* the visible signs of transformation – can be part and parcel of the expectations of both practitioners and clients.

Thomas Hanna's account in the late 1970s of Keleman and others at work captures the air of excitement and possibility that greeted these new forms of body practice, while unknowingly pointing to interpretive elements that to a later audience might ring some alarm bells:

> I think it improbable that anyone could watch somatic healers like Alexander Lowen or Stanley Keleman work with a patient and not be spellbound. Their ability to read an individual's personality in the lines of his posture is a special achievement. To see it done is at first mystifying. Then, with more familiarity, one begins to glimpse that the lines of that particular body say something about the habitual character of that person, and that by close attention anyone can

learn to read those lines. It is a question of noticing little things: the position of
the head, the curve of the neck, the slope of the shoulders, the cant of the pelvis,
the tension of the knees, the look of the eyes and mouth. When seen as a whole,
all these things add up to a single statement of who this person is. This reading
of the patient's body is, to a large extent, a diagnosis. (1977: n.p.)

Anyone who has worked with a skilled, experienced and sensitive bodyworker
knows just how exciting and *useful* such skills of observation and interpretation can
potentially be. Yet it is an easy slide into reductiveness, normativity and spectacle,
into the politically unpalatable vision of the practitioner's expert and authoritative
gaze fixing a body, drawing out its truths, summing it up as a 'single statement',
no matter how compassionate. The temptation of deciding – and revealing – 'who
the person is' proves too great for some practitioners, especially those who are less
experienced and/or more committed to a New Age metaphysics than their more
biomedically influenced colleagues. I am no stranger to this dilemma. In Chapter 4,
I will turn the analytical spotlight onto my own amateur practice of reiki, describing
my own wrestling with the dilemmas of interpretation, and it will become evident
that I am not a detached observer. I am thoroughly implicated.

Keleman describes his practice in California in the late 1960s as belonging to 'an
atmosphere of cultural revolution' (McClure n.d.). It is possible that the high-water
mark of therapeutic showmanship has passed. In any case, having not seen Keleman
at work, I make no claim that Hanna's account is an accurate representation of his
practice, and certainly not of his current practice. Even in the mid-1970s, his view
of the body was complex, its seeming structuralism counteracted by his insistence on
the dynamism, subtlety and multilayering of the human organism and his insistence
that the aim of bodywork is not normative:

> In speaking about emotional anatomy, it is important to avoid concepts based
> on either what is 'normal' or what is ideal. There is no ideal structure for humans.
> The primary concern should be how an individual uses himself to function.
> (1985: xii)

Even at this point, his debt to Reichian body typing was, clearly, somewhat ambiguous. He remained absolutely committed to the complexity, subtlety and individuality
of body patternings, insisting that they are always multilayered and hence resistant
to a simple scrutiny from the outside:

> The organism's emotional layering can be compared to the rings of a tree, each
> ring revealing age and experience. For example, defiance and pride may cover
> fear and sadness which in turn cover timidity and anxieties about abandonment.
> Each of these configurations is somatically structured. The outer layer may be
> stiff and rigid to cover withdrawal and contraction which further covers the

inflated expectation of an abandoned child who fears collapse. These examples illustrate the complexity of somatic reality. (1985: 149–50)

For those committed to less hermeneutic conceptions of embodiment, this may still be a little too neat. It sees the body as 'a text of the psyche' (Stacey 1997: 26) – albeit a complex, multilayered text, some of whose meanings might remain indecipherable. It acknowledges multiplicity and complexity, but nonetheless has at its core the search for a 'deeply lodged, dark or luminous, truth' (Stafford 1991: 7). This is hardly surprising, given Keleman's debt to mythological frameworks like those of Joseph Campbell, with whom he had a long professional association.

In recent interviews, Keleman has engaged with neurochemical theories of anxiety, panic and depression. For him, the discovery of chemical mechanisms involved in such experiences isn't an endpoint that rebuts somatic theories of mood disorders, but rather, further evidence of the complexity of embodiment:

> It's true there are illnesses that are biochemically induced. There are dopamine and serotonin based illnesses. What people leave out is that in a common response to a situation, like, having to control yourself when someone is shouting at you, you begin to shrink and hold yourself back. The body sends the brain two signals: compact, which stops the dopamine or serotonin, and, send some epinephrine to be charged and excited. So this muscular attitude starts stiffening even more to try to stop from being overwhelmed by its own epinephrine. This finally depletes the chemical that keeps us alert and aroused and you get exhausted and depressed. So, the chemical disturbance is not only caused on the inside by a mess up in the brain physiology, it's also a signal from the muscular attitude in response to a situation. (McClure n.d.)

I am unqualified to make a medical comment, but I want to note here the potential explanatory power of holistic models of embodiment, which see the brain as *part of* the body and of embodied life. In this understanding, neurochemical responses don't emerge from some invisible 'nowhere' but are produced as 'way[s] of using yourself', 'way[s] of being in the world' (McClure n.d.).

In this, Keleman stays true to Reich's fundamental claim that emotional and psychological responses are simultaneously somatic and psychic events, a claim I find intellectually convincing. Moreover, its therapeutic corollary – that forms of body therapy can be helpful in releasing blocked emotions and changing ways of being in the world – is highly enabling. To my current way of thinking, somatic psychotherapy is at its intellectually strongest and therapeutically most useful when it sees interpretation as only one component of a thoroughly bodily encounter. Keleman's own recent work is quite explicit about the limitations of pharmaceutical treatments in which the urge to narrativize overrides the invitation to 'rebody yourself':

I have a few people who are taking Prozac. They talk about their mood shifts, then you watch the content and the application of the insights. It's as if they went to an interesting movie. The urgency to have to rebody yourself is gone. What you get, since the urgency is gone, is pleasure in insight or being able to communicate. They're happy with that. Nothing has to reorganize itself. They feel better. They say there's a shift in their mood. 'I'm not well, but it makes it tolerable.' And this is the key sentence: to keep doing the things that they've been doing well, not to reorganize and relearn. I don't deny there are times that you need it. I only question what its long-term effects are. (McClure n.d.)

In Australia, those practitioners quite firmly embedded in the CAM paradigm – where alternative therapies seek credibility and interrelation with orthodox medicine through a range of professionalizing strategies – have often learnt to resist the temptation to speak the truth of the other and the easy slide from reading to diagnosis. In this cautiously professionalizing CAM environment, more mainstream manual therapists will want to be seen to avoid any form of emotional fundamentalism, where a posture definitely corresponds to a readily definable emotional state, and will tend to espouse – at least to an interviewer – more multifactorial accounts of body function and dysfunction. Bodywork practitioners working in the terrain close to mainstream manual therapies will typically be interested in functional as well as emotional accounts of biomechanics – not (only) what does this posture *mean*, but what can this body *do* in its current shapes, and how can it be reshaped to be less in pain, more mobile, and so on? Barbara doesn't discount emotional holding patterns but considers them more holistically – as part of a general life view that includes habits (like sitting at a computer) and accidents, and which, unlike New Age metaphysics, doesn't see such material matters as a coded spiritual message from the Universe. In any case, she takes it as an ethical principle that you start where the patient is rather than imposing an approach or a reading on the client. Rather than saying you are round-shouldered because you are protecting yourself (a classic Reichian reading) or simply saying you are round-shouldered because you sit at a computer too much (a classic materialist reading), she prefers to 'start with the shoulder'.

This is a commitment to starting with, and staying with, the body itself – to keeping the eyes wide open at some times and shutting them at others, giving oneself over to touch, silence and undecidability. This patient, body-centred, unshowmanly practice is less about putting acute observation skills in the service of narrative or even catharsis, than about trusting the body to do its own work, allowing it to reshape itself in a fashion that evades or exceeds interpretation. Naturopath Judy Singer calls this 'attending' to the body (2008: 145) – a term I like for the way it combines patience, perceptiveness and ministry. When the body unwinds on the massage table, who is to know what stories it is telling, what dramas it is undoing, what events – whether singular and cataclysmic, or daily, repeated and mundane – it is reliving, releasing or reshaping? In the words of one osteopath I visited: 'Never presume. Just observe.' This is a valuable precept, but also an impossible ideal. For, as we have seen, seeing is a set of physiological, cultural and professional trainings and cannot ultimately be separated from believing. But this shouldn't lead us to give up on the idea that in the right 'hands', precise seeing can be an opening into new knowledge. In a state of meditative stillness, the eyes can be used in 'non-habitual ways' (Milne 1995a: 83).

I cannot leave the discussion of bodywork, objectification and power without one final comment, reversing the line of sight and shining the Foucauldian spotlight elsewhere in the system in which bodies are made meaningful. While it is important to note the power invested in the bodyworker to judge the body and draw meaning from it, this shouldn't blind us to the other webs of surveillance and judgement in which we are all bound and from which, paradoxically, bodywork might allow us some respite or escape. For perhaps the most intense scrutiny in play in bodywork treatments is not the authoritative gaze of the medical authority, but a critical self-scrutiny made all too common by a culture whose hypervigilant policing of body norms arguably wreaks far more havoc than the clinician's gaze. Bodyworkers have repeatedly told me that the majority of their female patients start by apologizing for their body. Comments like 'sorry you have to look at my body' or 'sorry for my fat ass' are not, apparently, aberrant examples of female low body esteem but routine openings to a bodywork session. It can start young. The bodyworker I described at the start of this section, a sensitive and insightful practitioner, told me that he has treated thirteen-year-old girls brought in by their mothers, and seen them, in his words, 'pull back from their own bodies' as his professional gaze acts not (only) as a feared medical intrusion but as a trigger for a critical self-scrutiny internalized from our culture's broader web of surveillant gazes. Few people are exempt; most of us at same time experience our bodies as the wrong size, colour, age or shape – insufficiently beautiful, too evidently fallible, imperfect imitations of the artificial bodies they are meant to resemble. Perhaps these oppressive ideals are some of the bodily stories being undone and remade on the massage table.

CLAIRVOYANT SIGHT: THE ETHICS OF CLEAR-SEEING AND STRAIGHT TALKING

I turn now towards a mode of vision whose existence is highly contested: clairvoyant sight. In other times and places, such forms of vision have been deemed to rival or exceed the vision provided by ordinary sight (Soskice 1996). Medieval Christian theology accepted the primacy of vision but qualified it by a belief in the superiority of other forms of inner sight as ways of knowing God. Augustine had taught that physical visions come 'a poor third after spiritual and intellectual visions' (29). But in the modern West it is hard to imagine any more pointed example of the long-held association between images, fakery, delusion and unreason than the case of clairvoyant sight, nor any starker posing of the question of whether dreams, images and visions are deceptive and seductive phantasms or manifestations of the divine light. Clairvoyant visions undoubtedly fall within the category of images that are to be understood as empty and dangerous, in the way so vividly captured by Barbara Stafford, who claims that in the Enlightenment 'imagery, like the material body, became systematically drawn into a negative analogy with fraudulent apparitions, confounding dreams, and irrational delusions' (1991: 5). Within this regime, she claims, images were effectively divided from intellect (5) and sight itself became divided and gendered: the rational sight associated with scientific inquiry was mas-culinized and mystical sight was abandoned to women (Classen et al. 1994: 84). So much so, indeed, that even to *ask questions* (outside of history or anthropology) about this mode of seeing and the knowledge it claims to produce is, within the academy, to risk being contaminated by its feminizing powers – to be seen as a victim of nonsense and an instrument of unreason. The unspoken assumption is that only ancients or 'others' believe in non- or extra-rational capacities, or that modern people ought to have 'grown out' of such beliefs and practices. But of course they/we haven't.

Elsewhere (Barcan 2009a), I have written about medical clairvoyance in rela-tion to a contemporary popular fear about the resurgence of unreason, epitomized by trends as diverse as religious fundamentalism, the New Age, managerialism or postmodernism. I attempted there to complicate this binary picture of reason and its antagonists (nonsense, delusion, blind faith), arguing that many users of clairvoyance are not blind followers but self-reflexive and often strategic – often trying out beliefs rather than unreasonably applying them. Nonetheless, and despite a venerable tradition of feminist and anthropological critique of reason as itself a historically variable and occasionally limited mode of knowledge (Lloyd 1984), I find it easy to fall prey to the power of the contemporary rationalist narrative about the threat to reason and to feel foolish and anxious that I would take such practices seriously enough to bother exploring them. Clearly, the parallel tracks set down at the start of my twin induction into alternative medicine and post-structuralism are still there, and a sharp jolt can make me jump from one to the other. Still, I pro-ceeded with my ethnographical project of turning an analytical gaze onto practices even in the face of commonsensical ridicule, critique or dismissal. Once I began, there were many questions I wanted to ask clairvoyants, and did: systemic questions (What is it like to work as a clairvoyant or psychic in a Western context? How were you trained? How do spiritual forms of medicine interact with biomedicine?); political questions (Are we witnessing a rise of 'unreason' in the modern West, and if so, is that a cause for concern? What is the significance of the fact that this clandestine 'medical' system is so distinctly feminized?); and phenomenological questions (What do clairvoyant visions actually *look* like?) I have addressed some systemic and political questions elsewhere (see Barcan 2009b and 2009a, respectively). Here, I address the power relations and ethical dilemmas implicit in clairvoyant vision. I do not directly scrutinize the question of whether the 'clear-seeing' of the clairvoyant is part of the 'fakery of the visual' (Stafford 1991: 15). Rather, I approach that question in relation to *systems and practices* of truth-seeking and truth-telling – for example, via the question of the negotiation of professional ethics. My aim throughout this book is to take a range of practices, even unorthodox or marginalized ones, seriously. Taking them seriously often means suspending questions of belief or unbelief in favour of an analysis of the effects produced by systems of knowledge. But since I am interested in the therapeutic claims of alternative medicine as well as its socio-cultural dimensions I cannot fully evade the question of belief. My investment in alternative medicine as a therapeutic system means that I have a stake at least in the possibility that medical clairvoyance might occasionally, if not reliably, have some therapeutic value as well as being a culturally interesting practice. Therefore, and since the politics and ethics of disclosure and visibility are the themes of this chapter, it is important for the reader to know the extent of my own involvement –which is that as part of the participant observation underpinning this book I asked two of the clairvoyants to give me a medical reading and that I have intermittently consulted one of them over the succeeding years, with pleasure and interest. But there were also people I encountered with whom I would not have felt sufficiently secure to do so. I have experienced the genuine and sometimes significant value of the process, while remaining deeply aware of the potential of medical clairvoyance to induce distress and damage, and even, in the case of naive or dogmatic practitioners or vulnerable or naive users, to do real medical harm.

Chapter 5 is an extended discussion of medical clairvoyance. In this current chapter, I focus only on sight, and continue the discussion about the power relations and ethical dilemmas involved in seeing and interpreting another. Of course, clairvoyants (despite the etymology of the term) do not *only* see; they also claim to feel, smell, hear and, above all, to *know* in a way that integrates but also transcends other forms of sensory perception. But vision is the archetypal metaphor for a form of knowledge that is both truth-telling and seductive and deceptive, and hence an ideal type for the rationalist critique of clairvoyance.

In rather old-fashioned parlance, clairvoyants, mediums and channels are known as 'sensitives'. This term suggests that clairvoyant intuition has been conceived of as a form of *openness* to the full range of the visible rather than as an exceptional keenness of vision itself. For the Theosophists, clairvoyant intuition was about intense receptivity to the world rather than a phenomenological reaching out towards it. As the Theosophist Charles Webster Leadbeater put it, 'it is not in the least a question of strength of vision, but of extent of susceptibility' (1918: 10). In traditional Western philosophical terms, this framing metaphorically feminizes clairvoyant perception, which is to be understood not as a striving, capturing or mastery of a world 'out there' so much as an *openness* to the world. Moreover, for Leadbeater, this is true of *all* perception. He seeks to normalize clairvoyance by seeing it as an extension of the perception processes of everyday life, insisting that its most elementary forms (for Theosophy conceives of different varieties of clairvoyance) must be seen as an *extension* of the senses rather than as a separate capacity (1918: 12). As mentioned, the visual is only one part of what clairvoyants claim as special modes of perception. Their seeing is really a much more complex *knowing* that involves a range of senses, as well as sensations (e.g. chills, goose bumps) and judgements. It is a more holistic embodied knowing, irreducible to vision, or even vision supplemented or accompanied by other senses. The ultimate 'diagnostic' technique of spiritual healers and psychics is not vision but a form of *knowing*, and the aim of a 'reading' is less to pin down a body through a special mode of vision than to know a person in ways that exceed the control of both practitioner and client, and which not infrequently involve claims about what cannot or should not be made known at a particular juncture.

Nonetheless, clairvoyance is undoubtedly a practice underpinned by a desire to know the self, its histories and its futures, and which locates authority in a specially endowed figure, even though that figure understands herself[15] as a 'channel' or conduit rather than its author. Remote as clairvoyance undoubtedly is from the rationalist undertaking of the scientific or biomedical project, their underlying desire for truth and their aim of 'reveal[ing] nonapparent physical and mental experience' (Stafford, 1991: xvii) are, ironically, not dissimilar. Though they are radically different ways of 'visibilizing the invisible' (xvii), they are both structured by a similar desire – that of truth-as-unveiling. And rationalism has never yet simply trumped its opposites, even in 'high' modernity, supposedly the regime of arch-rationality. Paradoxically, the new visual technologies of the nineteenth century, such as the X-ray and the photograph, in making manifest many things that had hitherto been invisible – germs, bones, the spectrum of light, animal motion – did not simply advance the cause of science and eradicate belief in the supernatural. Rather, they could also allow belief in the supernatural to prosper, by revealing that the world was full of 'forces operating beneath and beyond the threshold of human perception' (Keller 2008: 19).

Clairvoyants claim to be able to see different things, and to see differently. Most of my interviewees claimed to be able to see entities or spirits. What is the nature of that seeing, I asked? Is it like seeing a person in the room? Most replied that it wasn't. When pressed to try to describe what it looked like, they used other visual metaphors, but ultimately couldn't fully compare it to everyday vision. Mary, for example, said:

Mary: Often I will do a reading and then notice that there's a spirit with the person. So I will say, 'Oh you've got so and so with you'. And I'll describe the spirit. And they'll say, 'That was my uncle', or brother, or whatever.

Ruth: Is that an image that you're seeing clearly in your mind or is it as literal as seeing that tape-recorder there?

Mary: Sometimes it's just like a light, like an outline, like a shape. And you just know that it's male or female – *was* when it was here on earth. Other times it's clearer than that and it can be like the picture of a man. It's hard to describe. I'm just trying to see if there are any other ways of knowing. Sometimes it's just like a vision. I don't know how else to describe it. It's just like a light goes on or something and you just see this being there. So you just know that that person has a spirit with them that wants to communicate with them.

What does it *feel* like to see this way? Mary used another visual comparison:

It's very draining being in tune. It's also very enlivening and enriching but it takes a lot of energy. It's like if somebody's watching a movie and they're describing every movement, every word; you get exhausted doing that all day. Well, that's what it's like.

Many clairvoyants claim to be able to see the human energy field, or auras, and believe that illness (or potential illness) is often visible as darker or stagnant colours in the aura. Some also see symbols or images in the client's body. Glen Margaret, for example, sometimes sees something quite literally anatomical (e.g. a piece of jagged bone if there has been an injury) and at other times something more evidently symbolic (e.g. a spider). These symbols are not universal metaphysics, nor are they simply visual 'translations' of illness, and they have a connotative or qualitative dimension. Thus, for Glen Margaret, the nature of the symbol may give some sense of the feel or quality of the illness, or of its causation, and hence imply the best kind of treatment. She carries out healing work in the same register, doing emotional release until the symbol disappears:

When I look at people who've got cancers I generally see the cancer as mushrooms or perhaps a bunch of grapes. On some people the cancer will show as red, really throbbing – an ethereal image – and it's a very emotionally 'charged' cancer. If

> you let go of the emotions the cancer will actually disappear. On others there is a
> black spot and you can actually feel the energy of it and you'll feel it like a piece
> of coal, and you'll actually see and feel a piece of coal.

So to whom do these symbols 'belong'? They evidently belong to a particular symbolic system, but are they brought into being by the practitioner or the client?

> The way it's presented is the way the person wants to represent it to you. Some
> people are very straight down the line and give you a shape of a bone, other
> people give you a spider, other people give you a bunch of grapes. They're their
> symbols rather than your symbols.

Clearly, relaying and interpreting other people's symbols to them involves starkly asymmetrical power relations and complex ethical, professional and legal questions, especially when it comes to medical matters, which are so heavily scrutinized in modern bureaucratic societies. Clairvoyance lies largely outside the scope of biomedical regulation, but there are certain legal frameworks, like a prohibition on diagnosis, that have become so recognized within the CAM field that most clairvoyants cannot help but be aware of them. In the following extract, the clairvoyant is careful to make the distinction between an act of non-biomedical diagnosis or prediction and her own practice which, she insists, consists of a faithful rendition of what she sees, without interpretation:

> I'm thinking of a particular client of mine and he is drinking a lot of alcohol
> every day and said to me, 'Is it having any effect on me?' And I said, 'Well, your
> aura is turning grey in that area', so he panicked and got all of these tests, cancer
> tests and all the rest of it, and he came back and said, 'Well, you're a heap of shit
> because you're wrong.' There is nothing wrong yet – but what I'm watching is
> that it's getting darker and darker; eventually he will have the problem there. He
> doesn't have it at the moment, but he will have it eventually. It's a very difficult
> one.

This judgement is very carefully and intentionally *not* conceived of as diagnosis:

> And of course you can't legally diagnose – so I don't diagnose. I just say, 'Look,
> what I'm seeing is this spot here. Let's just work until it's gone'.

The work referred to here is emotional release using visualization. For this practitioner, then, the visual is not only a set of prompts to action but also itself constitutes a *plane* of action – a terrain for intervention. This not only has its own therapeutic claims, it also allows the treatment to remain outside biomedical terrain.

The legal, ethical and epistemological complexities surrounding diagnosis are extremely complicated given the range of questions with which clairvoyants are commonly presented, and the often hidden or complex contexts in which they practice.

Like the iridologists I interviewed, many of the psychics and spiritual healers were well aware of the vulnerability of clients and the fact that they came to them in times of transition or need. This concern might be increased in the case of those who also practise other CAM modalities, like naturopathy, and whose clients may not necessarily come for spiritual guidance, but for something more mainstream. For example, an 'intuitive counsellor' trained in conventional counselling but also practising as a psychic told me that she mostly kept the roles quite separate, but was occasionally tempted to change gears and allow intuitive insights to bleed into a conventional counselling session. She was aware this was an ethical danger:

> We have to be very, very careful as to how you put that message across ... You've really got to be careful how you present that because you can frighten the hell out of them.

There is clearly an ethical danger in giving clients something they haven't come for – indeed, it is a rupture of the therapeutic contract. From the practitioner's point of view, there is also pressure coming in the other direction. The same intuitive counsellor also saw the ethical danger in being swayed by what the client evidently wanted to hear:

> Sometimes we do say things that we are hoping the person is wanting – so we are trying to placate them or give them what they want. So that's when you're projecting, and you're not really coming from that [intuitive] space. Sometimes [they want] answers to questions that you just can't answer, so when you [try to answer them] you are coming from the intellect and you are giving that person what they want – without *really* knowing intuitively whether that's right or not.

Equally, it is hard to provide an answer a client may *not* want to hear:

> People [sometimes] have a set idea in their mind that that is the answer that they want and they are not happy if you don't give them the answer that they want, so you try to plant a seed of doubt in their mind so that they actually look at another possible scenario other than what they're totally focused on. Say it's someone who really wants a child and you know damn fine that they are not going to have one, so how do you say that to them?

So, what *do* you say, I ask? I'll quote Darlene's answer in full here, because the complexity of the syntax indicates the muddiness of the ethical terrain:

Darlene: How do I? That's something I've really got to feel into as to whether there *is* [a baby] around, and what I say to them is that there is a possibility but that it may not happen and are you prepared for that? It's a very, very sensitive issue.

Ruth: I presume that most people would see that as code for 'no'?

Darlene: Yeah, so you start off in a very gentle way by saying there is a possibility; it just may not happen. Or else what I usually do – sometimes – (I don't always get the chance to because they always bring it back) but I'll focus on something else. I'll focus on the real issues that are going on around it – the relationship or something or other else – and then they'll say, 'We didn't get a chance to talk about the child.' 'Oh, time's up.' You know what I mean – so you can skirt around it by ... not necessarily creating a diversion but in some ways you are, you know, depending on their energy and trying to figure out what it is they are wanting here – how to get around a certain situation without actually donging them over the head with a sledge-hammer which you don't like doing. So there is some sensitive stuff.

These examples make it clear that clairvoyance does not always conceive of itself as a straightforward exercise in clear-seeing followed by clear-speaking. Seeing-through is obviously a significant element of the practice. (Darlene after all claimed that she might 'know damn fine' that there was no baby on the cards, and she made the distinction between what the client *thinks* he/she wants to know and what the 'real issues' are.) But the interviews also revealed that as an interpersonal practice, clairvoyance is much more ambiguous, situated and *negotiated* than the metaphor of stripping away to the bare truth might suggest. Both practitioner and client are likely to be mobilizing beliefs and belief systems in quite complicated ways – wrestling with contradictions, desires and fears, and picking up, putting down, modifying or testing out different modes of thought and belief, whether strategically or unconsciously. This is why clients try out different clairvoyants, or accept that the same clairvoyant may give them a different reading on a different day, or why they accept some bits as 'ringing true' and ignore others. This is undoubtedly a question of the ego defending and/or gratifying itself, but it also shows that even committed participants know clairvoyance to be fallible (or, to put it differently, they know it is situated, partial and contextual) and approach it not as a reliable exercise in clear sight but as encounters-in-context.

But there is no escaping the fact that the underlying metaphor of the stripping away of veils does structure the practice. The resulting ethical and power issues are in a sense quite obvious. It's all too easy to imagine the predicaments, abuses, dilemmas, unintended cruelty and sometimes the sheer danger of these largely invisible, very intense, and quite private transactions, which lie, moreover, beyond the scope of regulation, except, perhaps, under such tangential rubrics as consumer protection legislation. It seems that at least some unhappy clients seek protection not from outside the system but from within it; almost all my interviewees described (without my asking) having had to perform 'corrective readings' for clients who had come to them in a panic after having been to see *another* clairvoyant who had predicted dire futures of one kind or another for them.

Given the ethical and legal complexities, we might ask where clairvoyants learn their ethics. Most spiritual traditions place great emphasis on communities of practice, apprenticeship and the training or cultivation of perception. This gives some measure of legibility and protection to the members of that community, and binds clairvoyant practices into some form of ethical and regulatory framework. But in Western contexts, clairvoyance is often commodified and usually practised in isolation, though communities of practice do exist in particular ethnic traditions and spiritual contexts (like the Spiritualist Church). Outside of these traditions or communities, however, codes of clairvoyant practice are of necessity worked out in relative isolation.[16] When I asked Mary where she had learnt her ethical code, she replied:

> Well I think part of it is just my own basic nature. I'm very conservative and from a conservative upbringing. And very middle-class. Also I was a school teacher for many years. So you come with this set of moulds about what's right and what's not right. Ethically I stay within the conservative framework as it were.

In developing their own code of ethics, clairvoyants inevitably draw on the range of culturally available discourses. Spiritual, neoliberal, consumerist, medical and legal logics mix together but do not all tend in the same direction. Consumer rights, marketing, the New Age, social work, psychology and health care are all influences, sometimes working in harmony – as when neoliberal precepts about patient responsibility mesh with spiritual precepts about taking responsibility for one's spiritual journey, with consumer advice like caveat emptor, and with the neoliberal injunction to manage one's own health. But sometimes they are in tension – as when the *caveat emptor* principle collides with the spiritual-professional principle that one shouldn't practise clairvoyance until one is sufficiently spiritually evolved. As with most ethical thought, the result is a process of selection and combination from different traditions and discourses. So, for example, Suzie, a 'psychic masseuse' who is also a trained counsellor, considers full disclosure of any information she picks up to be part of her 'duty of care' to the client. Other interviewees, true to the spirit of the New Age, which teaches that we are '100% responsible for everything in our lives, the best and the worst' (Hay 1987: 7), believe that clients need to take responsibility for both their choices and their reactions. Here, neoliberal, consumerist and spiritual discourses coincide, commingled in some cases with a dose of everyday pragmatism:

> I think that people who come know that I'm not a medically qualified practitioner and that the advice is from a different sort of realm altogether. It's

> like a spiritual realm. So hopefully they will understand that it's not something
> which is scientific. (Mary)

Esoteric traditions teach that the intuitive gift is sacred, dangerous and to be treated respectfully – not to be used for self-aggrandizement or entertainment (Leadbeater 1918: 172). Many of the clairvoyants I interviewed believe that their special powers would shut down if they attempted to use them to gain power over another, or as a party trick. Some also believe that if they have managed to control or eliminate their own ego involvement then there will be in-built spiritual protection that will ethically guide the session. Mary, for example, believes that the suitability of certain kinds of information is actually part and parcel of what she picks up: 'I can kind of tell if it's not wise to go to some places within the client, so while I'm delivering information I'm also picking up other information.' I asked her whether this sense of what is or isn't appropriate comes from what we might call 'everyday' intuition (e.g. a combination of interpersonal sensitivity, an ability to read body language, or even professional training as a counsellor), or whether it too was psychically given:

Mary: It's more psychic information. Yes, I do read people. There's no question.
          I can sort of intuit what people are like. But most people can, so that's
          something separate. I'm talking more about I get psychic warnings as it were
          about not wanting to stir the pot.
Ruth: Do they come through as actual sounds or images?
Mary: Sometimes, but mostly feelings. It's like you just *know*.

(For a longer discussion of this distinction between everyday and spiritual intuition see Barcan 2009a.) Thus, within a spiritual logic, privileged access to the interior life of another is understood as not fully or ultimately under the control of the spiritual authority – who understands herself not to be voicing her own knowledge but to be a channel.

To its critics, this is self-evidently a get-out-of-jail-free card that enables charlatans, crooks and well-meaning fools to do incalculable damage underneath the regulatory radar. The paradigmatic remoteness and the social invisibility of clairvoyance make it resistant to all but the bluntest forms of professional and legal regulation. When I asked Mary whether she knew of any government attempts to regulate clairvoyant activity, she didn't, and she agreed that there are some benefits to being so much on the fringe that you don't register on the regulatory radar. She did, however, see this freedom as necessarily tied to an ethics of personal responsibility on the client's part:

> There are [advantages to being on the fringe] – yeah, absolutely. And there's
> the reverse of that, which is you've got to be very careful who you go to and

> you have to take responsibility ultimately for any information that you've been given. You decide.

Clearly this whole area is ethically fraught and one where the paradigmatic differences between intuitive medicine and biomedicine are at their starkest – and yet, thousands of people move between and across them every day, negotiating them in a form of everyday philosophical practice.

The clairvoyant claims for herself the power to see inside, and beyond, the body of another. But the bundle of different logics that contemporary clients are likely to bring to a clairvoyant session (from spiritual to consumer to neoliberal) means that this is no simple exercise in seeing-through. Perhaps the whole thing is an exercise in delusion; or perhaps the clairvoyant sees only what the client wants or allows her to see; or perhaps the client can 'practitioner shop' until she finally hears what she wants to believe? The clairvoyant no doubt also acts as a kind of provocateur or mirror whose reflections allow clients to sort out their own feelings for themselves.

The conferral of spiritual authority, however ambiguously, upon a paid outsider sits somewhat at odds with another contemporary spiritual injunction – that of seeking your own truth. The idea of seeking the truth inside oneself, so beloved of the New Age, has a number of precursors. In the Christian tradition, it has its antecedents in the 'privatisation of religion' (Carrette and King 2005: 37) brought about by the Protestant Reformation. This 'new sensibility' (37) emphasizing 'interiorised knowledge or experience of the divine' (38) in turn fed into the development of nineteenth- and twentieth-century spiritual movements such as Theosophy, where they blended with borrowings from non-Western traditions such as yoga. The Theosophist Leadbeater lamented the lack of formal and systematic training that characterized most European clairvoyants, claiming it made them 'fall very far short' of what systematically learnt clairvoyance can achieve (1918: 50). Today, the New Age treats intuition as a universal human potential, and one strain of New Age discourse advocates training people to develop their own powers of inner sight. This would eliminate the element of direct commercial transaction which so alarmed Leadbeater, who considered payment for clairvoyance to be a 'prostitution and degradation' (1918: 170) of a higher power and a 'sacrilegious folly' (171). (On the other hand, it has encouraged a whole other realm of commodity exchange, in the form of training CDs, courses on intuition development and so on.)

The injunction to develop one's own intuition also sits well with contemporary individualism and brings clairvoyance under the remit of the project of individual self-development that so typifies the New Age. One example of the genre is Susan Shumsky's book *Divine Revelation* (1996). Shumsky, for one, is adamant that the era of the guru is drawing to a close:

> You have within yourself all that you need. You do not need a guru or psychic
> adviser. You are the source of your own wisdom. (1996: 38)

Clearly this is intended as both democratizing and empowering:

> No one can tell you anything you don't already know. Be the power and the
> authority, take command over your life. (39)

Shumsky couches this democratization in an evolutionary framework: clairvoyance
used to be the province only of 'geniuses, saints and prophets. But now the vibratory
level of the earth has been lifted to such a degree that *anyone* can awaken his or
her inner genius' (35, original emphasis). It seems the new frontier for journeying
is inside the mind and the soul as well as the body, and both internal and external
guides are needed for safe travel:

> you will receive divine inspiration from deep within yourself. You need not fear
> this inner exploration … Once you make contact with the divine within, you are
> beginning a grand journey. There are many adventures ahead of you and many
> places to explore. But you need the proper map and the tools for navigation.
> For this reason this book contains all the techniques and procedures needed to
> ensure safety on this voyage. (33)

The governing fantasy of the body as a hidden world ripe for exploration (which so
suited the Enlightenment and colonialism) expands here to include other quests.

How liberating in practice is such a conception of the mind as a repository of
'unlimited possibilities' (Shumsky 1996: 34) waiting to be awakened? And what
are the benefits and dangers when persons take up these ideas in a medical context,
hoping to heal themselves, possibly from a serious illness? Is the idea of self-healing
kinder, more democratic, more effective – or does it just super-add the burden of
responsibility onto an already burdened self? These questions will be explored in the
next section, which looks at the healing power ascribed to inner sight, using creative
visualization as its major example.

In exploring the agglomeration of practices that go by the name of creative
visualization, I do not completely suspend my wariness about the uses to which
alternative medicine can put vision, especially since creative visualization is something of a blanket term and can describe quite different uses of inner sight. But I
also recognize the importance of looking at light and vision in their potentially more
positive guises and in so doing recognizing the potential of visual techniques to offer
up joyous, vibrant and healing experiences of light, colour or imagery.

THERAPEUTIC USES OF VISION: HEALING THROUGH INNER SIGHT

Underpinning the diagnostic techniques considered in the preceding part of this chapter is a metaphor of illumination as the shining of truth-bearing light onto the darkness of the body, the psyche or the world, a metaphor that informs biomedicine as well as the alternative diagnostic techniques described above. Hans Blumenberg (1993), in his history of metaphors of light in the Western tradition, dates this conception of illumination to the Enlightenment. In the latter decades of the twentieth century, much mainstream Western philosophy was wary of the metaphysical base of this metaphor and the authority it tacitly confers on the one who sees as well as on the 'givenness' of that which is seen. But positive meanings of light are foundational to many spiritual traditions. The Sanskrit word 'guru' embodies several aspects of the metaphor of enlightenment: the guru is the one who removes darkness and brings enlightenment ('Gu' = darkness; 'ru' = light) (Iyengar 1991: 28). As both guide and teacher, the guru is both 'a guiding beacon in the dark' and the instrument of 'an advancing dethronement of darkness' (Blumenberg 1993: 31).

Alternative medicine mobilizes metaphors of light in a variety of ways: as a metaphor for the divine source of truth or the guiding light; for our own mental faculties, which allow us to see and interpret the darkness of our psyches; or for the creative imagination that can be harnessed to manipulate our reality. In yoga, indeed, we are all imaginable *as* light – variegated and vibrating at different speeds and intensities:

> We humans are like a lamp that has five lampshades over our light. Each of the lampshades is a different color and density. As the light shines through the lampshades, it is progressively changed in color and nature. It is a bitter-sweet coloring. On the one hand, the shades provide the individualized beauty of each lamp. Yet, the lampshades also obscure the pure light. (Bharati n.d.)

In meditation and visualization, imagining white or golden light is often recommended as a source of protection from evil ('imagine your body enveloped in white light'), healing ('imagine your body flooded with white light') or connection with the divine ('feel yourself connecting with the Source of all light'). This metaphor of the healing power of light is also regarded unfavourably in modern anti-visual and anti-metaphysical philosophy, but it is a taken-for-granted motif in many alternative therapies, especially those influenced by the New Age.

The remainder of this chapter focuses on techniques of creative seeing – creative visualization, which uses the visual as both a set of tools and a plane of action. Creative visualization is a *cluster* of techniques, which all conceive of inner sight (the imagination) as a creative instrument, a bringer of change and a healing force. It may draw on older meditative traditions, modern psychotherapy or hypnotherapy. In some versions, light, including coloured light, is conceived of as intrinsically healing; in others, inner sight is used to better understand the self or the world. In its New Age guise it often takes this latter idea a step further, seeing inner sight as a tool of the will that has the power not only to illuminate the world but to *alter* the world and to bring new worlds into being. Seeing is thus understood as a form of making rather than taking.

CREATIVE VISUALIZATION AND HEALING THE SELF

Creative visualization is a general term that gained currency in the 1970s to describe a variety of auto-suggestion techniques involving the active, meditative contemplation or creation of mental images in the service of relaxation, self-development, spiritual revelation or the manifestation of desired goals. Examples are guided imagery meditations and New Age 'manifestation' techniques. Creative visualization adapts and combines techniques from older meditation traditions, including yoga and Buddhist meditation, as well as some of their Western derivatives and translations, such as hypnotherapy. It has been taken up to some extent within biomedicine, particularly in cancer care, where patients might be advised to use visualization as a tool in healing, stress relief, or assistance with chemotherapy. It is often used in combination with music.

Visualization techniques have an important place in meditative practices. Traditional yogic practice, for example, incorporates visualization alongside and intertwined with practices like specialized breathing (*pranayama*), concentration and withdrawal from the external world. *Yoga nidra*, or 'conscious deep sleep' (Bharati n.d.), is a form of relaxation and visualization practised at the end of a yoga session that has become well known to Westerners. It often begins with attention to sounds and then involves disconnecting from other senses by taking one's awareness around the body, systematically and in sequence. This practice of 'awareness rotation' (Goel n.d.) via the disciplined attention to the body promotes disconnection from external senses, known as sensory involution (Goel n.d.); with practice, you can't feel your body any more. As anyone who has practised yoga nidra knows, moving one's mind around the body, visualizing each part in turn, can have profound effects on respiration, hormonal activity, mental activity and mood. The practice is highly calming for both mind and body and in advanced practitioners it also helps cultivate insight and intuitive perception. Many Westerners, including myself, make regular use of it, whether as free-floating techniques or as part of a wider yogic practice.

Yoga nidra, based as it is on sensory withdrawal, is a practice of retreat. Such practices often subtly repose on metaphors of light. Blumenberg's (1993) history includes a fascinating analysis of the metaphor of the cave as an artificial world of 'screening-off and forgetting' (36). In Plato, the cave represents the condition of everyday life, in which we see only dimly, compared to the truth of the eternal Forms; in this cave, Being and truth are lacking (37). In the Platonic tradition, those who seek truth must turn away from the artificially lit world of the cave 'towards the sun as the origin of what can be known' (Vasseleu 1998: 3). As the metaphor evolves, however, the cave is comprehensively reworked into a place of dark retreat, such as the hermit's cave or monk's cell, in which truth can actually be found (Blumenberg 1993: 38). Many contemplative practices involve this metaphor of turning away from outer light towards inner light. In yoga, the cave is not 'out there' in the wilderness but in the 'innermost recesses of [the] soul' (Iyengar 1991: 21). The metaphor of turning away from false to true light can still be found in the modern West, as in the following modern yoga song:

> For the secret I long to know is hidden from sight
> When I turn my eyes away from this world's mirage to the inner light
> I can see that everything I long for I already have inside of me
> And in that place I know who I am
> I have no face; I am no one ...
> For I am free, living in a place outside of time. (Clapham 2006)

Traditional yogic meditation aims for transcendence – the elimination of the subject/object distinction: 'By profound meditation, the knower, the knowledge and the known become one. The seer, the sight and the seen have no separate existence from each other' (Iyengar 1991: 22).

Other traditional yogic visualization practices also have as their goal the development of subtle sensing. The traditional practice of *Tratak*, for example, involves concentrating on a candle flame, in soft focus and without blinking, for many minutes, in order to improve concentration and to learn how to develop inner sight. Concentration on an external object is seen as the initial stage of a mental training that can eventually progress to more subtle perception – for example of the *chakras*, an inner sound or an abstract idea (Srinivasananda 2003). This practice of concentration, visualization and subtle sensing is understood by some alternative practitioners to produce an ideal state for higher-order professional practice. The osteopath Hugh Milne, for example, considers a state of still receptivity to be the *sine qua non* of subtle perception (1995a: 10). Visualization is, he says, 'a foundational skill in healing' (83). But it needs to be cross-checked with other forms of subtle sensing to ensure that the practitioner doesn't slide into seeing 'what we want to see, what we expect to see, what is comfortable, or what will avoid rocking the boat' (82).

But seeing what we want to see is precisely the goal of another form of visualization – the New Age practice of 'manifestation'. The New Age uptake of traditional visualization techniques often involves their refashioning to fit individualistic, consumer and neoliberal values. Typically, these changes involve: the downplaying or elimination of ascetic elements; the detachment of visualization from a specified moral or ethical code; and the replacement of the life-long, patient, non-specifiable, uncontrollable aim of 'enlightenment' with particular, specifiable goals, including material ones. The relinquishment of desire and ego that typifies traditional yoga is replaced by the validation of desire/s and the promise that all desires can be realized, if only we rid ourselves of negative thoughts. In yoga, practices of retreat are inextricably bound up in a larger disciplinary context, including a moral code emphasizing restraint, austerity and the relinquishment of ego. In the New Age, the five universal moral precepts of yoga (known as the *Yama*) – purity, contentment, austerity, study of the self and dedication to the Lord (Iyengar 1991: 36) – give way to ideologies of self-fulfilment.

In recent decades, creative visualization has hybridized with currents in corporate, sporting and business cultures, where 'positive thinking' and the mantras of motivational culture have become pervasive popular philosophies: 'If you dream it, it will happen.' New Age and motivational cultures advocate the use of visualization for a whole range of goals. It doesn't matter whether one's desires are spiritual, emotional, financial or material, they are understood as responding to a single 'law' – the law of attraction. This law, 'the most powerful law in the universe', is the new-fashioned 'Secret', the title of the well-known New Age book and DVD by Rhonda Byrne (2006) in which the law of attraction is laid bare in all its simplicity for acquisitive Western consumers: that our thoughts and feelings attract all the experiences and events in our lives. Having sold several million copies,[17] the secret is, in fact, not a secret at all, but simply the same New Age axiom repeated again and again: 'Life is really very simple. What we give out, we get back. What we think about ourselves becomes the truth for us' (Hay 1987: 7). This axiom is underpinned by a 'belief in the unlimited powers of the imagination' (Hanegraaff 1998: 242) and by a number of interconnected ideas about the nature of the universe, some of which I described in Chapter 1: the idea that everything, including thought, is energy; that energy attracts (in Shakti Gawain's terms, that it is 'magnetic' (1978: 6); and that 'matter follows mind' ('form follows ideas' (6)). What you can consciously imagine in meditation, you will achieve in life. The imagination is creative, the universe is limitless, and all well-channelled desires can be met:

> Every moment of your life is infinitely creative and the universe is endlessly bountiful. Just put forth a clear enough request, and everything your heart desires must come to you. (1)

The imagination is not only visual. The 'Internet prospector' Max Steingart recommends activating *all* the senses:

> Decide what you want out of your life.
> Sense it before you have it.
> See it, feel it, taste it, smell it and imagine
> the emotions associated with the attainment of your goal.
> Pre-live it in your mind before you have it.
> Your vision will become a powerful driving force in your life. (2006: n.p.)

In similar fashion to Foucault's idea of the 'plurisensorial' medical gaze (2003: 202), which actually encompasses many senses, vision here is the arch-metaphor for the powerful, creative aspect of mind.

The general principle that 'What you visualize is what you actualize' has spread widely into Western popular culture. In this, the New Age not only reflects the materialist tenor of the modern West but also displays its links to the pragmatism and goal-orientation that characterized many of the nineteenth-century US spiritual movements that were its precursors and influences (Melton 1988: 36–9). It also reflects the pragmatism and adaptability of the Neo-Vedantic yogic schema, which was not a fully formed system picked up by the West, but was, rather, itself a result of the influence of Western ideas on Hinduism, and was then knowingly promoted, adapted and refashioned by pragmatic and entrepreneurial Indian masters like Swami Vivekananda to suit the Western ethos (De Michelis 2004: 119–23).

Underpinning creative visualization is a belief that the divine (or truth, or the source of power) lies within the self. This is not only an Eastern idea; it also has many Christian forms. Carrette and King note that the Protestant Reformation, with its emphasis on 'interior faith' (2005: 37) over 'conformist piety' (Bruneau, qtd in Carrette and King 2005: 37), set the scene for the interiorization of religion that characterizes modern spirituality. The Catholic Counter-Reformation also fostered the development of personal spirituality. For example, the founder of the Jesuits, Ignatius Loyola, designed spiritual exercises in which the mind was disciplined to focus on the object of meditation (2005: 37), as in much yogic practice. A century later, the revival of older Christian mystical traditions in which the object of meditation was to experience the divine *within oneself* continued this development (2005: 37–8). Carrette and King trace the ongoing evolution of this idea of the divine as within the self over the next few centuries, via German Romanticism, nineteenth- and twentieth-century spiritual movements and the rise of psychology. Today, the forms of individualism encouraged by consumerism and neoliberalism also form part of the New Age mix.

In the New Age schema, meditation is still framed as in Christian mysticism and yoga as a turning away from the distracting lights of everyday perception, and as a mode of connecting to a divine force that is interior to, but greater than, the self, but the effacement of self sought in yoga ('in that place I know who I am/I have no face; I am no one') is replaced by the quest to fulfil, magnify or express the self. One turns away from the world not in order to transcend desire, but in order to satiate it in the service of self. Some yoga practitioners lament what they see as the co-optation of traditional techniques whose aims were, they claim, more spiritually pure:

> Many people are now practicing all sorts of guided imageries in the name of Yoga Nidra so that they can make money, have better sex, or manipulate other people. There are CDs out which say Yoga Nidra is for 'this or that' named disease or other specific desire-based purpose. Yoga Nidra has been made to sound like 'The Law of Attraction', whereby you fulfill [sic] your desires through meditative techniques. Yoga Nidra was taught by the ancient sages for the purpose of exploring the deep impressions or samskaras, which drive our actions or karma. They taught this so that sincere seekers can purify the deeper aspect of the mind-field, which is accessed in the formless state of conscious Deep Sleep. (Bharati n.d.)

As with so much in New Age/alternative thought, which is typified by eclecticism, syncretism and hybridity (Hanegraaff 1998: 15–16), it is not so much that traditional techniques and aims have been replaced by late-modern, consumerist ones, as that they are to be found alongside and intermingled with each other, as alternatives and hybrids. Thus, visualization can be practised for different purposes and in various modes. It is, for example, still quite common to see visualization practised in a traditional mode, where the focus is on 'the lived experience of the images' rather than on their 'verbal processing' (Meadows 2002: 68). In this mode, visualization is a form of attentiveness, in which mental images are understood as something to be followed rather than manipulated. Here, the mind does not impose its will but acts as 'a witness, a spectator of your own internal drama: frame by frame, thought by thought' (Srinivasananda 2003). In classic yogic and Buddhist meditation, the procession of mental imagery is a flux to be observed without judgement or intervention: 'Never force the mind to be still. This will set in motion additional brainwaves, hindering the meditation' (Srinivasananda 2003).

Other contemporary visualization techniques, especially those influenced by psychology or psychoanalysis, focus on the *meaning* of the images. Psychotherapeutic techniques based on Jung's (1997) concept of active imagination are one example. These techniques often have a quasi-diagnostic or interpretive element – whether it be the meditating self asking questions of itself, or a hypnotherapist or psychotherapist mining the flow of visual data for meaning via interpretive practices, or a bodyworker opening an unspoken dialogue with the client during treatment (Milne

1995a: 83). These uses of creative visualization use inner sight as a mode of apprehending reality at deeper levels, with the aim of transforming it.

By contrast, the 'manifestation' mode that typifies the New Age and motivational cultures uses sight less as a tool for acquiring information than as a tool for transforming reality by implementing the will. In this mode, the imagination is understood as a tool of the will, and images are used 'directively' (Meadows 2002: 79), in order to bring a desired outcome into being. Speaking personally, I'm not fond of the manifestation mode, which often reeks less of hope than of despair, of fear rather than aliveness to unknown futures. As many critics of the broader social currents in which it partakes have argued, the urge to create ourselves – to transform our desires into reality – almost inevitably ignores all social determinants and their political correlates (have those who live in poverty around the world simply failed to practice 'abundance thinking'?). I am also uneasy at the absence of moral/ethical codes through which desire might be channelled or regulated, or rather, the reduction of ethical schemas to a banal ideology of individual fulfilment – such that one might equally well seek to manifest humility, a loving partner or a new Ferrari.

The problems of this approach are all the more stark when creative visualization is put in the service of health and healing, as it often is. In the most extreme New Age formulations, both healing and illness are conceived of purely as products of thought, often subconscious thought. Illness, therefore, is self-created (Hanegraaff 1998: 243). The logical corollary is that we can 'un-make' an illness. Shakti Gawain, for example, approaches healing with the philosophy that 'As long as you have an inner confidence in some form of therapy then by all means use it! It will work if you desire and believe it will' (1978: 61). Logically consistent, she applies this to biomedical treatment also, including surgery.

It's clear that this is intended as a democratization of healing – a shift away from the all-powerful medical authority with the power to name and foretell. And it has been welcomed by some patients in these terms. But, unsurprisingly, it has frequently been denounced by doctors, cultural critics and patients alike as sheeting home blame and responsibility for both the cause and the progress of an illness to the individual in ways that range from the unkind to the offensive (Sontag 1977; Stacey 1997). New Agers reply that responsibility is empowering, not guilt-inducing (Hanegraaff 1998: 243). One medical clairvoyant I interviewed responded to the critique using a distinction between causality and guilt:

> A lot of people – some of the doctors I've met – have said, 'If you say to somebody, "Oh, there's an emotional cause" or "there's a thought or some action they've done", then you're making them guilty of being responsible for a terminal illness.' Well they've thought that thought, they've done that action; but it's not guilt, it's just that it's a consequence.

A cancer survivor herself, she believed this approach had put her in control of her life:

> The first thing I did [when I was diagnosed] was [I kept] at it all the time: What emotions are there? What's happening? What have I thought? What have I done? And I changed everything that I found was associated with the cancer that I could either let go of or change. So who is in control of my life? I am in control of my life. If I die from the cancer or whatever, if I die I have done to the absolute maximum of my ability everything I can do to release it – but I'm not guilty of causing my own cancer … You see the difference? I don't hold guilt.

To its advocates, such beliefs are empowering; to critics, such as Stacey (herself also a cancer survivor), such theories are deluded and dangerous 'fantasies of invincibility and immortality' (1997: 28) that inevitably produce a sense of failure if the patient does not recover as hoped. She argues that metaphysical theories of illness and their associated practices of affirmation and manifestation construct narratives that 're-produce the conventional privileging of the triumphs of a few at the expense of the majority' (15), implicitly pitting the 'heroic successes' against the 'failed' visualizers. Stacey's critique doesn't sufficiently address the unpredictability and relinquishment of control implied in the alternative idea of 'healing' (Barcan and Johnston 2011). The subtle difference can be illustrated by returning to the quotation above: while the practitioner certainly desires control, she does not equate control with recovery. Her emphasis is on action and self-responsibility rather than on an inevitably successful result. Nonetheless, not every ill person wants healing rather than cure, and so Stacey's critique in my view hits the mark about the potentially devastating effects when fantasies of mastery and control are naively or simplistically invoked (Stacey 1997: 238). I agree with her concerns about the delusional and potentially dangerous effects when people are encouraged to believe that they can change anything, have anything and be anything they want through the process of imagining it.

It is instructive to contrast the contemporary neoliberal and individualist manifestations of the desire for control with the very different framing of control within traditional systems such as yoga, whose goal was *self*-control. As an ascetic practice, it advocated control *of* the self rather than *by* the self, with the aim, in stark contrast to the New Age, of freedom *from* desire rather than the manifestation *of* that which one desires: 'One who has conquered his mind, senses, passions, thought and reason is a king among men' (Iyengar 1991: 22). Indeed, 'steady control of the senses' is, for some, the very definition of yoga (Iyengar 1991: 20). Self-control leads to clear-seeing: 'He who attains it is free from delusion' (1991: 20). In the Yoga Sutras, desire, attachment and sensuality are obstacles to the practice of yoga rather than goals to be served (1991: 24). Ultimately, yoga is a victory *over* the self rather than the expression and fulfilment *of* the self:

To win a battle, a general surveys the terrain and the enemy and plans counter-measures. In a similar way the Yogi plans the conquest of the Self. (1991: 24)

The paradox is that one of the ways to conquer the self is not by trying to impose one's will through effort (itself a manifestation of ego and desire), but by patient attention. As the Buddhist monk Venerable Kittisaro put it: 'When you give attention to something without demanding that it be different, that very attentiveness has a profound transforming effect' (qtd in Geggus 2004: 67). Traditional meditation is thus inherently paradoxical: a making-happen based on the disciplined practice of letting-happen.

It is indubitable (and scientifically validated) that highly effective meditators create change through their disciplined seeing.[18] Contemporary brain science (e.g. Taylor 2006), as well as the emerging discipline of epigenetics[19] also point to the power of the mind to alter physical reality right down to the level of the DNA, and even intergenerationally (Church 2007). But it is hard for novices to meditate on their own, especially in the individualist popular contexts that are my focus. Many a mediocre meditator finds it easier to achieve results in a group setting, especially when led by a skilled guide. Therapeutic settings can certainly sometimes provide the intersubjective context that effective visualization so often seems to require, at least for those of us habituated to the fractured, rapid and multiple forms of consciousness that characterize modern urban life. Most Westerners *need* others to help us meditate and visualize, even if our visualization is aimed at serving our individual goals! But in the New Age context, visualization techniques are often learnt through books and CDs and visualization and meditation are often (though by no means always) practised in temporary communities (the workshop space) rather than as part of an ongoing community of practice. In the absence of community, many a 'manifestation meditator' fills his/her physical space with objects aimed at enhancing everyday visualization – classically, pictures of what he/she hopes to be or attain, or stickers on the mirror or walls bearing affirmations like 'I work at a fulfilling and creative job that rewards me amply'. But are these visual cues pathways to success or constant tacit reminders that one has *not* achieved one's desires, that one is *not* being amply rewarded?

This brings me to an instance of my own wrangling with creative visualization. When I was pregnant I embarked on a course known as 'Hypnobirthing',[20] run by a midwife who was also a hypnotherapist. The process involved an ensemble of techniques to prepare one for labour, including practising over and over a guided imagery meditation that involved visualizing a calm birth, and a suite of affirmations about the body's 'natural' ability to give birth. One of the fiercest, most frequent and most justified critiques of creative visualization is that it is framed individualistically. Hypnobirthing was a rare exception. The programme was explicitly social and political (and implicitly feminist) in its insistence that dominant cultural imagery, by setting up fearful expectations around childbirth, normalized expectations that contributed to the medicalization of birth and that were physically counterproductive during labour (stress hormones tightening those very muscles that need most to dilate). It stressed the role of discourse – the assumptions, language, stories and educative practices of midwives, doctors and other mothers – in helping to define and constrain women's perspectives and experiences.

It's hard not to embark on such a programme without being aware that one might be setting oneself for a crashing experience of failure. I didn't want to burden myself with expectations, nor to be perceived as naively believing I could control an unruly world. I found it necessary to say to those who would be present at the birth (and most especially, to the one among them who had gone through the experience of labour) that I wasn't an idiot, that I wasn't assuming I wouldn't need medication, that I wasn't seeing this as a panacea, that I knew things could go wrong. Clearly, something involving both intellectual pride and the complexities of bodily performance was at stake. I wanted to be a 'successful' visualizer but I also wanted others to know that I knew that 'success' has no guarantees – that nothing, least of all childbirth, is ultimately controllable.

When it came to the birth, the baby got stuck and I was on the verge of having an unplanned caesarean. I asked for a little time to accommodate myself, which I spent repeating one of the affirmations I had practised – the one about relinquishing control ('I am prepared to meet whatever turn my birthing takes' (Mongan 1998: 119)). It is entirely fitting that this, of all the affirmations, was one that actually worked. My entire mind-body must have let go, literally, and the baby was born without surgery – proof, it seemed to me, of the paradoxical power of relinquishing control. You cannot bluff the body *in extremis* – pretending to let go so you can really have your way. And the only reason I could genuinely let go of the illusion of control was, ironically enough, because I had spent so many months drilling myself in the affirmations. So there are a set of intertwined paradoxes here: disciplined, repeated visualization can indeed have an effect – even if that effect is to teach you that you cannot control everything. But for those of us who are not yogis, pride, naive faith and competitiveness do not absent themselves from the field, and I could certainly have set myself up for disappointment and 'failure'. A number of years later I met another woman who had done the same course; she told me of her own successes (two births, no drugs, no surgery) and did, it must be said, ever so gently hint that I could have done 'better' (that is, not needed pain relief) if I had tried harder.

It is indubitable that in the hands of a skilled practitioner, visualization techniques can be transformative. And I did promise that I would point to some instances of engagement with the visual about which I am unreservedly positive. So to conclude this chapter of wrangling with both the beneficial and deleterious effects of using visual methods in a therapeutic context, I turn to another hypnotherapist, one I have visited as a client on and off over many years: René Mateos. Biomedically trained – a doctor with qualifications in surgery – he is also trained in psychotherapy and hypnotherapy, and he combines the very best of rationalism – he is very smart – with something more: he is highly intuitive and empathic. His technique begins with careful listening – a detailed conversation that can last up to an hour in which he takes copious notes even while his eyes scarcely leave yours – followed by a guided meditation process in which he asks you to give visual form to particular feelings, issues or problems. In a technique he has developed by drawing on humanistic psychology and transpersonal psychotherapy, including Jungian active imagination,[21] he works with the images produced from the client's unconscious to produce resolutions that occur principally *as* visual phenomena. Some analytic work occurs at the close of the session (where the client is invited to offer up responses more than interpretations). But the primary therapeutic work is a drama that unfolds in, as and through the client's mental images, which remain invisible to the practitioner, and the client has some role in determining how much of the process is to be relayed to the practitioner. At the close of the session, the client is invited to concretize the process afterwards in his/her own time – classically, by drawing or writing. Over the last twenty years I have seen this practitioner for a variety of reasons: to help make a big decision; to help with chronic physical problems; even for something as vague, abstract and all-encompassing as when I decided I needed to adjust aspects of my emotional, mental and even intellectual approach to the world and to adopt a 'new paradigm'. Clearly, it must be that I buy into some aspects of the idea of self-determination – but I refuse a de-politicized idea of it.

René's professional practice is, to me, the pinnacle of integrative medicine: a highly trained, skilled, intelligent and empathic practitioner combines conventional and esoteric anatomy in a process in which cognition, interpretation and analysis have an important but not domineering role, and in which all the client's and practitioner's senses are activated: subtle, attentive listening, the production of mental images, dialogue with the practitioner and the possibility of crystallization in visual or narrative form in privacy later. Though I now visit him quite rarely (perhaps once every five years),[22] my life would be impoverished without recourse to the comforting, enriching, life-enhancing and effective techniques he offers. In a world in which the majority of people do not have access to clean water or sufficient food, such forms of solace are, I know, an immense privilege – available to me through sheer historical accident, the result of a string of material, familial, social and educational good fortune. This is true. And yet, the practice he offers relies on skill, intelligence, care and time. There is no technology whatsoever, except the pen and paper with which he takes his copious notes. What there is, rather, is an intense crystallization of time, in its many forms: the years of training invested in him by the state and at his own expense; the years of his own emotional and intellectual maturation and his professional and life experience; and the time of the therapeutic encounter itself, which in some cases may stretch even to three or more hours before a resolution is reached.

So when I say that only the privileged have access to this form of care, it is important to qualify this with the understanding that it is the economics of time itself – and their enmeshment in a particular medical paradigm – that helps create this practice – at once very simple, but requiring great skill – as a form of privilege. In my utopian medical future, such practices would be available to all.

3 SOUND: GOOD VIBRATIONS

> Like crystal, like metal and many other substances, I am a sonorous being, but I
> hear my own vibration from within.
>
> Maurice Merleau-Ponty, *The Visible and the Invisible*

In 1952, a stunned audience first 'heard' – or perhaps 'experienced' might be a better
word – a performance of the new work *4'33"* by the avant-garde composer John
Cage. A tuxedoed performer walked onto the stage, sat at the grand piano, periodi-
cally turned the pages, then rose, bowed and left the stage. The rest was silence. Or
perhaps not. During those four minutes and thirty three seconds, which must have
seemed interminable to both performer and audience, the audience were forcibly
made aware of a great deal of sound. Says one fan of the piece:

> You soon become aware of a huge amount of sound, ranging from the mundane
> to the profound, from the expected to the surprising, from the intimate to the
> cosmic – shifting in seats, riffling programs to see what in the world is going
> on, breathing, the air conditioning, a creaking door, passing traffic, an airplane,
> ringing in your ears, a recaptured memory. (Guttman n.d.)

4'33" was inspired by Cage's visit to the Harvard University anechoic chamber
(a kind of soundproof room), from which he emerged declaring that there is no
such thing as a state of silence. Even in 'silence' he had, he later wrote, heard two
sounds, 'one high and one low. When I described them to the engineer in charge,
he informed me that the high one was my nervous system in operation, the low one
my blood in circulation' (1961: 8). Just as well Cage couldn't *really* hear his body.
According to Diane Ackerman, it is 'merciful' that humans don't hear low frequencies very well: 'if we did, the sounds of our own bodies would be as deafening as
sitting in a lawn chair next to a waterfall' (1991: 189).

Sound is ubiquitous. Even if there is no external noise there are always the creaks,
sighs and gurgles of our own bodies and, perhaps, the inner chatter of our own
mind. This is why the ears are sometimes imagined as helpless (Bull and Back 2003:
6): 'We have no ear lids' (Schafer 2003: 25). But equally, there is much we *don't* hear.
Humans can hear sounds ranging from 20 to 20,000 hertz; homing pigeons can

hear sounds below this range; and bats and dolphins well above it (Weiten 2010: 161). And of course, we *learn* not to hear too; the sound of traffic, the computer's hum and the background television can disappear into the submerged soundscape of our everyday lives.

Despite the centrality of sound to our everyday lives, cultural analyses of sound and hearing, like those of smell, usually begin with a declaration that sound has been forgotten in social, cultural or philosophical inquiry, especially in comparison to sight. The phenomenologist Don Idhe, for example, points to 'a massive lack of [historical] philosophical attention to the phenomena of auditory imagination' (2003: 64); Murray Schafer to the striking indifference of early psychiatrists to sound in dreams, with both Freud and Jung having failed to 'realize the implications of the acoustics of the unconscious' (2003: 32); and historian of religion Leigh Eric Schmidt claims that accounts of surveillance have tended to focus on the visual and forget 'sinister modes of listening' (2003: 52–3). All this is, it seems, part of a broader neglect: 'The assumed eclipse of orality by the visuality of print has left hearing's complex history far more muffled than hearkened to, submerged under the reigning narrative of the eye's modern hegemony' (Schmidt 1998: 276).

These tales of sensory amnesia are not, of course, simple truths but one way of pondering the gains and losses associated with modernity. In his essay 'Hearing Loss', Schmidt describes two broad narratives that have characterized most academic discussions about sound and modernity. The first of these 'sprawling discourses' (2003: 41) is the story of the dominance of visuality, especially since the Enlightenment. As we saw in Chapter 2, this analytical line usually starts with the idea of a hierarchy of the senses, and with Aristotle's privileging of sight (2003: 43). The counterpart narrative to this tale of 'the eye's eclipse of the ear' (41) is a history of diminished hearing. Whereas smell is commonly argued to have been repressed in modernity because of its connection with animality, sound, it is said, has become vestigial (42). This analysis, made most famously by Marshall McLuhan and Walter Ong, is an evolutionary one – a story of the gradual movement away from the oral/aural modes of pre-modern cultures towards the dispersed, impersonal and asynchronous modes of communication that characterize print (and later, electronic) media. Both Ong and McLuhan characterize the print revolution as transforming oral cultures into cultures of private, silent reading. Although Ong claims that 'writing can never dispense with orality' (1988: 8), he nevertheless understands the decline of orality as part of the waning of entire kinds of civilizations – that is, of the oral cultures that preceded the 'Gutenberg galaxy', to quote the title of McLuhan's (1962) influential book. Today, says Ong, 'primary oral culture in the strict sense hardly exists, since every culture knows of writing and has some experience of its effects' (1988: 11).

The idea of modernity as characterized by a kind of silence – the transformation of external voices into inner voices – appears in histories of religion too. It has been claimed that after the Enlightenment, God 'became silent' (Schafer 2003: 8). The weakening of the authority of Christianity meant that sounds once recognized as divine voices (the sounds and voices of nature and of dreams) were no longer attended to as such. 'Various wonders of the devout ear such as divine calls, the voices of demonic possession, prophecy, mystical locutions, oracles, and even the sounds of shamanic spirits' (Schmidt 1998: 274) were opened up to sceptics and transformed from divine wonders into 'edifying amusement[s]' (1998: 275) via popular magic and showmanship. Rationalism, it is argued, 'extinguished the rich treasure of imaginary voices that once existed in Europe and still exist in many less civilized [*sic*] parts of the world' (Schafer 2003: 34). Moreover, even inner voices became more problematic, transformed from divine speech into a symptom of psychic disorder (34).

The idea of modernity as silent flies in the face of a third narrative about sound and modernity – the tale of an increasingly noisy world in which it is silence, rather than sound, that has been lost. Civilization, especially urban life, is characterized as an assault on the ears: 'Civilization announces its progress by a lot of noise, and the more it progresses the noisier it gets' (Dolar 2006: 13). Marx knew about the 'deafening noise' of the factory (1999: 262); so, too, do contemporary audiologists, who warn of the effects of industrial, background and contained noise (as in headphones and earbuds). Noise pollution is 'an all but inevitable consequence of economic development' (Sim 2007: 38). But the noisiness of modernity is an *idea* as well as a fact – after all, we reserve the idea of noise pollution for sounds produced by humans rather than nature (Sim 2007: 21). Tolerance to noise varies. Those who hate loud noises may well have recourse to the idea of ears as passive, as 'condemn[ing us] to listen' (Schafer 2003: 25): 'We are passive victims of this [urban] noise. There is no protection except to stay in bed with a pillow over our head' (Joudry and Joudry 1999: 16). The 'assault against silence' led Stuart Sim to write a 'manifesto for silence' – a plea for the recognition of the importance of silence to our philosophical, artistic and religious lives, and for a more stringent regulation of noise. Silence, he argues, is the essential precondition for thought (2007: 39), and hence noise is a danger not just to physical hearing but to 'our collective cultural health' (39). Noise is also, he argues, a political matter, since it is both the product of economic development and 'a signifier of ideological power, of an insensitivity to the natural rhythms of human existence' (2007: 39). Arguing that excessive industrial noise makes life a misery in an increasing number of jobs internationally (38), Sim conceives of his manifesto as a rebuttal to big business and 'the techno-scientific establishment' (2007: 40).

What, then, should we make of these three narratives about sound and modernity – this triple tale of the rise of visuality, the loss of hearing and the loss of silence – and how accurate is any of them as an empirical description of changes to the modern sensorium? Schmidt, for one, is critical of the tale of the post-Enlightenment triumph of eye over ear for two reasons. First, it oversimplifies the Enlightenment, reducing its 'multisensory complexity' (2003: 48) into too simple a tale of ocularcentrism. The modern sensorium is, Schmidt claims, more uneven and heterogenous than these narratives allow (48). His second criticism is that this account is politically compromised, dividing the world into an us and them (2003: 47) in which Western visuality is contrasted to a primal tribal orality and where the decline of the latter is assumed. To these empirical and political critiques, post-structuralism would add a third – a philosophical critique of the idea of presence. The work of the philosopher Jacques Derrida in particular offers an analysis and critique of the metaphysical tradition in which voice is prioritized over writing. Derrida uses the term 'logocentrism' (1997: 12) to describe the philosophical valuing of speech over writing – the idea that writing is a derivative, secondary form of communication that occurs, unlike speech, in the absence of direct contact. In this deeply embedded view of things, face-to-face speech is understood as a more authentic form of communication than print communication or the 'secondary orality' (Ong 1988: 135) of electronic media like radio and television. Sound, says Ong, 'is more real or existential than other sense objects, despite the fact that it is also more evanescent' (1967: 111), hence its importance in religious or spiritual systems. In the Christian tradition, God is imagined as both communicative and audient. He is a 'heavenly dictating voice' speaking directly or via mediators like the sounds of nature, or the voice of prophets, or the inner voice of conscience. But he is also listening – to our prayers, and also, more threateningly, to our deepest thoughts and deeds. Either way, the human relation to the divine can be conceived as a 'participatory encounter with divine speech' (Schmidt 2003: 53). When hearing 'dwindles' as a spiritual sense (41), religion loses its 'oracular power' (Schmidt n.d.), and divine speech is reduced to a 'lost presence' (Schmidt 2003: 41). For post-structuralists, the feeling that through the human voice 'one could get immediate access to an unalloyed presence, an original not tarnished by externality, a firm rock against the elusive interplay of signs' (Dolar 2006: 37), is an illusion, an example of what Derrida calls a 'metaphysics of presence' (1997: 49).[1] But from a spiritually derived position, particular forms of silence and noisiness are part of the lamentable condition of modernity itself – its 'alienation, disillusionment, and secularism' (Schmidt 2003: 41).

The idea of presence, then, connects the three seemingly contradictory themes about sound and modernity. As Sim's manifesto makes clear, the quest for silence is connected philosophically, but also through religious and spiritual *practice*, with the quest for the divine and with ideas of humanness. Some of the sounds we make, such as speech and laughter, have been used as definers of humanness; others, such as the scream or wail, we connect to animality (Dolar 2006: 29).[2] On the one hand, the power of speech is widely, if perhaps inaccurately, considered a marker that distinguishes the human from the rest of the living world; on the other hand, the importance of silence to thought and to religion leads Stuart Sim to conclude that 'a defence of silence is a defence of the human' (2007: 40). When understood less as empirical descriptors than as relations to presence it becomes clear that these accounts are not so much contradictory as different aspects of the same phenomenon. In spiritual world-views, loss of hearing and loss of silence are not incompatible: in the cacophony of noise that characterizes modern civilization we have lost the silence that allows us to hear the 'still small voice' of God (1 Kings 19: 12), or the conscience that we imagine as a voice in our heads.

As spiritually based practices, alternative therapies are bound up with this search for presence. They draw on a range of traditions in which sound, music or the human voice are seen as guarantors of that presence, in which the human voice is seen as intrinsic to individual distinctiveness, and in which sound and music are treated with respect for their power both to heal and to destroy.

THERAPEUTIC USES OF SOUND AND MUSIC

In his book *Healing Songs*, Ted Gioia delineates two key themes in studies of the therapeutic effects of sound – the influence of music, sound and rhythm on the physical organism, and music's ability to effect healing by reaching out beyond the individual (2006: xii). These two areas of inquiry he characterizes as an interior plane and an exterior one (2006: xii). Music's ability to reach both inwards and outwards – to enter the individual body and to connect bodies together – is at the heart of its therapeutic significance (Gioia 2006: 42). These two qualities of music are summed up in feminist philosopher Elizabeth Grosz's contention that of the arts, music is 'the most immediately moving, the most visceral and *contagious* in its effects' (2008: 29, my emphasis).

There exists a substantial literature on the therapeutic properties and ritual or magical uses of sound, especially music. Belief in the transformational power of music is so widespread and deep-seated that there is, claims Ted Gioia, author of a study of music and healing, some justification in considering it a universal belief (2006: 24):

> Wherever music has been found – which is simply another way of saying wherever people live together in society – its use in healing has been known and acknowledged. Long before music became an aesthetic activity, its efficacy as a change agent was paramount. This potency is all but forgotten today. (x)

This brief statement contains a number of themes that we will shortly see typify discussions of the healing power of music: the universality of music; its link to sociality; its therapeutic qualities; its potency (even to the point of danger); and the attenuation of these powers in modernity.

In alternative medicine, sound and music may be used in different ways: for relaxation, insight or healing. In some, clients *make* sound or music; in others they receive it. Some practices are for individuals; others take place in groups. Sounds may be loud, as in drumming, or gentle, as in crystal bowl therapy. Some therapies make use of vibrations so subtle that we wouldn't normally classify them as sounds, as in crystal therapy, in which solid crystals are placed in various locations on the body. Some techniques, like the playing of crystal bowls for meditation and healing, might seem to use sound as a purely physical vibration, especially when contrasted with therapies that make use of text, whether spoken, sung, chanted, toned[3] or even silently repeated (as in affirmations). But this is to oversimplify, for most alternative therapies intertwine physics and metaphysics. To a music therapist, a musical note is not just a sound with particular aesthetic qualities but a frequency with health implications; to a crystal bowl therapist, the frequency at which each bowl resonates corresponds to that of a particular *chakra*, and thus has particular qualities, effects and metaphysical significance. Sacred chanted syllables, such as the yogic OM, are also simultaneously physical and metaphysical. Underpinning and connecting most of these sound-based therapies – indeed, most alternative therapies – is the idea of a harmonious, humming, vibrating universe and a body made up of energy vibrating at different frequencies.

This chapter takes as its main example a sound-based therapy known as Psychophonetics. Before turning to this example though, I canvass a range of other sound/music-based therapies, including music therapy, and I read them in relation to some of the recurring historical themes about sound, music and healing: sound's connection to the body; its temporality; its role in sociality; its connection with order and harmony; its dangerousness; and its links to the divine.

SOUND AND THE BODY

The inherently rhythmic nature of the body is a common starting place in sociocultural approaches to sound. This is where Ted Gioia's study of the healing power of music and sound begins:

> Stop for a moment, and consider the rhythm within. Your heart pulsates at roughly the same tempo as Ravel's *Bolero*, an insistent seventy-two beats per minute, some thirty-eight million times during the course of a year. Twenty thousand times each day, you inhale and exhale, mostly oblivious to the process. Each day, your body's circadian rhythms run through a repeating cycle: the pulse rate and blood pressure rising upon wakening and temperature increasing during

the day, declining at night. Even your hours of sleep are comprised of repetitive cycles of around ninety minutes' duration. Your endocrine and immune systems run through their own diurnal cycles. Cholesterol, stomach acid, blood sugar, hormones – all ebb and flow at predictable points during the day. (2006: 1)

The body thus conceived is inherently and unalterably[4] musical, our own pulse 'a silent metronome' (Ackerman 1990: 180). Medical science agrees that at every level, starting at the molecular, 'biological life is a rhythmically organized process' (Spintge 1996: 5). This has often been couched poetically, as in the German Romantic philosopher Novalis's pronouncement that 'medicine is a musical art' (a precept beloved of music therapists),[5] but research into rhythmicity is now an established part of physics, mathematics and medicine, where rhythm is recognized by many as 'one of the basic governing phenomena, perhaps even the basic ruling phenomenon, in all biologic systems' (Spintge 1996: 5). A specific branch of medical research and practice has developed (known as MusicMedicine, to distinguish it from music therapy), in which the clinical effects of 'musical stimuli in medical settings' are subjected to 'scientific evaluation' (qtd in Spintge 1996: 3).

The body's rhythmicity is not closed; the body is open to influence from external sounds. As vibrating and dynamic structures, cells are capable of being influenced and altered by sound vibrations (Horden 2000: 6). Sound's impact on the body is commonly described as though it were more direct, more visceral, than that of visual stimuli: 'Light bounces off surfaces and conveys its message through a greater abstraction than sound', wrote the great violinist Yehudi Menuhin: 'Sound goes directly into our bodies' (1999: xii). Roland Barthes describes the impact of Schumann's piano music in a similar vein:

> Schumann's music goes much farther than the ear; it goes into the body, into the muscles by the beats of its rhythm, and somehow into the viscera by the voluptuous pleasure of its *melos* ... (1985: 295)

Sound affects not only the body but also the mind and brain. Aristotle connected sound to intelligence, but only incidentally – via the role of speech in learning (1906: 46–7). Today, it is known that sound affects the brain. Contemporary sound engineering techniques, alongside scientific research into brain function, have given rise to a range of auditory interventions to assist with learning and other difficulties. There exists a range of techniques (the Samonas method, the Berard method) that are used to help learning difficulties, concentration, memory or speech problems. The Tomatis method, for example, is a process of re-educating the middle ear and revitalizing the brain via daily listening, through headphones, to music specially filtered to remove the low frequencies. The underlying belief is that low frequencies exhaust the system while high frequencies, those between 3,000 and 20,000 Hz, recharge and energize it (Joudry and Joudry 1999: 19).

Music therapy shares with these forms of sound therapy a belief in the importance of music to cognition, memory, motivation and learning. In addition, it focuses on music's role as a modulator of emotion or affect and its connection with personal and cultural memory. The practice emerged in the US and the UK in the first half of the twentieth century, mostly centred on hospitals or psychiatric institutions. It began to professionalize around the middle of that century (Tyler 2000: 379). After the Second World War, some musicians attempted to ease the trauma of hospitalized war victims. Today, music therapists may work with the dying, the socially isolated or disadvantaged, the elderly or children. From the start, music therapy has made use of mythical and historical tales of the healing power of music, at least as a rhetorical strategy, but it has also worked to bolster its academic credibility via a theoretical and research base. Today, music therapy research papers tend to combine humanist or spiritual discourse about the power of music to lift the spirit with social scientific, evidence-based data, including the clinical research of MusicMedicine. For example, one of my interviewees, Kirstin Robertson-Gillam, who trained and worked for many years as a music therapist, was able to move fluidly between talk of emotion, memory, spirit and hertz cycles. She moved between the familiar discourse of music's power to stir and uplift and an appealingly physiological appreciation of music:

> Pachelbel's Canon is absolutely wonderful for moving bowels, in somebody who's constipated because they've got cancer and they've had morphine. And Pachelbel's Canon is also often used for women in childbirth, to help them get the rhythm of it, to get their uterus actually working in rhythm. It's very good for heart disease where the music actually goes sixty to eighty beats a minute, which is the heart rhythm and it can help to stabilize that – but then so can shamanic drumming! Shamanic drumming is very good for migraines. Believe it or not. You wouldn't think so but it is.[6]

Robertson-Gillam can work the discourses in different directions. She can construe the laxative effects of Pachelbel in more musically technical terms ('a steady ground bass which is hypnotically repetitive and can act as a powerful catalyst for slowing down the body's rhythms' (2004: 3)), and the heart-warming effects of music more medically ('music using cardiac units – appropriate music – will help to slow the heart rate and stabilize the heart rate, and hopefully help the person gain more control of their heart condition').

She can also use the language of vibrations, since she is among those music therapists who incorporate subtle anatomy and a spiritual conception of the person into their professional world-view. For although music therapy is quite an academic discipline (with courses in universities, and reliance on an evidence-based paradigm), there are nonetheless some music therapists who combine a scientific understanding of the body with subtle anatomy. For those practitioners, it is not just a question of the physiological effects of sound on the body, mind or emotions; rather, sound is in a very crucial sense *of* the body itself. Living beings are vibratory (Grosz 2008: 33). Sound is the quintessential form of the stuff of the universe – vibration itself: 'Ancient teachings and modern science agree: you, I, all living things, all things in existence are made up at their most essential level of vibrating, pulsing energy' (Gordon n.d.). The universe *hums* – at between 4 and 50 Hz (Montiel et al. 2005: 65). The average of this so-called Schumann Resonance is 7.8 Hz – a frequency that corresponds to the alpha waves in the human brain (2005: 65), which are the waves most associated with meditation. I first read these claims in a music therapy website and confirmed them in a physics text. Perhaps we should not be surprised that both spiritual and scientific discourse agree on this; Ted Gioia claims that the history of healing music as a body of thought in the West is saturated with the mystical, Orphic tradition and the rational Pythagorean tradition (2006: 89–90). Both of these schools of thought 'represent different, if related, attempts to reconcile primitive magico-musical beliefs with the classical world's desire for more systematic and analytical approaches' (90).

Whereas New Age-style sound therapists tend to speak in universals, music therapists are aware that the production and reception of sound are culturally mediated and that each culture produces its own sounds and its own arts of listening. They are thus caught between a scientific understanding of sound as soundwaves – in which sound may seem to have universal physiological effects – and a cultural model in which its connections to memory, emotion and mental states are understood in sociocultural terms. Music therapists' training (e.g. in ethnomusicology) makes them deeply aware of the cultural variations in music, but the scientific aspirations of their discipline (at least as a body of published literature) also make them open to a seemingly more neutral, universal understanding of sound. At their best, both music therapy and science recognize the *interplay* of culture with perception and re-sponse. Nonetheless, reconciling an appreciation of sound as physics and music as a cultural practice can be a vexing problem. As we will see later, the recurring thematic of beneficence and danger (the healing potential of sound and music versus their potential to do harm) clearly interweaves the physiological, the moral and the social.

The poetic and the literal are also not easy to disentangle. For music therapists, Novalis's idea that 'Every disease is a musical problem' is not just metaphorical; the body in pain is a body that has literally lost its rhythm: 'loss of rhythmicity is the characteristic feature of states of high physical or mental strain, such as anxiety or pain' (Spintge 1996: 10). 'But what is cause and what is effect?' ask the makers of a British television programme on Healing and Harmony: '[I]s disease damaging musicality, or is damaged musicality – being "out of tune" – making people ill?' (Paul Robertson, qtd in Horden 2000: 11). Presumably the answer is a predictable 'both', but my point is rather to propose that these embodied metaphors of being out of tune, out of time or out of step all suggest music's fundamental connection to temporality and to sociality. The music physician Ralph Spintge hypothesizes that music and dance are essentially a sociocultural projection of 'the essential rhythmic components' of the central nervous system and other biological functions (1996: 7). Rhythmicity is, he claims, the missing link needed to understand the impact of music on human biology (7–8). If true, this hypothesis might give a biological grounding to the social realization of the connection between time, rhythm and the social.

SOUND AND TEMPORALITY

Rhythm connects the biological, the social and the temporal; cycles like night and day, the seasons and menstruation helped early humans organize the perception of time and the socialization of individuals (Spintge 1996: 3). In a phenomenological sense too, 'sound has a special relationship to time' (Ong 1988: 32). The most temporal of the senses, it exists 'only when it is going out of existence' (32):

> It is not simply perishable but essentially evanescent, and it is sensed as evanescent. When I pronounce the word 'permanence', by the time I get to the 'nence', the 'perma-' is gone, and has to be gone. (32)

Sound is not only phenomenologically temporal; it is deeply connected to historical time, via memory. It takes you back. But back where? Songs and chants connect the generations, and also have a formative role in individual development, beginning *in utero*. The foetus can respond to sound from twenty-four weeks onwards (Abrams et al. 1995: 315), and the foetal environment contains 'an impressive array of sounds that vary in pitch, loudness, and pattern' (Ronca and Alberts 1995: 335). The infant is not only born into but *created within* these ebbing and flowing rhythms of life: the uterus is an acoustic and rhythmic world of the mother's heartbeat, pulse, digestion, breathing, walking and other sounds of life into which external sounds (voices, music, noises) enter. Unusually intense or loud noises provoke foetal responses, and there is scientific concern about the potential developmental impact of particular types or durations of noise, especially low frequencies and vibrations of the same frequency as the body's natural resonant frequency, which may occur in some work environments (Abrams et al. 1995: 319). The foetus hears and recognizes the voices it will later connect to people in the world. The mother's speech is of particular significance; foetal heart rates consistently decrease during maternal speech (Fifer and Moon 1995: 362). The idea of the sonic womb echoes throughout the literature on sound, from academic books to pregnancy manuals. For example, the mother's heartbeat is described as 'perhaps the ultimate cradlesong of peace and plenty'; the womb as 'an envelope of rhythmic warmth' (Ackerman 1990: 178–9). Once born, the baby emerges into a world which we love to idealize as one of soothing voices, lullabies, rocking, patting and walking, though it also of course includes unexpected bangs, shouts, barks or bumps and, for some, industrial or other forms of urban noise. Sound, rhythm and touch are interwoven, as in the rocking of babies during lullabies, which provides auditory and tactile stimulation simultaneously (Montagu 1986: 146).[7] In this conception of the baby's sensory landscape, the singing of the mother becomes an archetypal figure for the therapeutic power of the voice: 'the song of the mother is, in fact, our first healing song' writes Gioia (2006: 7). When sound or music take you back, then, they are often imagined as taking you back to the maternal, to infancy, or to the pre-linguistic.

SOUND AND SOCIALITY

Maternal songs are instruments of connection, bonding and socialization. Sound moves *between* people. It 'connects us in ways that vision does not' (Bull and Back 2003: 6). This makes it important in rituals and ceremonies that affirm community. In fact, 'keeping together in time' was, according to a hypothesis advanced by William McNeill, an important component of human social evolution; collective forms of singing, moving and dancing were part of the organizational mechanisms of early human groups, allowing forms of bonding and co-operation that enhanced their chances of survival and prosperity (1995: 4). Drawing on McNeill, Paul Filmer argues that all societies integrate physiological time (which regulates the body) and social time ('a necessary condition of culture' (2003: 92)), and that the 'active, conscious use of the voice' is a 'central feature of concerted human action' (2003: 92). Your body is like a musical instrument, 'synchroniz[ing] its performance to the contrasting and complimentary [*sic*] rhythms surrounding it' (Gioia 2006: 1). Some of these synchronizations are rhythms learnt from the surrounding society – habits and patterns that are inherently social, ranging from broadly shared rhythms like calendars, school hours, timetables and TV schedules to the specialized synchronizations shared by smaller groups, such as in military drills, synchronized swimming or choral singing.

This then is the ground of the second theme identified by Gioia about music and healing – namely, music's ability to effect healing by reaching out beyond the individual and 'shaping and interacting with the societal, communal, familial, and attitudinal structures in which healing takes place' (2006: xii). It reaches out, unpredictably and invisibly, for sound, like smell, 'is no respecter of space' (Bull and Back 2003: 8). Music can break down the boundaries around the individual in different ways. For example, in some conditions it can effect a kind of 'dissolving' of the self. As phenomenologist Don Idhe puts it, it may sometimes

> lead to a temporary sense of the 'dissolution' of self-presence. Music takes me 'out of myself' in such occurrences. (2003: 62)

This is the effect of some music designed for relaxation or meditation, especially that of the 'space music' genre that is the signature tune of the New Age. Interestingly, a number of reviews I found of a CD by one of the foremost composers in that genre, Constance Demby, wrote of the dissolving of the self: 'Prepare to be shattered and then reconstructed', wrote one reviewer. Another wrote:

> [T]his music will dissolve you ... On a dozen listens, I sensed I either dropped through a trap door or got 'gonged' out of this universe ... Perhaps she's found a way to make time reverse. (Demby n.d.)

Of course, many forms of music can do something like this for those who appreciate them.

Sometimes the self dissolves not into the cosmos but into the collectivity. A musician or singer may connect with and move an audience of thousands, a process which the violinist Yehudi Menuhin, in his foreword to a book on Tomatis sound therapy, construed as a physical resonance, a movement across time, and a merging with others: 'When we hear music we are actually vibrating with the whole audience, and with the performer, and we are thereby put in touch with the composer's mind and heart' (1999: xi). Some composers have aimed for this type of union. At the time of his death in 1915, the Russian composer Alexander Scriabin, for example, was working on a piece called *Mysterium*, in which he intended to bring together music, colour (projected onto a giant screen behind the orchestra) and fragrances wafting through the concert hall. The aim of this synaesthetic work was to connect humans and the divine via a 'loosening [of] the bonds which held their true selves in their physical encasements' (Tompkins and Bird 1974: 144–5). Moreover, Scriabin made it clear that there was to be no distinction between spectator and performer: 'All are celebrants somehow as a boundarylessness prevails, a union and merger of participants' (Garcia 2009: 478). This was an experiential embodiment of an ethico-spiritual desire for oneness:

> The Mysterium, in action and intended result, would join all peoples together, obliterate disparities, erase conflict, eliminate gender, and bring humankind to a form of ecstatic union or 'oneness'. (478)

This is precisely the appeal of many forms of popular dance music. Rave or trance music, for example, are celebrated by their fans for their ability to reduce or dissolve differences between people and generate a sense of collectivity, a sensation often enhanced by recreational drugs.

Some quasi-therapeutic sound practices aim for connection or union, even if in less grandiose terms, for they are only *possible* when performed with others: laughter clubs, choral singing or sonic baths.[8] In choral singing, numbers are needed to generate volume, mass and harmony; in laughter clubs, others serve as instruments of contagion; in sonic baths, they generate vibrations; and in some psychotherapeutically framed sound practices, they externalize inner voices, as when a group sings out your name to you.[9] But connection need not always be harmonious. Crystal bowl therapist Susie, working within a New Age paradigm, believes that the healing or damaging properties of a musical frequency can be interfered with, for example by the *intention* with which they are played.

Music therapy deploys sound's connections to the social in a number of ways. First, it actively works with an understanding of cross-cultural variation and of music's relation to memory, sociality, ritual and healing. Whereas New Age sound practices are often described in terms of the channelling of 'universal' energies, and will appropriate techniques from a wide variety of contexts often with scant regard for their original contexts (from shamanic drumming to Tibetan bowls to chanting or didgeridoo), music therapists will tend to be much more aware of the cultural embeddedness and specificity of music. After all it would be impossible to be a contemporary musician and remain unaware of the enormous historical and cultural variety in music (whereas a colour therapist might more easily assume a universality of colour and colour perception). So music therapists actively work with sociocultural factors like ethnicity and generation, choosing music that is appropriate to the age and ethnicity of their clients:

> We tend not to speak in universals. There's a stereotype that says music is a universal language. Music is a universal *communicator*. Music is a universal stimulator of emotions, but each culture has its own musical language. (Kirstin)

Moreover, music therapy is frequently a social *practice*. Although clients can come for individual sessions, much music therapy is practised in groups. Choirs, drumming and chanting aim to generate a shared experience greater than the individual, and much of the therapeutic effect is derived from a commingling whose physiological, affective, musical and social dimensions are hard to separate. Kirstin described working with a man with Parkinson's Disease whose swallowing reflex had diminished to the point where he had to be fed through a tube; her description of getting in sync with him is at once material (a question of sound waves), musical (a question of harmony) and existential (a question of intersubjective communication):

> He joined the choir to be able to communicate better and he's having lessons with me and that's what I talk to him about – let's find a note where we can resonate together and you can feel the sound flapping between us and we'll know that we're on the same level and we can resonate.

This resonance between people, this literal 'wave flap' (to use Kirstin's term) has ethical implications:

> There's this total connection between one person and another and I don't see myself up here and the person down there. We're on the same plateau; everyone's equal as far as I'm concerned.

This democratic commitment to *relationship* is one of the features that distinguish post-War music therapy from its nineteenth-century precursors (Tyler 2000: 385) and that make it an essentially *social* mode of therapy. With music, the social, the recreational and the therapeutic are not always easily separable and are often a matter of framing (when does a choir become choir therapy? Is a laughter club the same thing as laughter therapy?). In Kirstin's description of group sound work, sociality is both a therapeutic mechanism and an outcome:

> Often in my workshops I do toning as a group exercise, and we start off and I encourage people to just explore their voices within the group. But it always works out in the end we're all singing in harmony, because it's the resonance factor; we *want* to be in harmony with each other and they end up saying, 'Oh, we didn't know we could sound so beautiful', and then they all feel in harmony with each other because they're resonating together through sound.

As a group called 'Toning for Peace' put it:

> When we tone with a group, something emerges from our coordinated breathing. We con-spire (breath together) to evolve higher. We give what Hazrat Inayat Khan terms 'vitalized breath' our full attention, exercising it with unbending intent to express ourselves creatively. That expression frees us, and we enter a world of unlimited potential. (n.d.)

Con-spiring may produce entrainment (a form of synchronization in which differences attenuate and individuals move towards 'oneness') and/or harmony, in which differences are orchestrated to produce beauty.

SOUND, ORDER AND HARMONY

This theme of harmony resonates with a long-standing philosophical and religious analogy between 'personal and cosmic order' (Horden 2000: 8), in which music serves as an exemplary instance. Novalis, for example, believed 'that the rhythms of the body move in harmonic order, and disease can be detected as a dissonance in the harmonic ordering' (Schafer 2003: 33). Every disease is, he claimed, 'a musical problem'. It is also, perhaps, a mathematical problem, at least for philosophers like Pythagoras, who were interested in the mathematical underpinnings of music and who saw a scientific understanding of music as the necessary basis for its therapeutic use. Music may stir our natures, but nature, it seems, 'uses maths'.[10] Pythagoras influenced Plato, who saw music as a tool for personal and social harmony.

Platonists 'understood audible sound to be an echo of the perfect concord in the heavens' (Voss 2000: 156). Earthly music, by closely imitating the music of the spheres, could be used to bring the soul and the body back into harmony (159). This Platonic idea of correspondence between heaven and earth (summed up in the Hermetic axiom 'as above, so below') also underpinned the natural magic of the Renaissance philosopher, musician and physician Marsilio Ficino. It referred both to the correspondences between microcosm and macrocosm and to the idea that intervention in any one plane of existence (physical, mental, spiritual) resonates across the others. It was thus a question not just of mirroring (of one world in another or one body in another), but of a universal field of vibrations through which any action resonates. Influenced by the neo-Platonic thinker Plotinus and the Islamic philosopher al-Kindi, Ficino believed, like many of his day, that 'all realities emit vibrating rays which together compose the harmonious chorus of the universe' (Sullivan 1997: 2). When the string of an instrument is plucked, another 'trembles' in accord and the 'carry-on echoes' continue to reverberate throughout the entire cosmos (2). Ted Gioia describes the common analogy between social and musical harmony as a 'seductive idea' (2006: 94). Yehudi Menuhin, for example, claimed that:

> Good music is the harmonization of all the vibrations of which matter consists, and it restores us to ourselves and to our universe. It is the bond that we have between our own frequencies and those frequencies which vibrate millions of light years away. (1999: xi)

Most sound therapists, even those trained in conventional medicine, do not see the question of harmony as merely metaphorical. Oncologist Mitchell L. Gaynor for example, who uses Tibetan crystal bowls and chanting as an integral part of his practice, understands illness as 'a manifestation of disharmony' and sound therapies as tools for 'restoring the normal vibratory frequency of the disharmonious … part of the body' (1999: 17).

For obvious historical reasons, twentieth-century European philosophy tended, in general, to be less trusting of order and harmony, and more focused on randomness and chaos, whether bleakly or in celebratory mode. Drawing on a celebratory lineage, via Darwin, Nietzsche and Deleuze, contemporary feminist philosopher Elizabeth Grosz agrees that the natural world can be understood as 'musical' (2008: 39), but she does not construe that musicality as order. Rather, she understands the arts as an engagement or struggle with chaos. She describes music (and other cultural forms like dance, and even philosophy) as taking with it 'little shards of chaos through which it wrenches a consistency, an intensity or a predictability in order to set itself on the other side of chaos' (28). In the process art does not generate harmony so much as 'intensify life' (39).

Chaos and discord spoke to many European composers of the twentieth century, many of whom experienced the turbulence of revolution and war. Stravinsky and Schoenberg, for example, wanted their music to shake audiences out of familiarity and complacency. Even a twentieth-century Theosophist, English composer Cyril Meir Scott, drew on his belief in subtle anatomy to argue that only musical discord could be strong enough to combat moral discord. Dissonance could 'break up estab-lished thought forms' (Tompkins and Bird 1974: 144); harmony, Scott thought, was too rarefied for that purpose (144).

New Age philosophy, however, pulls more towards order, despite this potential prompt from Theosophy, and its science of choice is not Darwin but quantum physics. Physicist and healer Jude Currivan, for example, points to string theory, which postulates that the 'fundamental building blocks of the physical world' (2005: 21) are one-dimensional oscillating strings rather than point-like particles (21–2). Whereas in Grosz's formulation this ceaseless vibration might signal the essentially *creative* impetus of natural chaos, to a New Ager it reflects harmony – both in nature and in knowledge. Thus Currivan sees string theory as pointing to a potential rec-onciliation between contemporary science and the 'essentially harmonic' theories of the cosmos that typified the ancient world (2005: 21). In this typically synthetic and holistic New Age conception, the music of the spheres is updated into the 'unheard hummings of atoms and molecules' (Gordon n.d., summarizing Joseph Campbell). Cosmic energy 'is said to manifest in our hearing awareness as a humming vibra-tion around and within everything else' (Gordon n.d.). In the Sanskrit tradition, this sound is called the *Anahata Nada*, or the 'unstruck ["unmade" or "uncreated"] sound' – that is, a sound which, unlike ordinary audible sounds, is not made by striking two things together, but is, rather, the primal sound of the energy of the cos-mos (the Zen image of the sound of one hand clapping is another well-known figure for this). In yoga, the OM is understood as the audible sound that most closely resembles this primal, divine energy and that leads one to it (Gould-King n.d.). It is comprised of four quarters, of which three are audible phonemes (A-U-M) and the fourth is silence. In this silence, the individual is unmade; 'beyond the reach of ordinary transaction', the self experiences 'the cessation of the visible world' (Olivelle 1998: 477).

SOUND AND DANGER

In the popular imagination the word 'vibrations' so typifies the New Age that it has become a shorthand for all that might be risible in contemporary Western spirituality. 'Vibrations' may conjure up images of dolphins-and-crystals style New Age practitioners, but they also make an appearance in the pseudo/scientific techno-wizardry of so-called 'resonance' or 'electro' medicine. These controversial technological forms of vibrational theory conjoin traditional ideas – such as the life force and the potency or dangerousness of sound vibrations – with the imagery and technology of modern electronics. Every organism, it is believed, resonates at its own unique frequency, which can be used against it in a process known as 'audiopathy'. Sound frequencies and electrical currents, generated by, for example, Rife machines,[11] are believed to destabilize or even kill pathogens. Some practitioners believe you need to know the precise life-force frequency of the pathogen, and for this purpose a shared database of frequencies is being collaboratively established; others are a bit more hit-or-miss in their approach. Either way, electromedicine situates vibrations within a similar cultural imagery to that of the laser guns of sci-fi, in which sound waves are used to kill unwanted aliens. Its advocates often make a comparison with medical ultrasound. Thus, electromedicine replays in a technological form an age-old theme – that of the fundamental duality of sound (Gioia 2006: 13): its power to both harm and cure.

In the Western tradition, the two key mythic representatives of the power of music are Orpheus (who charmed wild beasts with his music) and Apollo, the Greek god of medicine, music and poetry (Gioia 2006: 90–1). Sound, then, can evoke both order and harmony, disorder and dissonance. The idea that the individual can be unmade through sound – the self dissolving into the cosmos – has less benign faces, like that of a self dissolved irrecoverably, a self harmed by damaging sounds, or a social body rocked and disturbed by the 'wrong' kinds of music. Music, according to Ficino, can not only carry away 'certain diseases of the soul and body', but also bring them on (1980: 162).

There are plenty of quite literal ways in which sound and music can be damaging to the body, most obviously the damage to ears caused by loud or close noises. The intensity, duration and frequency of a sound, coupled with the length of exposure and the susceptibility of the individual, all influence a sound's potential to cause hearing loss (Bess and Humes 2003: 178). Music, too, can be a literal source of danger, a form of physical (tactile) shock. It can be precise and targeted – the soprano shattering glass[12] – or it can be an experience that can make whole bodies, and whole roomfuls of bodies, thrum with its power, as in Japanese Taiko drumming or heavy metal music. Music of all forms has the power to affect the body, including its heart rate, blood pressure and muscle tension.

Perceptions of physical danger are also often bound up in fears of social and moral danger. Does the following quotation from a music therapist, which emphasizes the violent *physicality* of rock music, shade into a fear about the plight of young people today?

> With a lot of the loud music it feels like it's just crashing into you and you've just got to take it in, but it's got a knock-you-over sort of feel. I know a lot of the young people like that. And I read somewhere that they – to get it into their body they need it really loud so it gets right into their physicality. For some reason it needs to bash right through their bodily cells and that's how they take the music in.

Certain forms of music are widely held to damage not only the individual body, but also the social body. It is not uncommon to assume a 'causal link between music and moral decay' (Lynxwiler and Gay 2000: 64). In its time, the Romantic music of the nineteenth century 'mesmerized' legions of females, who were rendered either manically excited or deeply melancholic by Franz Liszt's virtuosic piano concerts in the 1829s and 1830s (Kramer 2000: 341). But these 'toxic' effects were also countervailed by its 'tonic' ones; Liszt himself was invited to play the piano to a woman in an insane asylum, who 'vibrated to every chord struck by the young musician' (qtd in Kramer 2000: 343). Today, Romantic music's toxic qualities have been safely inoculated by the passage of time, and it is other forms of music that trigger fears of the disintegration of the social body. Rap music, for example, may trigger fears about the rise of black culture, as in one white critic's description of rap music turning its audiences into a 'single-minded, moveable beast' (qtd in T. Rose 1991: 286). Or, to take another example, heavy metal is feared to encourage anti-social, sexist and illegal activity (Lynxwilder and Gay 2000: 67). In both these examples it is hard to disentangle fear about the music itself from concerns about its social *practice* (that is, its contexts, settings and demographics).

At their best, cultural studies of music remind us that cultural context and the physical experience of music cannot be separated. They make it clear that there is no universal human perception of sound. Tolerance of noise, for example, is 'not just a matter of decibels but of expectations of what one's environment should by like' (Sim 2007: 20). Sensitivity to noise is 'often class and culturally based' (Bull and Back 2003: 9). There are connections between our experiences of space and of sound: 'Cultures with strong notions of "private space" as a form of entitlement are more prone to complaints about noise' (9). And yet, I am also cautious about the discipline of Cultural Studies' tendency to embrace the physiological only at moments when it suits politically. We might be prepared to accept that a rock concert is damaging to hearing (120 dB as compared to 140dB of a jet engine at takeoff (Bess and Humes 2003: 43)), but Cultural Studies' emphasis on music as a cultural process bound up in signification, identity and social regulation can make it somewhat programmatic in its tendency to sidestep questions of physical response except when they can be used for resistive political purposes.

For music and sound therapists, of course, the intricacies of the physiological effects of music are core business, and therapists have their own repertoire of ways for thinking about how sounds may damage the body. Kirstin, for example, talks in terms of the 'toxicity' of particular frequencies:

> There are certain sounds that are extremely toxic to a person – particularly low wave sounds, white noise. Low brain wave sounds can be very toxic. They found that oxygen has a frequency of the note C. So does hydrogen, but lead, which can be very toxic to us, has a frequency of the note D sharp. Well, for some people who are very allergic or sensitive to that kind of metal that might be a very bad thing for them to have. There are different types of sounds that affect different types of people. And there are associations too with those sounds.

The reference to 'associations' points again to the difficulty (indeed the impossibility) of disentangling physiological, moral and social claims. What I find interesting here is Kirstin's refusal of an ultimate separation between physiology and meaning, as well as her recognition of the question of individual difference in receptivity and experience. Such an approach is multifaceted, combining numerous perspectives: the '"psychologization" of musical experience' that characterized the nineteenth century; earlier philosophies that linked music to physical states (Kramer 2000: 39); ancient philosophies that ascribed metaphysical significance to particular sounds; and scientific accounts of perception and sensory stimulation. This may not, of course, always be a comfortable reconciliation.

Even studies purporting to describe sound as a purely physical phenomenon are inevitably mired in (or, ideally, enriched by) sociocultural subtleties. For example, Peregrine Horden describes a scientific experiment on the effect of sound on cells *in vitro*. In this experiment, normal and cancerous human cells were subjected to Ayurvedic 'primordial sounds' and to rock – AC/DC to be precise (2000: 6). Since the experiment occurred *in vitro*, it was an attempt to study music in its purely physical form – as pure sound vibration without 'benefit of psychosomatic mechanism, cultural expectation, placebo effect and so on' (7). So why were the results so culturally predictable (the rock music increased the rate of tumour growth, of course)? Does this reflect a brute physical reality about the effect of sound on cells and/or may there have been an impact, procedural or esoteric, of the intentions and assumptions of those involved in the experiments?

That physical, moral and social danger blur into each other is even more suggestively hinted at in a series of studies recounted in Tompkins's and Bird's book *The Secret Life of Plants* (1974). They describe various scientific experiments, first in India and later in the US, on the effects of music on plant growth, crop stimulation and pest reduction (1974: 135–42), which were prompted in the first instance by the familiarity of an Indian botany professor called T.C. Singh with ancient Hindu legends about Krishna making plants grow by singing devotional songs to them (135). Reporting of these experiments prompted a chain of others in North America. In 1968, biology student Dorothy Rettallack studied the effects of classical and rock music on various vegetables and flowers. Haydn, Beethoven and Schubert made them flourish; rock music caused them to use more water, to be stunted, or to grow abnormally tall. Acid rock music caused them to grow on a measurable lean in the opposite direction. I first found a report of this study on a website with the URL hinduism.co. Why? Because the same study found that while the plants enjoyed their classical concert, they positively relished classical *Indian* sitar music!

> The plants gave positive evidence of liking Bach since they leaned an unprecedented thirty-five degrees *towards* the [organ] preludes. But even this affirmation was far exceeded by their reaction to Ravi Shankar. In their straining to reach the source of the classical Indian music they bent more than half way to the horizontal, at angles of more than sixty degrees, the nearest one almost embracing the loudspeaker. (Gould-King, n.d., original emphasis)

Some New Agers and yoga devotees would respond that such findings are evidence of an ancient wisdom – that particular musical traditions best reflect a physiological reality. Some claim a special spiritual status for the phonological base of Sanskrit.[13]

Some music therapists – advocates of the Bach-Vivaldi-Mozart school of thought – base their own series of claims around the complexity of Western classical music, arguing that it is not a cultural bias but an objective truth to note that the symphony orchestra uses many more instruments simultaneously than many non-Western musical forms and thus has a greater power to trigger complex and multifaceted emotions than, say, the Indonesian gamelan. But more cross-culturally aware music therapists are suspicious of such universalist claims, focusing instead on the importance of selecting music that is culturally and personally appropriate for the client. After all, we have heard tales of the universal and beneficent powers of European culture before. In a discussion with the music therapist Kirstin about the frequency with which Bach, Vivaldi and Mozart are cited as having inherently healing properties, I described to her a video I had seen depicting a pregnant woman playing not the expected soothing music to her unborn baby but rap music, loudly. The voiceover described how later this baby was soothed to sleep by rap. Kirstin responded, reasonably enough, in terms of acculturation and habituation. These learned affective responses are, of course, only part of the picture. To approach a full understanding of the power of music to move and affect us, we need to be open to many different forms of understanding: scientific information about the effects, including *in utero*, of vibro-acoustic stimulation;[14] musicological analysis of the differing musical properties of different musical instruments and forms; psychological awareness of the links between music, affect and memory; and cultural understanding of cross-cultural differences and the use of music to represent broader social hopes and fears (Lynxwilder and Gay 2000: 64). So while rap music lullabies and cells *in vitro* 'disliking' AC/DC and liking sitar music ought to remind us that it is difficult to disentangle physical dangers from moral and social ones, it is important not to throw the baby out with the bath water. We need to recognize not only the different physical properties of different forms of music and their effect on, for example, the immune system, heart rate, brainwaves, breathing and the production of endorphins (Gaynor 1999: 18), but also to keep exploring the role of habit, expectation and context in modulating these very effects.

SOUND AND THE DIVINE

Music's ambiguity extends to the domain of religion, where it can act as both stirrer of the flesh and 'the agent of the sacred' (Dolar 2006: 31). Music is 'not essentially a *cognitive* mode' (Finnegan, qtd in Filmer 2003: 94, original emphasis); it can stir emotions and bypass rationality. For this reason, it has had a historically vexed relation to sacred texts. As Mladen Dolar puts it, singing is 'a flourishing of the voice at the expense of the text' (2006: 30). Singing 'turns the table on the signifier' (30); it lets 'the voice take the upper hand' (30). This was historically part of its seduction and its danger. Dolar gives a brief outline of the problem of music for the Christian Church. On the one hand, music 'elevates the soul to divinity'; on the other, it is a sin, 'carnality at its most insidious' (48). The singing voice is both flesh and non-flesh, 'both the subtlest and the most perfidious form of the flesh' (48). It has the potential to overtake and unbind sacred text, to undo the boundaries of self, and to unleash emotions, not all of them holy, in the hearers. The history of church music is thus a history of repeated attempts to codify and regiment sacred music – in particular, 'confining the voice to the letter, to Holy Scripture' (48), often via the principle of keeping one syllable to one note. Departures from text, in the form of vocal flourishes and ornaments, or even in the form of polyphony, where different simultaneous melodic lines threatened the singularity and intelligibility of the sacred text, embodied awe and jubilation, but also threatened 'moral ruin' (49). There was a fine line between 'redemption and catastrophe' (47).

Singing's focus on the voice over language is paradoxical, a 'structural illusion' (Dolar 2006: 31):

> The voice appears to be the locus of true expression, the place where what cannot be said can nevertheless be conveyed. The voice is endowed with profundity: by not meaning anything, it appears to mean more than mere words, it becomes the bearer of some unfathomable originary meaning which, supposedly, got lost with language. (31)

For a Lacanian[15] like Dolar, transcendence is an illusion bound up in 'the long history of the voice as agent of the sacred' and in music's traditional links both to nature and divinity (2006: 31); the primordial state of wholeness we often seek is 'always a retroactive construction' (31):

> The voice as the bearer of a deeper sense, of some profound message, is a structural illusion, the core of a fantasy that the singing voice might cure the wound inflicted by culture, restore the loss that we suffered by the assumption of the symbolic order. (31)

While the voice may not be able to make us whole, some have argued that it can at least bring us *closer* to bridging the gaps. The phenomenologist Maurice Merleau-Ponty, for example, considered the human voice to be a marker par excellence of individual distinctiveness: 'My voice is bound to the mass of my own life as is the voice of no one else' (1968: 144). Yet through the proximity of breath and sound, the voice is also a means by which we can *almost* – though never quite – bridge the gap between self and other:

> But if I am close enough to the other who speaks to hear his breath and feel his effervescence and his fatigue, I almost witness, in him as in myself, the awesome birth of vociferation. (144)

For Merleau-Ponty, the sounds of one's own speech are 'heard from within' (144), but sound's ability to move between people saves us from solipsism, and reminds us of reciprocity and of connection; the other person's speech sounds 'have their sonorous inscription, the vociferations have in me their motor echo' (144). In Merleau-Ponty's formulation, human sounds' connection to the intimacy and mobility of breath is a phenomenological fact with ethical import. We are not discrete, separate or bounded. The act of breathing, which sustains us, connects us to others; and the act of speech, which might seem to symbolize and confirm our individual separateness, since we hear ourselves from within ('I hear myself with my throat' (1968: 144)), can work as a bridge to bring us closer to others, for the speaking other resonates within us.[16]

Some sound-based alternative therapies share this idea. Typically, they mobilize the intimacy and the sociality of sound, its connection to the body and its ability to move across space, to try to bridge gaps, whether they be gaps between present and past experience, between self and other, or between self and wider cosmos. Bridging such gaps may be understood as achievable only momentarily, or only after a lifetime's discipline (as in yoga) or as an ideal rather than a possibility. But – and this is where the gap between these therapies and contemporary philosophies like post-structuralism (and its psychoanalytical affiliate, Lacanianism) is unbridgeable – in those therapies based on a vibrational model, there is as I have noted no absolute ontological distinction between mind and matter, self and world, even self and other, for they are ultimately composed of essentially the same stuff. This stuff is differentially and hierarchically organized across a number of planes, and some differences (e.g. that between self and other) matter a great deal in some planes of reality, but not in the oneness in which the search for transcendence culminates in this energetic model of the universe – known in yoga as Samādhi, that state in which 'the individual aspirant (sādhaka) becomes one with the object of his meditation' (Iyengar 1991: 21). In practices based on this model, sound's relation to sacred text is thus not a dualistic battle for supremacy, as in the historical Christian tradition, so much as a search for perfect resonance. Text and sound are different aspects of the one phenomenon.

In such traditions, sacred sounds are associated with particular parts of the body. The *bija* mantras, for example, assign single-syllable sacred Sanskrit sounds to different parts of the body (principally the *chakras*) (Gaynor 1999: 14).[17] In the sacred yogic syllable OM, for example, the materiality of the sound is inseparable from its meaning. As noted earlier, the single sound 'OM' (or 'AUM') is broken down into four components – the A, the U, the M and the silence that follows. Each of these components both *means* (represents, symbolizes) something, and *does* something (activating particular parts of the mind and body). The 'M' resonates predominantly in the chest, while the 'Ah' is in the throat and the 'Or' in the head.[18] Ultimately, then, the distinction between physical and metaphysical ceases to hold; mantras are not just symbols, they are 'energy encased in [a] vibrational structure' (Prattis 1997: 248). The influential yoga teacher B.K.S. Iyengar discusses OM in terms that suggest it is a *symbol* or *representation* (of a variety of triads (e.g. past-present-future; mother-father-guru; speech-mind-breath of life)). But he also states that 'as water takes the shape of its container, the mind when it contemplates an object is transformed into the shape of that object' (1991: 51). Thus, uninterrupted contemplation of this 'symbol' of oneness will mean that one is 'integrated in the object of his contemplation' (51). In Prattis's formulation, metaphors both represent and embody their symbolic meanings: 'When the OM mantra is chanted these cosmological metaphors of Universal energies [the forces of creation, maintenance and destruction symbolized by Brahma, Vishnu and Siva] enter the body directly, because different parts of the breathing system are affected through its vibration' (1997: 250).

The different sounds have different physiological effects. As Simon Borg-Olivier, who is a molecular biologist, a physiotherapist and a yoga teacher, speculates, in response to a query I put to him:

> We know from studying different systems that, for example, bone density can be affected by vibrations. So you affect on one level your bone density and the bone mass just by vibrating one part of the body. So also you generate a bit of heat with vibrations in one point. So as the heat builds up in one area it will send blood up, radiating heat from that one point. So I can imagine on a physical level that if you chant a specific sequence of sounds you'd affect your circulation, you'd affect the deposition of the minerals in different parts of the body. You can imagine how it could happen. But it's not really understood.

In the form of Bhakti yoga known as Hare Krishna, one of the ways in which Krishna incarnates in the contemporary age is in the form of sound vibration: 'Sound is one of the forms which the Lord takes. Therefore it is stated that there is no difference between Kṛṣṇa and His name' (*Chant and be Happy* 1982: 95). This is reminiscent, perhaps, of the anthropological claim that among oral people language 'is a mode of action and not simply a countersign of thought' (Malinowski, paraphrased in Ong 1988: 32). In such a system, words, especially names, have power, functioning less as 'tags' than as dynamic and potent operatives. Hare Krishnas believe that chanting the holy name has powerful effects; it 'acts like fire' (*Chant and be Happy* 1982: 94). Moreover, they claim that this action occurs irrespective of comprehension. The spiritual sound vibration of the holy name 'surpasses all lower strata of conscious-ness' (xv) and hence there is no need to understand the language of the mantra or to engage in intellectual or mental speculation about it. It is, rather, 'automatic' (xv). Other branches of yoga might elaborate on the physiological mechanisms somewhat more. Some of chanting's transcendental effects are believed to occur by virtue of the eighty-four meridian points on the upper palate, which act as 'a keyboard for the tongue' (Shannahoff-Khalsa 1996: 352). Different sounds require the tongue to move in different patterns across this keyboard, and hence induce different effects. The achievement of a transcendent state is thus in part a matter of physical patterns: 'What is required for the development of the transcendental mind is the correct code' (352).

Yogic mantras are spiritual texts, and that spirituality is understood in very mate-rial terms. Borg-Olivier noted the specificity of Sanskrit in this regard. The sounds are produced from different places – the nose; the base of the throat; the back, top or front of the mouth. Some are aspirated; others not. Speech sounds not only mean different things but also make the muscles do different things:

Each of them has a slightly different effect on the way your muscles have to work. Your larynx, for example, and the pharynx, as they operate in different ways, different muscles pull against the skull and the spine. So you can imagine how by making the voice-box move in different ways you affect your spine. So I can quite rationally see how mantras have a very potent effect on the body. But it's fascinating to see how Sanskrit is formed. A very cursory regard to how to make Sanskrit sounds, this is quite remarkable. This is quite a science. Like if you place the tip of the tongue just behind the teeth and you make a sound. And you place the tongue on the roof of the mouth and you make the same sound. Then at the back of the throat. And each of them sounds slightly different just by positioning different parts of your tongue in different places. And in yoga we know for example that the tongue positioning affects the secretion from different glands to the brain as well.

In contrast to these thoroughly embodied, holistic theories, interpretive disciplines like semiotics, or for that matter psychoanalysis, seem insufficient vehicles through which to fully understand the bodily transformations associated with alternative therapies, based as these academic disciplines are on extracting meaning from experience. The ability of both these disciplines to get at the 'meaning' (personal or social) of bodily events is an important start, but the distinction between a bodily event and its meaning is ultimately difficult to draw. This is especially the case with practices drawing on non-modern cosmologies in which, as the anthropologist Alfred Gell says in relation to magic, 'matter and meaning become miscible fluids' (1977: 27) and the distinction between metaphor and metonymy, or sense and reference, becomes an 'irrelevance' (Howes 1991: 135). This is, as Gell notes, 'a scandal ... from the point of view of scientific method' (1977: 27). It is also hard to find a find a contemporary language that can do justice to this holism.[19]

The final example for this chapter is a form of psychotherapy based on a paradigm in which meaning is inescapably physiological. And it reserves a special place for sound in the encryption and experience of that meaning.

PSYCHOPHONETICS

Psychophonetics is the name of a mode of embodied psychotherapy developed in Australia in the late 1980s by a psychotherapist named Yehuda Tagar, now based in Cape Town. Originally known as Philophonetics ('love of sound'), and based on Rudolf Steiner's Anthroposophy and Psychosophy, Psychophonetics combines elements of counselling, coaching and personal development, with applications for healing. Anthroposophy is Rudolf Steiner's humanistic elaboration of Theosophy. As such, its fundamental anatomy is a version of the subtle anatomy schema described in earlier chapters. According to Tagar, 'Steiner's unique contribution to psychology' is the claim that memories are stored in what Theosophists call the life body (also known as the etheric body, or the *chi* body) in the form of sound vibrations. Hence sound work is a major tool of this technique, although it is embedded in a wider context of non-verbal modes, such as visualization, gesturing and body awareness, as well as in a broader cognitive context. (Psychophonetics sessions proceed only after a great deal of preliminary negotiation between client and therapist.)

My own encounter with Psychophonetics occurred over a decade ago, when I did a one-off workshop with Tagar. When I came to consider forms of sound healing for this book, my recollection of this workshop was dim yet compelling. All I could re-member of the theory underpinning it was that sounds resonate meaningfully in the child's body well before they are cognitively patterned via language. What I *could* recall was a man with a powerful and precise voice alternately bathing, spraying, assaulting and caressing participants with speech sounds. I could remember little of his person. (In fact, I mis-remembered him as a giant, Dickensian character with a stentorian voice, when actually he is fairly short, with a soft speaking voice.) What I remembered most vividly (and accurately, as it turned out) were explosions like B! B! B!; murmurings of MMMM; the sound 's' whispered then hissed; strange but vivid combinations of sounds (KTCH! BRRNG! XXT!). When I interviewed Tagar in 2007 and heard those sounds again, it was as if my body itself remembered them. According to one of Tagar's colleagues, Robin Steele, it had: 'you carried whatever the meaning of the experience was from 1993'.

Tagar claims that there is little academic literature on the connection, both theo-retical and applied, between the sounds of speech and psychotherapy. There is, he claims, a gap between the psychological disciplines and those of phonology, phonet-ics and linguistics. This might seem odd given that Freudian psychoanalysis – 'the talking cure' – was based on talking and listening. It is true that Freud considered the voice to give clues about the patient's unconscious and he described the special-ized arts of listening necessary to the psychoanalytical method.[20] The patient's voice was certainly attended to *as a voice* – stuttering, pausing, coughing and so on were carefully noted – but since psychoanalysis was ultimately a quest to uncover mean-ing, and the analyst not just an interlocutor but finally a translator and analyst of the patient's symptoms, in the final instance such vocal signs pointed elsewhere. They were important clues to be deciphered – signs of a drama elsewhere. The materiality of the voice is left behind once it has done its job and pointed to the meanings hidden below or inside the speech.

This is, after all, what we ordinarily expect language to do for us. The human voice is distinguished from the cacophony of sounds and noises that constitute eve-ryday existence by an *expectation* of meaning:

What singles out the voice against the vast ocean of sounds and noises, what defines the voice as special among the infinite array of acoustic phenomena, is its inner relationship with meaning. The voice is something which points towards meaning, it is as if there is an arrow in it which raises the expectation of meaning, the voice is an opening toward meaning. (Dolar 2006: 14, original punctuation)

For Mladen Dolar, this understanding of the voice construes it as a mere tool. In this commonsensical understanding, the material voice is a vehicle, an instrument, of meaning; it does not contribute to meaning so much as enabling it. It is, indeed, 'that which cannot be said' (15). According to Dolar, the question of the materiality of speech trapped both traditional phonetics and post-Saussurian linguistics. Phonetics, he claims, became inextricably mired in the physical and physiological properties of the sounds of language (17); but the Saussurian solution, a search for the 'fleshless and boneless entity' (17) it called the phoneme led it back into 'a certain theology of the voice' in which the voice precedes and is subsumed by the Word. In the Saussurian model of signification, the signifier is essentially arbitrary, important only as a means of distinguishing one word from another ('bat' is not 'cat' only by historical linguistic convention, as we Cultural Studies academics famously tell our first-year students).[21] Phonemes are defined negatively in what is, for Dolar, ultimately a 'theological' conception of language, in which the voice is a mere carrier for meaning. Dolar's wonderful book is an attempt to work backwards, as it were, from word to voice.

In its own, very different, way, Tagar's Psychophonetics is also about the materiality of the voice and the refusal or deferral of interpretation. Psychophonetics is 'not interpretive; it's not instructive; it's not didactic; it's not analytical', says Tagar. Psychophonetics draws on an understanding of sounds and words as *events*, a conception which, according to Walter Ong, typifies oral-aural cultures, for whom 'A word is a real happening, indeed a happening par excellence' (1967: 111). While, as I noted at the outset of this chapter, some contemporary thinkers shy away from (or indeed critique outright) this way of characterizing societies, Ong's description of the word as an event is an apt conceptual frame through which to approach Tagar's therapeutic practice, pointing, as it does, to the relative lack of interest in interpretation in Psychophonetics, in stark contra-distinction to the psychoanalytical tradition. For perhaps the most distinctive feature of Psychophonetics is that it uses the sound of human speech as a significant, meaningful materiality in its own right rather than as a vehicle for cognitive or narrative meaning. Psychophonetics aims not to discover an inner truth about the client – to search for meanings – but to transform the client:

> We 'meaningfy' experiences. We don't fix, we don't cure, we meaningfy. The
> core of healing for us is that a new meaning is given to old experience. It's
> not just cognitive stuff. It's experiential. But we regard meaning not as an
> intellectual construct. Meaning is deeply experiential. Even when it is cognitive
> it is experiential. You cannot give meaning. It has to be created individually.

The subtle body schema, with its focus on the interrelations between and inter-effects of different bodies – implies that there are many potential starting points for therapeutic intervention. For example, a therapy might intervene on the plane of emotions and produce effects on both body and mind. Another might intervene on the plane of cognition, and through that gradually have an impact on the body. Or it might intervene in the body and have effects on the mind. There is a theoretical reciprocity – for example, breathing affects thoughts and controlling thoughts via meditation affects breathing – but in practice different individuals often respond to some starting points more than others.

Psychophonetics's particularity is that it intervenes on the plane of physical vibra-tions. Words and speech sounds are used for their sound rather than their meaning – or rather, their meaning lies in how they resonate in the body. In this schema the body is not merely a vehicle for the expression of sound; it is *made* of sound. To be more specific, in the Anthroposophical framework in which Psychophonetics is conceived, *one* of the four human bodies – the life body or etheric body – is made of sound. In Anthroposophy, there are four bodies, of which the life or etheric body is one. The life body is a body of vibrations, and is comparable to *chi*, *prana* or mor-phogenetic field energy in other subtle systems.[22] As in all subtle anatomy, this body is understood as real and tangible, but invisible to normal sight. All living things, humans, animals and plants have such a body, which is 'the organizational principle of the physical body and the basis of our existence'. That body, known variously as the life body, the *chi* body, or the *pranic* body, is understood to be made of sounds:

> The way the psyche lives in the body is organized in sounds. The way our
> biography is stored in us is organized in sounds. The way our learning lives in us
> is organized in sounds. In the way that memory in a computer is organized in a
> digital system which is encoded in some way that can be scanned. In the same
> way, our memory is stored in sound vibrations.

The meanings embodied in sound are primal, bodily, and beyond the reach of con-scious access. But in the process of everyday life we continually make older experi-ences resonate. When we encounter sounds heard in a meaningful way in earlier times, they chime in the body. The entire body (physical, sensory and energetic) is thus conceived of as a 'centre of communication, a reflector and a resonance cham-ber for experience'.

I have already remarked that the metaphor of the body as a centre of communication surfaces in a range of alternative therapies; it is, after all, a metaphor that makes cultural sense in the age of the internet. Another of Tagar's metaphors is that of the computer, used to describe the workings of memory. But whereas the metaphor of the brain as a kind of hard disk is commonplace, Tagar, in keeping with many in alternative medicine, decentralizes the brain in favour of the body as multiple, and he sees memory as dispersed, both spatially and temporally. All memory is stored in the life body, not the brain, he claims. The brain is not a storage device but a transmitter:

> The brain *is* a scanning mechanism to a certain extent, and it *is* a communication between embedding and restoring. You know, memoriz*ing* or remember*ing*. This mechanism needs a system, sure. But it's a transmitter – it's not where it is stored.

The connection between random memory and deep memory is much more fluid and continuous than that on a computer, where archived memories are either 'up' (on-screen) or 'down' (on the hard disk). It is, to use Tagar's term, 'alluvial', since all memories vibrate in the life body all the time and are, in that sense, never really fully 'in storage' and are able to be triggered accidentally, mundanely, or subconsciously.

I said earlier that sound, especially music, is widely believed to take you back in time, often to infancy. While this is the case in Psychophonetics, the movement back is not a regression, or a recovery, for in the subtle body schema the past is never, in fact, past. All experience is still present in the body; body-time is not linear but simultaneous: experience 'is simultaneous in the body. It happens all the time; it's not like it happened in the past'. All memories vibrate in the life body all the time. Psychophonetics is thus not about searching for the lost object, so much as searching for frequencies that resonate in ways that might transform you in a liberating way:

> We don't deal with the past; we deal with patterns in operation. They may have been formed in the past, but we don't dwell on the past; we just look at the forms.

It is also less focused on cognition and narrative than other forms of psychotherapy, and hence relatively immune to the contentious problems of truth and falsity that plague debates about memory.

If memory is stored in sound, then with sound we can access memory. Tagar estimates that there are around two hundred basic sounds in human languages, which can then be combined in an infinite variety of ways, and intoned in different manners:

> It's beyond count. If we had to write our sound possibilities in a materia medica, it would break a database. So we don't even try. We rather train the intuition.

I'm travelling around with my medicine cupboard; if this were homeopathic, I would need a whole train. But I don't need a train because I make it on the spot and test it on the spot.

Psychophonetics counsellors thus have thousands of sound combinations at their disposal, and they use them as medicines in a quite literal sense, with the therapist 'prescribing' a dose of a particular sound at the end of a psychotherapeutic process in which the client has already gestured, visualized and sensed the issue that they are working with. Tagar elaborated this with a metaphor from naturopathy:

There is sound hidden there – they just don't *know* that their body is desperately trying to do 'D!'. So the 'D!' is not an imposed form – it's like saying you need more haemoglobin, you need more liquids, you need more iron.

On reflection, though, he decided it was more like homeopathy than naturopathy, since the 'remedy' being 'prescribed' is vibrational: 'If you were a homeopath you would prescribe some form of remedy. If you are an aromatherapist you would prescribe some oil. So we prescribe "hmmmmm".' It takes precise sounds to access precise memories:

Compare doing 'BRRRR! D!' with 'D! D! D!' [If a client's body needs 'D'] they prefer the sound because it just does it better. It's like doing a job with bare hands and doing a job with proper tools. You can dig the ground with your fingers, but, you know, take a spade! So we give them the right tools to do the job.

CONCLUSION

Sound, in this esoteric conception, is a tool, like a spade. But this tool is not just a pathway to meaning. It does not just represent or signify; it *does* physical things. What it does, what it is and what it means cannot be completely separated. Moreover, sound is the fundamental stuff of which everything is made: the stuff of the body and the stuff of the cosmos. Social, connective, penetrative, sound makes and re-makes bodies, and can be used to draw them together.

Sound, this meaningful materiality, is also dynamic. It *moves*. Hearing is a physical movement in which 'waves of sound roll like tides to our ears, where they make the eardrum vibrate', which moves the tiny bones, which press the fluid of the inner ear, which brushes tiny hairs, which triggers nearby nerve cells (Ackerman 1990: 177). In that sense, sound is like a form of subtle touch, with actions that are akin to the subtler forms of therapeutic touch, which will be examined in the next chapter.

4 KNOWING TOUCH: BODYWORK

Touch is, they say, the closest sense, available only in proximity and dispersed throughout the body. It is a mode of contact, exploration and communication (Rodaway 1994: 45), a means of establishing not just particular physical relationships but also an underlying emotional bond between self and world (44). Touch is primary. The first sense to develop (from six weeks *in utero* (Montagu 1986: 4)), it is the 'foundation upon which all the other senses are based' (4). Touch, says Ashley Montagu in his beautiful book-length study, is 'the parent of our eyes, ears, nose, and mouth' (1986: 3). Primacy and primality, though, are two sides of the same coin, and touch, like smell, has traditionally been feminized – associated with animality, servility and the unconscious (Chidester 2005: 72).

Since touch is the basis of all sensory perception (2005: 73), losing our sense of touch would mean losing our sense of being in the world (Rodaway 1994: 41). It would also curtail our emotional life, since touch is connected to a broad range of emotional experience. Our tactile engagements may be delightful, disgusting or painful, or they may scarcely register, passing unnoticed as sedimented or subtle body habits, or bypassed in the body's drive towards unreflexive functionality (Leder 1990). While certain forms of self-touching escape our notice (our hair falling on our necks, our watch on our wrist, our glasses sitting on our nose), other forms of touch are highly charged, and a whole evocative vocabulary serves them. Caressing, stroking, cradling, rocking – even the words themselves are deliciously, or perhaps uncomfortably, or even dangerously, intimate. This intimacy provides a frequent starting point in philosophical and cultural accounts of touch, which commonly see its 'proximal' nature as marking it out from more distant senses like vision, smell or hearing.

Both the primacy and the proximity of touch make it seem inimical with deception (Tuan, in Rodaway 1994: 44); it is 'perhaps the most truthful sense' (1994: 44). Mark Smith starts his chapter on touch with a reminder that the saying 'seeing is believing' is a contracted version of 'seeing is believing but feeling's the truth' (2007: 93).[1] Touch, then, has been understood as 'an authenticating sense' (2007: 97), which cannot, unlike sight, be deceived (Benthien 2002: 195, summarizing Condillac and Berkeley). Yet both Aristotle and Plato considered it 'radically inferior to sight' (M. Smith 2007: 93), as did Augustine, who claimed that 'the objects ... that we touch, taste, or smell, are less like truth than are the things we see and hear' (1964 [387–395] II xiv: 147).

Debates about the effectiveness of touch in conveying reliable information about the world can slide into claims about its moral qualities. Sander Gilman stresses the 'ambiguity inherent in the physiology of touch' (1993: 198): touch is assembled from diverse and relatively undifferentiated receptors (199); it is linked to both pleasure and pain (200); and it calls us up both as subject and object (we can touch ourselves as well as others) (199). Touch is, he claims, arguably 'the most complex and the most undifferentiated of the senses' (199). For this reason, and the fact that it spreads out far beyond the noble head (Benthien 2002: 197–8), it is ambiguously valued in cultural terms: it is both 'the highest and the lowest of the senses' (Gilman 1993: 199). There is a thread in Western culture in which tactility has been denigrated (Chidester 2005: 72) – for example, a recurring association in Western thought and iconography between touch, sexuality and disease (Gilman 1993). But not all touch is devalued; rather, all societies divide touch into different categories: good, bad, acceptable, prohibited and so on. Its regulation through prohibitions and social rules reflects its power – sometimes symbolic, sometimes literal, sometimes both – to bring pleasure, or to wound, corrupt or threaten. For the subtle, variegated and proximal nature of touch makes it continually open to suspicion. We may touch heaven when we lay our hand on a human body, as the poet Novalis claimed (qtd in Carlyle 1846: 181), but touch can also spell danger.

A contemporary example in the West of anxiety around touch concerns the touching of children. Here, the moral division of touch into 'good' and 'bad' forms seems obvious – maternal caresses versus child abuse – but between these two extremes there is of course, ambivalence, with many forms of touch, such as smacking and corporal punishment, remaining contested. Suspicion of touch is also matched, especially in the late twentieth century, by a rise in the cultural value of touch, especially with regard to child-rearing (Synnott 1993: 161). It is now widely understood that touch is essential to physical health, emotional wellbeing and intellectual development (156–7); in order to prosper, the infant needs to be 'handled, and carried, and caressed, and cuddled, and cooed to' (Montagu 1986: 99). The role of touch in stimulating the brain and building neural pathways is now so well established as to be a staple of popular child development activities. A leaflet from an Australian kindy gym, for example, emphasizes the importance of tactile play

of self-perception' (Benthien 2002: 200). Later, it functions also as a site of identity-for-others – including as a cultural marker of race, age and gender. So skin has served in much cultural analysis as a metaphor for an 'inscription' model of the body according to which culture 'writes' its stories on our bodies like tattoos on skin, or ink on the page. This inscription model has been conceptually and critically useful, foregrounding the 'unnaturalness' of the body and the role of culture in determining how different types of bodies are to be understood and valued. Unfortunately, at its peak it all too often produced an overly textualist account of the body, implicitly thinking of skin only through the lens of vision rather than that of touch, which might have produced more lived analyses of the powerful role of the skin in embodied experiences of race and racism.

For the skin can be 'viewed' through a much more complex sensory lens than just that of vision. In Michel Serres's work, for example, it stands as a metonym for the complexity of embodied life. In stark contrast to the inscription model, Serres uses skin as a metonym not for a surface that gets written upon by culture but for a model of embodiment in which there is no strict division between inside and outside, and in which all the senses are conceived of as thoroughly intermeshed. For Serres, skin is not a simple surface dividing inside from outside. Rather, it is itself variegated – topological not topographical. Skin, like touch itself, 'could be called variety, in a precise topological sense: a thin sheet with folds and plains, dotted with events and singularities and sensitive to proximities' (2008 [1985]: 61). Serres claims that each sense originates in the skin and is 'a strong individual expression of it' (70). Skin is not the barrier between self and world – not even a barrier conceived of as permeable or leaky – but a site and means of contact with the world into which all the senses are 'wired'. The senses 'haunt the skin' (60). In Serres's difficult poetic evocation:

> The skin hangs from the wall as if it were a flayed man: turn over the remains, you will touch the nerve threads and knots, a whole uprooted hanging jungle, like the inside wiring of an automaton. The five or six senses are entwined and attached, above and below the fabric that they form by weaving or splicing, plaits, balls, joins, planes, loops and bindings, slip or fixed knots. The skin comprehends, explicates, exhibits, implicates the senses, island by island, on its background. (60)

For Serres, skin is both a heightened example of, and a metaphor for, 'the way in which all the senses in their turn also invaginate all the others' (Connor 1999: n.p.). This tallies with Montagu's account of the development of the embryo. *In utero*, the ectoderm (or outer embryonic cell layer) is like a kind of proto-skin that also gives rise to the hair, teeth and all the sense organs (1986: 4). The nervous system develops from the same embryonic cell layers as the skin (4): 'The nervous system is, then, a buried part of the skin, or alternatively the skin may be regarded as an exposed portion of the nervous system' (5). So there is both poetry and accuracy in conceptions that trouble the simple idea of the skin as the 'outside' of the body. Thus Montagu cites the anatomist Frederic Wood Jones, who declared that 'he is the wise physician and philosopher who realizes that in regarding the external appearance of his fellowmen he is studying the external nervous system and not merely the skin and its appendages' (qtd in Montagu 1986: 5). For Montagu, it is a physical fact, not merely a cultural truism, that the skin, and especially the face, records 'the trials and triumphs of a lifetime' and 'carries its own memory of experience': 'On our skin, as on a screen, the gamut of life's experiences is projected: emotions surge, sorrows penetrate, and beauty finds its depth' (6). Skin is a two-way medium: site of cultural inscription, but also screen for the inner depths of the body.

The idea of bi-directionality occurs in a second persistent example in discussions of touch – that of the hands. Culturally speaking, the hands are highly symbolically charged. Intertwined, they may be metaphors for care, reciprocity or connection; raised, they may signify violence or aggression; stretched out to another, they may be a show of welcome or friendliness; or they may activate fears of dirt, germs and contagion. As vehicles for contact with and exploration of the world, the hands are instruments of knowledge. They can also be understood as communicators, whether through primal tactile 'communication between person and world' (Rodaway 1994: 44) or codified into gestures and actions (such as handshakes or kisses) that signify and cement social values and relationships. The hands have also provided a metaphor for the relationality, power and reciprocity involved in touch. Touch is the most reciprocal of the senses (Rodaway 1994: 41): 'to touch is always to be touched' (1994: 41). Merleau-Ponty saw tactile experience as involving a certain *enmeshment* of self and world; touch doesn't allow us the illusion of unsituatedness, as sight can (1962: 316). Whereas sight is stereotypically understood as 'pained by the sight of mixture', to use Michel Serres's beautiful phrase (2008 [1985]: 67), touch is typically understood as inevitably more *involved*: it 'apprehends and comprehends, implicates and explicates, it tends towards the liquid and the fluid, and approximates mixture' (67). Or, to put it more simply, 'touch is participation, passive and active, and not mere juxtaposition' (Rodaway 1994: 44). Touch only 'works' if the thing we touch 'finds an echo within me … and if the organ which goes out to meet it is synchronized with it' (Merleau-Ponty 1962: 316). Reciprocity is at the heart of touch,[3] but reciprocity is not symmetry (Rodaway 1994: 45), and questions of intention and power thus remain at the heart of tactility.

Such themes – power, knowledge, reciprocity and communication – thread through this chapter, whose subject is therapeutic touch, using the case of bodywork practices, which were examined in Chapter 2 through the lens of vision. Both hands and skin will feature, but so too will less visible parts of the tactile network – the fascia that 'weaves its way through the body like a gossamer blanket' (Grimm 2007: 1234); the cerebrospinal fluids that pulse almost imperceptibly through the body; and the subtle energies that, according to alternative medicine, constitute and animate the body. In bodywork, claims are made about the ability of touch to get to sedimented emotions and experience, whether through the movement of a masseur's active hands skilfully dynamizing the body's hidden histories, or through the patient, motionless hands of the reiki practitioner acting as channels for a more-than-human healing agent and as conduits for the flow of information. The reciprocity of touch has therapeutic significance, for in therapeutic touch the hands are charged with both diagnostic and therapeutic potential, and can function as channels, receivers, conduits or transmitters of energy. The skin's function as a 'perceptual system' (Rodaway 1994: 43) is also amplified in these practices, since the 'energy' that is mobilized, dynamized, transmitted or channelled in bodywork is understood as 'imbued with intelligence' (Milne 1995a: 4). For many bodyworkers this energy is another way of talking about 'spirit' – the 'ordinarily invisible energy field whose activity gives us life' (Milne 1995a: 4), known in yoga as *prana* and in Traditional Chinese Medicine as *chi*. But what is meant by 'intelligence' and how might it relate to 'information'? Can the hands detect 'information'? These questions bring me back to my recurring fascination with the exciting yet problematic potential for interpreting and narrating the body. Do the questions raised in Chapter 2 about the possibilities and ethics of information gathering and interpretation look any different when revisited through the lens of touch?

Before exploring these questions, I will give an overview of some of the bodywork practices that will be canvassed in this chapter. As noted in Chapter 2, bodywork refers to a large cluster of manual therapies, each of which has its own internal schools, traditions and variations, and which are in any case very often practised in different combinations and styles, often in hybridized forms. These techniques are interesting not just for their medical significance,[4] but also for a raft of cultural, conceptual and intellectual ones – for example, that they sometimes incorporate pleasure and indulgence into the realm of the medical; that they conceive of the body as a dynamic field of subtle energies that can receive, store and express 'information'; and that many bodywork researchers and practitioners combine biomedical, scientific and esoteric knowledge.

The main examples used in this chapter will be: massage, myofascial release (MFR), craniosacral therapy (CST), Zero Balancing (ZB) and reiki, each of which I will briefly explicate here. Massage is no doubt the most well known manual therapy in the West. It has been part of diverse healing traditions over many centuries. In India, it formed part of the Ayurvedic tradition, which dates back to 2500 BC

(Govindan 2005: 366); in the West, it was used by Greek and Roman physicians. An indication of the diversity of different schools and styles of massage was given in Chapter 1. Myofascial release (MFR) is a form of manual therapy that focuses on the fascia – the connective tissue that surrounds and penetrates all the tissues, organs and bones of the body. The fascia is a filmy substance like that seen surrounding a chicken breast – a multilayered network of fibrous connective tissue whose function is to support, insulate and protect the body and its organs, and which carries nerves, lymphatic vessels and blood vessels to the muscles, bones and organs (Tortora and Grabowski 1993: 239). It is not only extensive, it is richly innervated (Grimm 2007: 1235). In contrast to mainstream science, whose interest in the fascia has until recently been quite low, a number of bodywork modalities hold 'the fascia in high regard' (2007: 1234).⁵ Rather than focusing on localized restriction, weakness or tightness, MFR approaches the body holistically, releasing tension in the fascia in order to remove symptoms and, ideally, to correct the causes of pain or dysfunction (Chaitow 2001: xii). MFR is a descendant of the 'structural integration' technique developed by Ida Rolf, known as Rolfing, which used direct force on muscles, fascia and ligaments to release tension and restriction. As it has evolved, however, and particularly under the influence of the physical therapist John Barnes, it has developed another strand, in which the fascia is not so much forced to release as gently held, directed and followed. According to several of my interviewees, the more direct style is dominant in Australia, especially in sports medicine, but the more subtle style is growing in popularity. This latter style is often practised concurrently with craniosacral therapy (CST), a form of subtle bodywork derived from cranial osteopathy and developed by the osteopath John Upledger. CST is based on serious attention to the lifelong, subtle mobility of the articulations joining the cranial bones (Giaquinto-Wahl 2009: 76). It involves an extremely subtle intervention in the flow of cerebrospinal fluid via holds at the base of the cranium and the sacrum, which allow the body to 'self-correct and reorganize' (2009: 79). In this chapter I also make passing reference again to the modality called Zero Balancing. Although this is not a widely known therapy, its founder, Fritz Frederick Smith, writes in interesting ways about the energetic body. An MD, trained in osteopathy, Rolfing, acupuncture and Eastern meditative techniques, Smith typifies the figures working in the points of intersection between seemingly incompatible medical cosmologies.

The final technique discussed in detail is reiki, which is a form of therapeutic touch in which energy is directed through the hands of the provider to stimulate the body's own healing mechanisms. Here, too, there are different traditions and styles of practice. For some practitioners, it involves very still hands – putting their hands on the body and waiting as long as seems to be required at each part of the body, whether that be ten minutes or more, with a total treatment lasting between sixty and ninety minutes. Others practise a much more mobile style, in which the hands are moved frequently around the body, every few minutes. Still others work *off* the body – moving their hands above the body according to their own intuition. This intuitive practice is in stark contrast to the first, much more regulated, style, where the body is usually attended to with a protocol: hands on particular parts of the body, in the same sequence each time, until all the major organs have been covered, along with key points in the endocrine, lymphatic and circulatory system. This use of a protocol reflects reiki's status as a 'nondirective' healing modality (Singg 2009: 262) – that is, one in which the practitioner allows the body to make its own 'decisions'. The energy being channelled is understood as a universal life force, like *prana* or *chi*, and thus understood to have its own intelligence. The recipient's body is believed to respond according to its own needs, rather than the practitioner's will (262), and hence is able to reject, as well as accept and direct, the energy.[6]

Bodywork treatments can involve quite diverse and intense experiences of touch, including the subtle, the painful, the mechanistic and the utterly sensuous. They provide rich experiences of touch all too rare in a culture in which individuality is asserted and protected in part through sanctions on touch. Part of their appeal, then, is the different types and registers of touch they offer up – often to a privileged demographic with disposable income, but also, importantly, and especially in the case of massage and reiki, to those who have formed networks of unpaid, reciprocal care. Reiki in particular is often carried out by groups meeting at regular intervals in a home. Women usually predominate. Other forms of touch, like Touch for Health, have been developed specifically for amateur use at home.[7]

Personally, I find bodywork modalities to be the most intellectually exciting of the alternative therapies; their difference from, yet close proximity to and collaboration with, more mainstream physical therapies puts them, to my mind, at the forefront of integrative medicine. Experientially too, bodywork modalities are my favourite therapeutic cluster; I find them therapeutically very effective and I gain pleasure from them. They also mark the point where I enter the picture not only as a researcher and consumer of alternative therapies, but as a kind of practitioner – an amateur reiki practitioner for around twenty years. As I noted in the Introduction, I took up reiki at the same time as I took up a PhD in Cultural Studies – an unusual and disconcerting conjunction. Reiki and post-structuralism ran like parallel train tracks in my mind and life for well over a decade, forcing me slowly to find possibilities for living and thinking them together. So I bring years of sometimes painful reflection to this chapter. I include my experiences for another reason, though, and that is an ethical one. It seems only right that I turn the tables and shine the analytical spotlight onto my own practice as part of the give and take of intellectual work, exposing my own practice to the analytical gaze.

TOUCH IN BODYWORK

Touch has traditionally been understood to have therapeutic or healing potential, whether through supernatural or natural means (Classen 2005: 348). The exemplary instance in the Christian tradition is Christ himself, who healed by the laying on of hands. English royalty appropriated this idea through the tradition of the King's Touch, a belief in the healing power of the royal hand that developed in thirteenth-century England and peaked in the seventeenth century (Thomas 2005: 354–5). Belief in specially endowed touch was also accompanied by a powerful folk legacy in which the hands were credited with healing power, a belief found in many cultures around the world. Roy Porter (1993) says that in the UK the tradition of the healing hands was more or less obsolete as an active belief by the Enlightenment, though it persisted a little longer in France. Despite this decline, the tradition of healing through touch remains powerful in the West as a remnant or symbolic idea, and one which contemporary practitioners of therapeutic touch are keen to draw on, as in the opening of Fritz Frederick Smith's book *The Alchemy of Touch*: 'Touch is perhaps the oldest and still most reliable healing modality that we possess' (2005: 1). To the extent that the idea of the healing power of touch persists or is revived in contemporary bodywork, it may invoke a number of ideas about the natural and/or magical power of the hands: folk or popular belief in the innately healing power of touch; religious or magical belief in the special endowment of particular individuals; and modern scientific interest in the psychological and physiological benefits of touch. It may also be at the threshold of new scientific ideas about the physiological mechanisms by which the body converts mechanical pressure into chemical energy (Davis 2009: 13).

The fortunes of touch as a valued diagnostic and therapeutic instrument have ebbed and flowed over the centuries in the West. Roy Porter's (1993) history of the physical examination in medicine makes it clear that some periods have considered touch the backbone of medical diagnostics while others have considered it far inferior to other methods, such as the taking of a case history. Though the idea of diagnosis without a physical encounter probably seems foreign to many Westerners, touch has undoubtedly had to cede a little ground in contemporary biomedicine. It may still be a frontline technique, but it is less likely to be the ultimate arbiter of medical truth, edged back by an ever-expanding battery of technological diagnostic procedures. Physicians Drew Leder and Mitchell Krucoff (2008) consider that in contemporary medicine the role of touch falls into two major categories. The first they call objectifying touch (analytical, information-gathering forms of touch like being palpated, measured or weighed); the second, absent touch – that is, touch mediated largely by technologies. This retreat has left only a minor role for touch that is intended to be something other than instrumental – that is, empathic and/or actively therapeutic. Bodywork fills this breach; its touch is at once analytical and compassionate, and is increasingly valued by those who seek relaxation and/or a sense of connection as part of the medical encounter.

A number of lineages of conceptual practice have found their way into contemporary forms of therapeutic touch in the West. The first is an anatomical line – the result of developments in biomechanics, especially the rise of physiotherapy (physical therapy). Many bodyworkers (John Barnes, for example) were originally trained as physiotherapists. A second informing tradition is the embodied psychotherapy line that draws on the psychoanalysis of, among others, Wilhelm Reich, who saw repression as a physical as well as a psychical event. Such 'somatic psychotherapy' takes it as a given that there can be no effective therapy without touch (see also Synnott 1993: 176–7). A third line is a spiritual tradition – the energetic conception of the body, influenced by the subtle body models of India (*chakras*) or China (acupuncture meridians), and given currency in the West via, among other things, the New Age. Like the psychotherapeutic tradition, this lineage understands all significant and habitual experiences to be 'lodged' in the body.

Different forms of bodywork privilege different parts of the body as sites of focus and intervention – in massage, the muscles, ligaments and tendons; in MFR, the fascia; in CST, the cerebrospinal fluids. But it is not a matter only of modality but also of the tradition in which that practice is framed. In the Ayurvedic tradition, for example, massage is no mere manipulation of muscles and tendons; it also works to improve the flow of *prana* (life force) in the body (Govindan 2005: 367). As the osteopath Hugh Milne notes, any art can be practised in different ways (1995a: xii) – whether technically or intuitively, at the centre of a practice or as an adjunct, in pure forms or in fusion, 'scientifically' or 'spiritually'. Practices are not just techniques; they involve *philosophies* of practice. For example, one of the major polarities in bodywork practice involves a distinction between those who 'oblige' the body to release and those who 'wait' for it to release, a distinction that one of my interviewees characterized as a continuum ranging from 'getting in and bulldozing' to 'holding and slow release'. What makes things difficult for consumers and commentators alike is that quite different things can occur under the same name. Moreover, it is difficult to tell from the outside what paradigm a practitioner makes use of, not only because the same label may describe quite different forms of practice, but also because a practitioner may vary his or her practice (or the way he or she talks about it) to suit different clients.

One of the features that mark out 'alternative' bodywork modalities (or practitioners) from more mainstream manual therapies like physiotherapy is a commitment to deep holism, alongside an interest in the communicative dimensions of the body. Though particular modalities may choose different parts of the body as their 'entry point', bodyworkers of all kinds understand the entire body to be a responsive and expressive network and a site of memory. Rather than focusing on localized areas and symptoms, or on the musculoskeletal system only, the forms of bodywork described in this chapter are far more holistic – interested in structure, function and energy, and attending to both 'remote and local interactions and influences' (Chaitow 2001: xii). Thus, rebalancing the sphenoid, for example, might equally well correct a headache or an internally rotated foot (Milne 1995a: 3); or vertigo might be traced back to an old knee injury, as in Upledger's celebrated successful treatment of a US Olympic diver (described in Giaquinto-Wahl 2009: 78). Holistic practitioners are alert to the signs sent from the entire body: in MFR, for example, when you work on one area of the body, another area altogether might go red, or another area might tingle. For some bodyworkers, the pattern for this holism is the hologram (Milne 1995a: 6); for others, it is the network, an intricate web of inter-connections along energy meridians or fascial 'trains' (Myers 2001). Most bodywork therapies incorporate the entire body-mind-spirit – whether by physically traversing it as in massage (which in its alternative framing is never just a localized treatment of painful spots) or by stimulating and catalysing the entire system through a touch that may be localized but that is understood as operating in relation to the entire body system (as in MFR and CST). The physical touch used may be very mobile (as in massage) or very still (as in CST and some forms of reiki).

Different modalities and styles of bodywork involve different forms of touch. Some techniques have their own names, and can be taught – *effleurage*, *tapotage* or *petrissage* in massage, for example – while others are less formalized, more intuitive or idiosyncratic. Some tactile taxonomies emphasize not the type of strokes but the level and style of inter-involvement; Smith, for example, identifies four ways in which touch can be used therapeutically: blending, streaming, channelling and interface (summarized in Geggus 2004: 67). Some practitioners approach the body with a set protocol, but others approach each patient individually.

Contemporary bodywork often characterizes the body in terms of fluids and energy, seeing it as a dynamic energy system rather than a solid mass of bone, muscle and viscera – understanding these more solid structures either as a denser form of energy (Milne 1995a: 5) or as structures in complex interplay with energy (F.F. Smith 1986, 2005). Barbara, the MFR teacher quoted in Chapter 2, recounted a portrayal of bones given by one of her teachers: '[He] always says, if all our bones were taken out, our connective tissue would hold us up. And so really the bones are like spaces in the connective tissue'. This is a body metaphorically softened and aerated, one which recognizes the vibrancy of even the most 'structural' of the body's features. In this understanding, bones are not symbols of death; they are 'living twigs' (William

Sutherland, qtd in Milne 1995b: 10), alive and responsive to the bodywork encounter: 'Touch them, and they respond: they know you are there' (Milne 1995b: 10). Even those bones seemingly most inert – the cranial bones, which until recently were believed to have been fixed after childhood – have been found to change shape 'minutely and meaningfully' with every cranial wave (Milne 1995b: 8). A traditional osteopathic belief in the continued motility of the cranial bones after childhood was confirmed in the 1970s when Upledger, the founder of CST, worked with a team of researchers and discovered that the material in the cranial sutures contained blood vessels, nerves and connective tissue (Giaquinto-Wahl 2009: 76). Other researchers have used ultrasound to confirm the existence of cranial movement and intracranial pulsations (2009: 76). It is hard for those brought up in a metaphorical tradition in which bones are imagined as 'white, hard and breakable' to visualize them as 'slightly pliant', 'malleable', 'plastic' and 'saturated with blood and blood vessels' (Milne 1995b: 8). So Hugh Milne advises his students to try visualizing bone as a plasma field, or a 'jellyfish pulsating through a kelp bed' or 'a tired puppy slowly squirming in its basket' (1995b: 8).

As these descriptions indicate, bodyworkers often describe – indeed, rejoice in – this dynamic, rhythmic and fluid body via metaphor. They do not necessarily see science and poetry as incompatible registers. Thomas Myers, for example, describes his book on fascial meridians as 'a work of art in a scientific metaphor' (2001: xiii). The metaphors evolve over time, of course. Stanley Keleman's early work, for example, evokes the body in somewhat mechanical terms as a series of pipes, tubes, pumps, pouches and bellows; nonetheless, even thirty years ago he was arguing passionately for the processual nature of anatomy. Today, mechanical metaphors have largely given way to metaphors of the web or network (especially in MFR) and of fluidity (especially in CST). Reich's vision of the body as solidified history (1969: 146) now extends beyond the idea of muscular armour into metaphors of fluidity. John Barnes, for example, apparently likens the body to a saucer full of water that needs to be rocked without spilling it;[8] John Upledger describes CST as like 'removing stones from a river so the flow is not impeded' (qtd in Giaquinto-Wahl 2009: 75).

Bodywork 'honors motion' (Milne 1995b: 31). Practitioners of CST, for example, learn to detect and interpret the ongoing rhythmical movement of cerebrospinal fluid, which is continually produced and reabsorbed (Giaquinto-Wahl 2009: 75) and pulses through the body in a 'cranial wave' (Milne 1995a). Indeed, movement continues even after clinical death: Milne claims that the cranial wave continues for twenty minutes after physical death (1995a: 5). The body is inherently rhythmic – pulsing with life – its many different layers of energy bodies subtly and complexly interacting. In this way, the 'physical' therapies of bodywork and the sound-based, vibrational therapies explored in Chapter 3 are actually in proximity, for they both conceive of the body as rhythmic – a series of waves, pulses and vibrations. In this conception, hearing and touch are ultimately just different modes of perceiving the movement of energy.

Thus, MFR practitioner Tim Bone describes his approach to the body as a form of listening with his hands in response to muscle movement:

Ruth: Do you have a set way of approaching the body?

Tim: I have a set way in that the body will direct you. The body has its own inherent treatment plan, but it's whether or not the practitioner is actually able to
sit and listen to the body. Palpation skills from a remedial therapist's point of
view are just, 'Oh that muscle's tight. We need to relax it'. But when you start
getting into fascial work and deeper levels of structure and tissue, you actually
are directed by the *movements* of the tissue. So [as a masseur] you might put
your hand on an area of restriction and you say, 'Well, the fibres go this way;
I need to massage this way', but when you go in to do fascial work, it's like
taking the scenic route. You don't take the direct route because you end up
confronting the body – and to confront the body is adding more fuel to the
fire. So you need to be a counsellor in a sense for the body. A counsellor sits
with somebody and they listen. And they reflect back what the person has
said and the person learns more about themselves through the listening and
through continuing to go over their material and each time they go deeper
into their state and they go deeper into their levels of consciousness. Same
with fascial work.

I have quoted this at length because I want to illuminate the way physiological understanding and ethical precepts are, in this account, bound together, and professional expertise is inextricably bound up in the project of self-cultivation – both the patient's ongoing attunement to her own situation, and the practitioner's own need to develop qualities of patience and selflessness and increasingly sensitive modes of perception.

TACTILE TRAININGS, SENSITIVE TOUCH

Such modes of perception are a trained sensitivity developed over many years, requiring skill, attentiveness, training and practice. Smith's book *Inner Bridges*, for
example, contains exercises for Zero Balancing practitioners to train their perception of energy flow and quality by, for example, assessing energy currents and flows
within the bone (1986: 86–7); assessing skeletal energy through 'joint play' (the
subtle aspects of joint movement (1986: 93)); or assessing soft tissue energy. Hugh

Milne's books (1995a, b) on CST likewise contain exercises for developing appropriately subtle and centred perception.

A bodywork treatment typically begins with an initial period of assessment (via dialogue, visual examination and sometimes some elementary palpation) but after the first consultation this period is often relatively short, for every treatment is itself a process in which assessment and response are intermingled and ongoing. The practitioner detects, understands and responds to minute changes in the patient's body, alerting all his or her senses to responses that may include eye movements, tummy rumblings, twitchings, changes in temperature, skin colour or breathing, and even in the patient's voice or odour (F.F. Smith 1986: 112–26). The changes being tracked are often minute. Craniosacral therapists, for example, are trained to 'locate and evaluate the quality of a person's craniosacral rhythm anywhere on the body' (Giaquinto-Wahl 2009: 77). Hugh Milne claims that the measurable amplitude of this wave ranges from forty microns to 1.5mm (a sheet of paper being 100 microns thick) (1995a: 5).[9] One might well respond to this claim by supposing that this level of subtlety is undetectable, but Milne uses examples from patients' experiences of dental treatments to refute this.[10]

To access this kind of subtle perception, the practitioner may need to enter a meditative state (Milne 1995a: 4). Hugh Milne describes a form of touch, available only in such a state, in which perception and intention are intertwined: 'From [subtle, meditative] perception springs accurate, meaningful and vectored touch – touch that reaches the source' (1995b: 82). As I understand this, this refers to the ability of a skilled and sensitive practitioner to concurrently perceive the patient's energy fields and to direct his/her own intention to mobilize those fields in particular ways. Milne's books include meditation and visualization exercises aimed at helping the practitioner develop the necessary practical and intuitive abilities. To return to the questions about power and capture raised in Chapter 2, this perceptive mode makes it explicit that though bodywork involves 'seeing how a person really is' (Milne 1995a: 83), it is ideally not a capture from the outside, but rather, a sensing born of subtle, empathic, non-ego-based perception. As suggested in Chapter 2, there are forms of 'empathic vision' (J. Bennett 2005) that combine the visual, the tactile, and the intuitive. This form of visualization is 'a foundational skill in healing' (Milne 1995a: 83). It may *begin* with seeing, but it ends up with holistic sensing: 'You have to learn a thousand techniques in order to understand a single one. Then you only need one' (Milne 1995a: 9).

Practitioners use a variety of sensory and intersensory metaphors to describe this process of active receptivity. Some describe it as a form of 'listening'; others talk about 'seeing with their hands'. Smith talks about training the fingers, as well as the mind, to recognize the distinctive but repeatable 'feel of things', which he calls the 'signature' of such things as bone vibrations, ligament tension and so on:

> Regardless of the words we use to describe the palpatory sensation, it has a specific feeling in terms of touch. Once you have identified this for yourself, it will feel the same to you everywhere you find it. (2005: 72)

Barbara uses the phrase the 'fascial voice' to characterize the way areas of the body remote from where she has placed her hands might start to tingle: the fascia is talking to you, she says. Your hands are your eyes, 'because a lot of the time, you don't see what's happening, because it's happening deep within the body – so your hands are telling you what's happening'. But vision is important too; Barbara sometimes works with her eyes closed but at other times keeps them open,

> because someone might be grimacing or … I always like to check and I watch for rapid eye movement. That's a sign that they've gone into an emotional process and they may be sighing. I like to see what's going on as well as feel.

In contrast to the worst-case scenario of vision-as-capture I explored in Chapter 2, then, it is clear that for most bodyworkers the diagnostic eye is one that sees feelingly rather than purely objectifying, and one that is often closed in order to give way to the hands that detect the subtle waves, pulses and twitches of the body on the table, the ears that hear gurgles, yawns and sighs, and even the nose that sniffs out change. Indeed, in its highest forms, it is a form of synaesthetic perception.

What, meanwhile, does the *client* perceive during a treatment? Regular receivers of bodywork are themselves engaged in a form of tactile and proprioceptive training, becoming ever more sensitive to the nuances of therapeutic touch and to their own preferences and responses:

> All the while the therapist is involved in his or her work, the client is perceiving the therapist, his or her adeptness, touch and interest. Whether the client does this consciously or unconsciously, information feeds into the client's personal data bank of experience and affects the degree of trust. This in turn directly affects the availability of the client's energy body to the therapist and the therapeutic process. (Smith 1986: 82–3)

Some of the sensations detected by the practitioner will exceed the patient's perception, whether because they lie outside frames of understanding, knowledge or expectation that would render them perceivable, recognizable or meaningful, or because the patient's consciousness is engaged elsewhere – in deep relaxation, reverie, curiosity about the process, reflection, or sometimes anxiety or distraction. They may well have their *own* sensory images to evoke what is going on. Barbara recounted having had a client who described her own tissue releasing as being like having lots of worms crawling under her skin, or another for whom it was like glue moving. A person who regularly receives massage or some other form of bodywork may become quite discerning – able, for example, to distinguish a deep holistic experience from a more 'technical' massage; able to tell whether a practitioner is engaged or has her mind elsewhere; and likely to move between different practitioners, different modalities and different levels of 'immersion' according to their own perception of what they need at a given time. Barbara describes having been for a massage 'where they just lay you on the table like a slab of meat and go through their routine'. She teaches her students that 'your client will know if your focus goes out the window because your touch will change'.

Some bodyworkers make big claims about the contemporary social significance of the forms of tactile awareness and training able to be brought about by a serious commitment to bodywork. Thomas Myers, author of the book *Anatomy Trains*, argues that the social and environmental problems of the twenty-first century require the contemporary cultivation of new modes of perception, especially 'a more thorough and sensitive contact with our "felt sense"' (2001: xiii). Myers extends the now-popular language of IQ and EQ (emotional intelligence)[11] to something he calls KQ (kinesthetic intelligence), a deep connection with 'our kinesthetic, proprioceptive, spatial sense of orientation and movement' (2001: xiii). He very explicitly connects this non-mechanistic anatomy to the social world. Deeper connection with our felt sense is, he claims,

> a vitally important front on which to fight the battle for a more human use
> of human beings, and a better integration with the world around us ... Only
> by re-contacting the full reach and educational potential of our kinesthetic
> intelligence (KQ) will we have any hope of finding a balanced relationship with
> the larger systems of the world around us. (xiii)

Such an argument recognizes, as phenomenologists have done, the fundamental importance of touch in establishing an individual's ontological grounding and wellbeing. It recognizes that being-in-the world is a fundamental, unconscious *orientation* – that it is both a physical and an emotional bond between self and world (Rodaway 1994: 44). And it develops this insight into a larger thesis about social relations. The fascial web becomes, in essence, a bodily metaphor for a new mode of sociality, one in which empathic connection with others and the environment is predicated on a thoroughly *embodied* knowledge of self.

I will return to connection later in the chapter, but I want first to think about questions of will and power, since the intimacy and bi-directionality of touch make it a potential vehicle as much for exploitation as for empathy. As I have indicated, one of the current points of difference within bodywork is between the making-happen and the letting-happen approaches. In this latter style of practice, while the practitioner's touch might be imbued with intention (as in Milne's concept of 'vectored touch'), its aim is to *allow* the body possibilities for release and transformation, rather than to impose them. This philosophy is accompanied by a professional ethic in which practitioners strive not to require visible cathartic displays that bear witness to their own effectiveness. Barbara, for example, says:

> I try to impress on the students that a lot of the time – if they have to see that dramatic result, then it's only their ego that's needing feeding. And they don't need their patients to feed their ego.

It's not only about ego, of course. As partners in a commercial exchange, neither a professional practitioner nor his/her client can be immune from the logic of the market, which naturally enough incorporates the expectation that something can be seen to have happened in exchange for the fee paid. This commercial logic may not tend in the same direction as either a therapeutic or a spiritual logic, according to either of which, 'healing' may not always be visible, immediate, or tangible (Barcan and Johnston 2011).

Those who adhere to the principle of non-imposition see it as simultaneously an ethical and a therapeutic precept. Certainly, Smith, who studied with Ida Rolf, believes force to be counter-productive. He instructs bodyworkers

> not to let our expectations get in the way and 'force' the person's subtle body to respond in a specific way. Each person will have his or her own way of responding to energetic stimulation, and it is our job to observe what this is. If we attempt to create a breath cycle or a REM when there is no inclination for it to occur of its own accord, we are imposing our will and energy on the person. If we override the natural response, we can actually create imbalance and chaos. (1986: 126–7)

For Smith, forcing the body to respond is thus not only ethically dubious, but therapeutically counterproductive.[12]

This is a conclusion I came to myself after enduring a series of deep-tissue massages, which typically use strong and painful pressure to relieve muscle restriction and which not uncommonly brings about emotional releases in the form of tears. At first I found this form of massage appealing, because I felt certain that this must be an effective way of 'digging out' muscular tightness. Finally, one time lying wincing on a massage table, I realized that I was experiencing this as a type of assault and my body was, in fact, tightening itself up to fend off the practitioner's touch, rather than releasing tightness through receptivity to touch. I have heard other women complain of a kind of forced spectacle of catharsis, where a male masseur has kept 'digging' until the desired result was achieved – a (supposedly) cathartic emotional release.

But of course, some clients desire, seek and enjoy such cathartic releases, and much depends on the nature of the relationship between therapist and client.

Just as there are different personal attitudes towards, and even national styles of, emotional display and release, so too there are different levels of comfort with diverse forms of touch. Many clients (typically, according to my interviewees, men) are uncomfortable with subtle, energy-based approaches both because they want to see evident results and because of the feminine and feminizing associations of light touch. Tim Bone, whom I quoted above, began his career with 'heavy' modalities like deep tissue massage and has gradually extended his practice into the subtler, more energetic, modalities like CST and MFR. He is intrigued by the power of the lighter energetic work, but recognizes that different forms of touch will work for different styles of person:

Tim: I find you'll get some people who need the confrontation of muscle tissue work. They need deep tissue trigger work …

Ruth: To feel that something's happening?

Tim: Exactly. They feel comfortable in that. They feel comfortable in their pain. They believe in no pain, no gain. Whereas you get a lot of other people who are extremely sensitive and very responsive to subtle energy work or subtle contact and tissue work. These are the people who are usually very sensitive to their surroundings. Whereas the people who need the deep tissue work – you could whack them with a baseball bat and they just do not get the message. So there is no point in me going in there sometimes doing really subtle work unless I've attuned their body and gotten them a little bit more sensitive to what's going on.

This practitioner believed that the heavy physical touch is less confronting for macho types:

> Quite often [with] these guys it's just the façade they create – internally they are very sensitive. But they have created that façade to keep people at a distance. That's the bravado – the typical egotistical male bravado. 'Ah, I'm all right.' But inside they're a quivering mess, and their biggest fear is they will be found out that they're like that – so these are protection mechanisms. Now, if I came in and went subtle with those people, sometimes they actually just break down.

His first professional task is to serve his clients' priorities, rather than imposing his own idea of what they might need. Like the iridologists described in Chapter 2, he was well aware of how easy it is to frighten people. And, like many CAM practitioners, he recognizes and respects medical pluralism as both a social reality and a spiritual principle.

PLEASURE AND DANGER

Bodywork can be understood as a culturally licensed revelling in touch of many kinds. In bodywork, touch may be intimate, gentle, painful, subtle or obvious – pummelling, stroking, stretching, kneading, compressing, caressing, cradling, rocking. A good bodywork treatment can help us reconnect with our ignored, over-familiar or tired body parts – feet, calves, scalp, ears – and in so doing to weave the body together, reintegrating the body image. Some bodywork techniques are similar to yoga nidra, in that they achieve the relaxation effect by a process of sensory implosion, in which one loses sensory awareness of the body. The body is systematically traced, using awareness and imagination. Other techniques, such as holistic massage, relax by a more obviously physical retracing, remaking and reintegrating of the boundaries of the body, including, of course, re-marking its prohibited zones. As a sensory experience, this is very intense, and can involve a variety of sensations – not only tactile ones like tingles, warmth, goosebumps, friction, energy flows, 'good' or 'bad' pain, but a host of others brought about by such features as lowered lights, a warm environment, the scent of essential oils, gentle music or the luxury of an hour of almost complete silence. For a particular client demographic, among whom I include myself, there may be pleasure in pure receptivity. Relieved of the responsibility of doing anything, even talking, the harried professional may delight in a passivity rarely experienced in the frenzy of late modernity; or the overworked mother may rejoice in the pleasures of receiving rather than giving; or the person whose mind is always active may allow it to be still.

Many clients have a long-term professional connection with 'their' masseur or osteopath, who knows their body well. The experience of receiving bodywork from a practitioner one trusts is quite different from an initial or one-off encounter; the body sinks into deep relaxation fast as the practitioner's hand and the client's body renew a familiar meeting through touch. Naturopath and masseur Judy Singer recognizes this deeply touching power of trusted and patient touch, calling it 'deep care' (2008: 144). To acknowledge the possibility of deep care is not to romanticize bodywork as a place of perfect connection, reciprocity or pleasure, or to exempt it from questions of power. The tradition and the potential of therapeutic touch and the sensitivity of skilful practitioners do not mean that touch, or particular forms of touch, will always be experienced as helpful, or welcome, or pleasurable. Many factors, including cultural and family background and personal life history, influence the types of touch that are acceptable and/or pleasurable. Even within the privileged demographic of people who have material and economic access to bodywork, people take pleasure in different things and have different cultural backgrounds and life histories. The sociocultural literature on touch emphasizes the role of gender in conditioning the meanings of touch, receptivity to touch, and the forms of touch prescribed and proscribed in a given society. As Synnott puts it:

> Men and women live very different tactile lives, as givers and receivers, as to who touches whom, where, and why; as to how they understand the meanings of touching and being touched, holding and being held. (1993: 164)

Gendered parenting practices 'socialize [sons and daughters] in different tactile directions' (1993: 165), influencing such factors as comfort or discomfort with touching others, and producing particular bodily habits and aptitudes. These all take place within differentiated and dynamic social rules governing gender, sex and tactility, including rules about same-sex and opposite-sex touching. Gender plays a significant role in the modes of touch we develop, as well as our responses to touch.

The anxieties discussed at the start of this chapter about touch, contagion (symbolic or literal) and the erotic can never fully be dismissed from bodywork practice. The often intimate nature of physical therapies makes them a particularly loaded site for experiencing both the pleasures and the anxieties of gendered touch, particularly around the erotic, whether it be same-sex or opposite-sex touching. A man uncomfortable with having his naked flesh touched in a caring fashion by another man might opt for a massage performed not in classic 'alternative' mode but by a sports physiotherapist, where both environmental and paradigmatic features – fluorescent lights, commercial radio, electronic devices and a relatively mechanistic body paradigm – might work together to mitigate the perceived threat of same-sex intimacy. This style of practice contrasts with the typically more feminized space of the therapeutic massage in its alternative guise, with its dim lights, soft music, lavender burning, gentler and more variegated touch, as well as a therapeutic paradigm in which the emotions are given a significant role.

However the erotic is managed (whether downplayed, indulged or incorporated as something to be witnessed), bodywork therapies are undoubtedly examples of a contemporary commodification of tactility – paying others to touch in intimate, pleasurable or restorative ways. In the professionalizing climate of CAM, advocates of bodywork have sought to repel the popular image that bluntly aligns therapeutic touch with the erotic (e.g. the clichés associated with 'Swedish massage'). To do this they have developed codes of practitioner behaviour and linked them to practitioner registration. In Australia, for example, one of the major professional associations for alternative therapies, the Australian Traditional-Medicine Society, requires that to be registered with them as a massage therapist one must agree to no 'unprofessional' touch, including, specifically, touching the genitals or the 'mammary glands' (Australian Traditional-Medicine Society Code of Conduct, 2006, 5.3). While most therapists recognize the rationale and need for such restrictions, some also lament what they perceive as a therapeutic diminishment that may accompany them (for example, some practitioners believe that breast massage is an important component of lymphatic drainage, a technique designed to remove toxins from the body). But in the struggle to divide good touch from bad, appropriate from inappropriate, in a publicly legible and enforceable manner, such nuances are almost inevitably lost.

Professionalizing protocols rightly recognize the potential emotional and physical vulnerability of the client. There are some forms of somatic therapy in which the client remains clothed and upright, but in most, she or he lies down, often covered only by towels. Lying still and receptive, the bodywork client is thus *prone* in all senses – lying down, open, vulnerable to the actions of the person standing by (or over) them, and to their own fears, desires and memories. Tucked in bed, mimicking sleep, ready for love, fearful of violence – all these are experiences, shapes and postures clients may re-embody as they present either their vulnerable front or their blind back to the hands of a licensed authority standing above them.

Aware of the difficulties, pleasures and anxieties of intimate touch, most bodyworkers allow the client some role in determining what kind of touch they are prepared to accept. For example, an osteopath might ask whether a client is happy to have any spinal manipulation, and a masseur will typically ask how much pressure the client seeks or enjoys, and which parts of the body they do and don't want to have touched. In very difficult circumstances, such as when working with people known to be traumatized, especial care is required. Judy Singer, for example, describes with great sensitivity her naturopathic and massage work with refugees, explaining how in the right circumstances careful, gentle touch can acknowledge the lived bodily experiences of traumatized people and provide a space where they can 'allow their bodies to speak to the complexity of their circumstances' (2008: 147). Such practices also help rebuild connections – between past and present, homeland and new land. The art of connecting helps re-make the self (157).

TOUCHING, CONNECTING, BLENDING: BODYWORK AS AN INTERCORPOREAL EXPERIENCE

In bodywork, we are taken back to the 'reassuringly basic experiences' (Montagu 1986: 99) of touch enjoyed by the infant – being rocked, caressed, even held. We are tended to physically by another, with no obligation to reciprocate, nor sometimes even to speak. Perhaps we have never, since our infancy, been ministered to like this – we lie, wordlessly perhaps, on the table, while someone lifts our arms for us, repositions us, cradles us, strokes us, or simply sits by us, with their hand on us. Some forms of touch evoke this childhood body more than others. A rocking movement used in an MFR procedure known as rebounding, for example, recalls the rhythms of infancy, especially, says Barbara, as adults have only infrequent experiences of being rocked by another person. Another example is when a masseur gently palpates my hands and fingers and I am transported back to the finger games of infancy – as though I were engaged in a therapeutic version of the children's rhyme round and round the garden. The masseur's hand on mine, her fingers pressing gently on my fingers, I lie face down on the table, like a middle-aged baby.

This type of connection with the practitioner is, in essence, a means of reconnecting with our own earlier bodily life. But bodywork involves other forms and experiences of connection as well as disconnection, since the practitioner's touch may provoke or catalyse a whole host of bodily and emotional responses – anxiety, anger, resentment, yearning or erotic desire. Perhaps unsurprisingly, some bodywork discourse focuses on the ideal of harmonious connection. The Ayurvedic practitioner S.V. Govindan, for example, considers a 'feeling of oneness and harmony' with the receiver to be the 'essential ingredient' of massage in its traditional forms (2005: 366). Clearly, this ideal may not always be realized, but this certainly doesn't mean that a deep and comfortable connection between practitioner and client is impossible. Barbara, for example, describes working with a woman who is 'so finely tuned and in touch with her body [that] she knows exactly where I am working'. In other words, the woman is aware not only of Barbara's hands on her physical body, but also of where Barbara is directing her focus. For example, she may be holding the client's head but the client says, 'I can feel you in the sacrum now'. Such meetings – rare because of the degree of sensitivity, focus and concentration required of both practitioner and client – are highly effective therapeutically, because the intention and awareness of both practitioner and client are engaged synchronously. Other bodywork experiences involve not so much the synchrony of two intentions as a profound letting-go generated by deep trust. The patient may drift into deep relaxation or even sleep; or conversely, the practitioner may drift into reverie and the client be exceptionally aware of even the most minute sensation in his or her body.

The connections generated by bodywork can also involve something a bit more disconcerting, something resembling an actual bodily *mingling*. In my own practice of reiki, which I will describe in more detail in the final section of this chapter, I have observed over many years that sometimes my hands feel as though they have sunk right into the recipient's face or body and I literally cannot feel where I end and they begin. These experiences have always felt especially significant, but having only my own years of amateur experience to fall back on, I have not known what to make of them. So I asked Barbara whether this sensation was well known:

Barbara: Yes that's what you are looking for and that's called melding. You become part of their tissue.

Ruth: In what sense?

Barbara: You are sinking – you are sinking so far in it's as if you are ... I don't just think you're on top of the skin. (original ellipsis)

For bodyworkers, the idea that one is doing more than touching the skin of another – that one is actually entering the energy field of another, and hence transforming both it and one's own self – is quite normal. Legitimately, different practitioners have different ideas about how best to work with the meeting, synchronizing or mingling of bodies that is intrinsic to bodywork. Barbara, for one, likes to harness the client's intentions and awareness, using visualization as a co-operative imaginative endeavour, not an asymmetrical capture:

> If I'm working somewhere and the restriction is really strong I'll say to the client, 'Now, try and bring your thoughts to where my hands are. So bring your awareness to under where my hands are. So we'll see if we can get this to move'.

In Smith's Zero Balancing too, 'both practitioner and client pay attention to their experience in the moment' (Geggus 2004: 67). But awareness is not the same thing as mental engagement, and Smith likes to keep the client's mind from getting too involved, lest it interfere with the process:

> My basic instruction to the person on the table is to just relax and enjoy the session. I want as little of their mental engagement as possible. To the extent that the person is in their left brain, thinking or tracking the session, the working signs are blocked. (F.F. Smith 2005: 26)

I mentioned earlier that Smith distinguishes between four different types of energetic connection between practitioner and client: blending, streaming, channelling and interface (Geggus 2004: 67). This latter form of touch involves the practitioner making a conscious effort not to 'blend' with the client's energy – remaining 'very sensitively "in touch" and yet distinctly separate' (2004: 67). This form of contact, in which the boundaries between the two people remain consciously intact but subtly dynamized, is one of the core components of Zero Balancing. But the depths and styles of practitioner-client interaction vary according to modality, therapist and client wishes. As one masseur told me, different therapists work differently, but 'I tend to work beneath the skin level'. Not all clients want this, of course, so he also works with people who 'just want a rub'. When he massages them, 'we haven't made contact at that deeper level'. While this masseur recognizes the value of the physical assistance given to muscles in massage, he personally values the broader emotional and spiritual possibilities of massage: 'it's more the nurturing, the deeper level stuff, that I think has a longer term effect', since people who experience nurturing can learn to nurture themselves.

Are such experiences of connection, melding or synchrony the kind of thing the phenomenologists mean when they write about touch as a sense where the fundamentally 'implicated' and 'fluid' nature of all sensory perception is most evident, and most heightened? For Michel Serres (2008 [1985]), whose book *The Five Senses* is subtitled 'A Philosophy of Mingled Bodies', *all* of our senses allow us to 'mingle' with the world rather than to stand before it, and each sense is itself not singular but a 'nodal cluster, a clump, confection or bouquet of all the other senses, a mingling of the modalities of mingling' (Connor 1999: n.p.). A few decades earlier, Merleau-Ponty was also developing a phenomenology based on participation and mixture rather than separateness and objectivity. He used the term 'intercorporeity' (now usually translated as 'intercorporeality') to describe the way humans share perception and thus can mutually comprehend and function in the world (Crossley 1995: 144). For Merleau-Ponty, this shared perception of and operation in the world mean that self and other share a unity that is philosophically prior to any division or conflict between individuals and groups (1995: 143). Merleau-Ponty's phenomenology was based on a 'radical' intersubjectivity, in which subject and object are understood as 'relationally constituted' terms (Crossley 1996: 27) rather than as two autonomous entities in dialogue: 'I am all that I see, I am an intersubjective field, not despite my body and historical situation, but, on the contrary, by being this body and this situation, and through them, all the rest' (Merleau-Ponty 1962: 452). For Merleau-Ponty, then, the self is not a separate unit peering on the world and other people from inside its secure shell; rather, self and other help bring each other into being through their shared participation *in* the world. This conception of the self as inherently interrelated helps explain how it is that separate individuals can share – and function in – a seemingly privately perceived world. Another person is, in that sense, not a threat to one's subjectivity but an *extension* of it, since another's perceptions help confirm one's own (Kruks 1981: 14).

How relevant are these phenomenological ideas about intersubjectivity to bodywork? Is the idea that bodies together co-create a 'practical-perceptual space' (Crossley 1995: 144) sufficient grounding for understanding these experiences of deeply mingled bodies? Certainly, bodywork seems an excellent illustration (and extension) of the concept of intercorporeality, and of the power of bodily experiences of reciprocity and interconnectedness. Most obviously, the practitioner's touch is used to affect and dynamize the patient's body. It facilitates responses right across the body systems (e.g. nervous, muscular and endocrine) – muscle relaxation, eye movements, twitches, tummy rumbles, changes in breathing patterns, heart rate and so on – as well as in the patient's energy fields, which may 'elongate', 'extend', 'contract', 'stream' or 'rebound' in response to the therapy (F.F. Smith 1986: 83–5). For this to occur with any depth, the client needs to be receptive. As one masseur put it:

> For me, when someone *accepts* the massage – in other words, they're really getting into the feeling – there's a nice flow of energy. It's a two-way flow. Whereas with the other person it's like there's this shell. I can work maybe the first quarter of an inch of the skin and that first layer of muscles, but to touch the soul, if you want to call it that, it takes time to do that.

The reciprocity of touch means that changes in the patient's body may produce changes in the practitioner's own body, as their energy fields intermingle and the process triggers bodily memories for both of them. For example, Barbara notes that the MFR rocking movement mentioned above also sets up a rocking movement in the practitioner's own energy fields.

In this two-way process, the practitioner's hands act as both transmitters and receivers simultaneously: the heat they generate helps soften up the tissues and at the same time their hands are receiving information about where to move next. Indeed, CST practitioner Hugh Milne considers that at the highest level of practitioner mastery and the deepest levels of bodywork, touch comes, ultimately, from the *client*. In the hands of true masters, says Milne, there are unlimited forms of touch since, ultimately, a deeply connected practitioner derives his or her touch *from* the client: '[E]very touch is a fresh technique, the world has never seen it before, yet it is perfect, coming as it does from the client' (1995a: 9). Such hands, he says, have access to unlimited forms of touch. Healing, therefore, is not a one-way, top-down process, but something more reciprocal, a process that loosens, ultimately, the commonsensical division between practitioner and client, healer and healed. As the reiki practitioner Sharron put it:

> When I'm giving a reiki treatment the healing is mutual. I'm receiving reiki too.
> So I'm getting healing for some grief [for example], [and] so are they.

Therapeutic touch, then, transforms both the toucher and the touched. But bodywork extends the idea of the porosity of the body, whereby energy and emotion can cross its boundaries and move back and forth between practitioner and client. It also extends the phenomenological concept of intercorporeality as the co-creation of a shared perceptual realm. For most bodyworkers recognize the possibility of 'absent touch'. The practice of distant or absent healing – where people attempt to heal others remotely, whether via the use of intention, ritual or proxy objects – is commonplace in alternative medicine. Phenomena such as absent healing or the coincidence of mental phenomena are commonly reported. The subtle body schema grounds such phenomena in an anatomy – one that, unlike dualist conceptions of the body, does not make an absolute ontological distinction between matter and spirit (Johnston 2008: 2). In this esoteric anatomy, which comprehends but exceeds the Merleau-Pontian anti-dualism, it is logical that there can be such a thing as effective touch-at-a-distance, an intercorporeality produced across space and time.

Even a face-to-face bodywork encounter is, however, inherently intercorporeal. It is patterned yet singular. It couldn't occur without the presence of the other, nor can a particular experience be repeated at a different time, or a different set of persons substituted. The hopes, fears, expectations and experiences of both client and practitioner cannot be excluded – they are part of the back and forth of the encounter. The process also continues after the event: sometimes, says Barbara, 'the connection has been so strong that, even after you've finished the treatment and they've gone home, they can still be having movement within their tissue for two or three days'. Movement can also *precede* treatment, as the experienced client's expectant body decides to start the job ahead of a scheduled appointment, using its memory of the practitioner's hands to anticipate a future touch. In the alternative paradigm, all these possibilities, like that of absent healing, are familiar, grounded as they are in the anatomical schema of the subtle body, which takes the multiplicity, fluidity and inter-implication of bodies as a given. Such a radical intercorporeality is threatening to any philosophical or social system based on a conception of a discrete self, and it is one of the reasons many Westerners – disenchanted (at least partially)[13] with what they see as the rampant individualism of modern culture – seek out and enjoy alternative medicine (see Barcan 2011, forthcoming).

Much of the New Age literature romanticizes this intercorporeality as a harmonious oneness, but there are of course both upsides and downsides to the conception of the body as porous and of touch and healing as reciprocal and intercorporeal. Aside from the obvious question of the possibilities for physical and psychological exploitation that any intimate tactile encounter in private opens up, which are dealt with in the discourses and practices associated with the professionalization of CAM, there are also a set of dangers that belong more to the spiritual paradigm in which bodywork is embedded. Despite the preponderance of romantic discourses about oneness, harmony and transcendence, the healing literature is also replete with its own version of the traditional theme of touch as potentially contaminating, in the form of warnings and guidance about the potential physical, psychological and even spiritual dangers of blending. Most bodyworkers report the potential dangers of the two-way flows between practitioner and client. On a physical level, many report feeling clients' pains or emotions during a treatment and having to learn to distinguish between when they are receiving somatic information about the client's own pains and emotions and when the process is triggering their *own* emotions and bodily responses. Most report the potential for 'contamination' or contagion (commonly known as picking up 'stuff' from your client) and have developed mechanisms (physical, psychological, spiritual or ritual) for avoiding it – keeping the boundaries between self and other distinguishable despite the intercorporeal mingling that goes on in bodywork. Some clients are, apparently, worse than others – more prone to dumping their 'stuff' onto the practitioner and/or to drawing needily from them. As one practitioner put it, 'I believe there are energy grabbers in the world who come and suck all of your energy'. (Perhaps professionals of many stripes – teachers, doctors, academics – can testify to this!)

Despite these physical, psychological and spiritual risks (which are canvassed through a variety of discourses, ranging from spiritual discussions to protocols about professional ethics), the mutuality, reciprocity and intermingling experienced in bodywork (as in many other forms of alternative medicine) are, finally, among the greatest attractions of bodywork, and indeed other forms of CAM, whose regular users prefer it to what they see as the clinical detachment of biomedicine. Enthusiasts of bodywork welcome its ability to open one out to another person and to a larger world co-created with the practitioner. In the words of Fritz Frederick Smith, therapeutic touch is 'alchemical' (2005: 2).

The metaphor of alchemy implies a ritual in which a melange of ingredients is transformed into something greater than its constituent parts. In this, I am reminded of an example used by Merleau-Ponty – that of the conversation. Arguing for an idea of the world and of experience as bigger than our individual capacity to grasp, reflect, translate or explain it, he gives the example of a 'genuine conversation', which, he said, 'gives me access to thoughts that I did not know myself capable of, that I *was* not capable of' (1968: 13). A bodywork encounter can be thought of as this kind of conversation. Bodywork is a singular experience. It is something that happens and cannot be repeated, nor reduced to a definitive 'explanation'. It is familiar and patterned – bodies sink under the weight of familiar hands on familiar tables in familiar rooms, and it is likely to involve similar protocols of preparation, commencement, practitioner style, and to utilize previous sessions as a tacit bodily history and repertoire. Yet it is also profoundly singular, unrepeatable. Like sex, it is the same-but-different – infinite variations on a limited set of bodily themes; it is potentially profound or pleasurable, but not always. Like sex, it can be transformative, creative and seemingly unscripted, or mundane, repetitive and technical. Like meditation, it can 'work' at different degrees and levels, offering experiences of the utmost profundity or completely failing to 'take'. And also, like Merleau-Ponty's concept of the conversation, the bodies in bodywork function as conduits for a knowledge that is bigger than the individual participants – that gives access to thoughts, experiences and sometimes even knowledge itself that one didn't know oneself capable of. For me, the most miraculous and intriguing part of bodywork is the way not just affect, or even intelligence, but sometimes even *information*, can be part of the material that flows back and forth between practitioner and client, and it is to this possibility that I turn next, through an account of my own encounters with reiki.

TACTILE INTELLIGENCE: TOUCH AS A FORM OF KNOWING IN REIKI

I need to state from the outset that I do not know what reiki energy actually 'is', even though it is a familiar part of my life. Within the healing literature, reiki is described as a universal energy, which some writers use almost synonymously with terms like *prana* or *chi*, and others label simply as a 'higher' energy. This energy is, as I have stated earlier, understood as having its own intelligence, so reiki is usually practised as a non-directive modality – that is, the practitioner conceives of herself as a conduit or channel for a healing energy, rather than as a 'healer' per se. Inevitably, though, things are more complicated in practice – both because there are many variants and schools of reiki and also because an ideal of disinterested engagement is, for most of us, hard to live up to. Moreover, the practice of reiki can, for some people, open up an intuitive capacity of hitherto unencountered depth and precision – practitioners and recipients may see images, or pick up information – and so the channelling of energy may become caught up with the relaying of this information, and hence with curiosity, desire or anxiety, and so with affect, ego and power.

How can the flow of information be so readily bound up in the flow of energy? To have any hope of broaching a question as complex as that, we need to start with the idea – axiomatic in reiki, as in so many alternative therapies – of a knowing body. This concept accords with, but exceeds, a conception of the body articulated within phenomenology by Merleau-Ponty. For Merleau-Ponty, the body is not just an object of knowledge but rather the means by which knowledge is possible; it is *in* the world and gives us access *to* the world. His argument that knowledge begins in the body was a radical challenge to much Western philosophy, especially to Cartesianism, which had construed the thinking mind (the *cogito*) as the bedrock of identity, in the famous formulation 'I think therefore I am'. For Merleau-Ponty, a whole form of knowledge – bodily knowledge – precedes the development of cognitive knowledge. This repertoire of preconscious bodily knowledge, which he called the 'primordial layer' of being (1962: 219), is, in the first instance, 'perceptive' rather than conscious (Kruks 1981: 10). It doesn't arise through contemplation or reason but through action in the world (10).

One way to think about bodywork is as an intervention into this accreted bodily knowledge. Changing the primordial schema that orients us in the world and preconditions our conscious thought can be remarkably transformative on a range of levels. Precisely because bodywork intervenes below or before or outside the level of language, the changes it enables can be deep, even foundational. And although the flows are occurring outside of language, they can bring about revelations of many different kinds – some that can be translated into language, many that can't. In the words of Richard Beaumont, energetic techniques 'can facilitate a flow of extraordinary non-mental content that comes from subtle energy changes, and in such moments portals of inspiration and truth are opened that can never be closed' (2005: xi).

But bodywork takes the idea of bodily knowledge further than either a commonsensical idea of bodily experience, or a phenomenological idea of primordial being or, for that matter, a sociological idea of accreted embodied experience (such as Pierre Bourdieu's concept of *habitus*)[14] – all of which it comprehends but exceeds. Drawing on esoteric anatomy (and increasingly on contemporary biomedical science), it extends the concept of bodily knowledge as the 'prethematic sensory grasp' (Leder 1990: 7) that allows us to know and function in the world into a more thoroughgoing and more temporal concept of bodily (or cellular) memory. Almost all alternative therapists believe that in addition to the cognitive memories stored (perhaps) in the mind, the entire body also stores memory. A masseuse I interviewed claimed that the body knows/remembers 'everything':

> The body stores everything. At a cellular and a neural level, it knows everything: emotional memories – sometimes even future stuff … The body remembers everything. Everything.

Theories about how and where the body stores experience and memory vary. The Reichian tradition, which saw 'character' as the functional sum total of past experiences (Reich 1969: 146), inspired a tradition of somatic therapies that focused on structure – muscles and bone – as the mode by which we embody history. Other therapies, drawing on spiritual rather than psychoanalytical precepts, have more esoteric ideas of how experience is stored in the body and (re)activated in everyday life. As we saw in Chapter 3, Yehuda Tagar, drawing on Rudolf Steiner, sees the brain as essentially a processor for memories that are actually stored in the *chi* body and encoded in sound. Smith claims that 'body memory' or 'tissue-held memory' may be held locally or globally within the body (2005: 45). In MFR, the focus is on the fascia, which is seen as undoubtedly implicated, if not in the storage then certainly in the transmission of bodily memory. At one point in my research for this book I got very excited about the fascia. Whereas early bodywork tended, perhaps, to see the muscles and bone as harbouring history, perhaps the fascia might legitimately be the hero of the new digital era – a fitting embodied metaphor for an age that prefers process to structure and which is fascinated by flows of information. The fascia, after all, is by its very nature dispersed, networked and communicative. Criss-crossing the entire body, this 'ubiquitous, elastic-plastic, gluey component … invests, supports and separates, connects and divides, wraps and gives cohesion to the rest of the body' (Chaitow 2001: xii). Perhaps, indeed, the fascia was the embodied unconscious! I ran my theory by the MFR practitioner Tim Bone, who rapidly reminded me that things are never that simple:

> Well, I have to call on non-myo [i.e. non-MFR] and go more into cranial [i.e. CST] on that level. Because I don't believe the physical body of structure and tissue holds consciousness. I believe it's deeper than that. And I'll go down to the cerebro-spinal level, which is fluid, and intelligence, which is even *within* the fluid.

From there, he talked about life force, and embryology, and I was duly reminded that metaphor is our way of making the mysteries of the body legible to new audiences, and creating new ways of seeing, imagining and experiencing it. The network is the metaphor *du jour*, and I am not alone in being excited about the communicative possibilities of the fascia,[15] but the network metaphor will no doubt be replaced as technologies change and science moves on. In the words of another MFR practitioner on whom I tried out my theory, 'It would be lovely to think that it's as simple as that. Yes'.

Still, however it does it, the body does seem to store memory, and when bodies are put in proximity through bodywork, somehow they are catalysed into releasing memories and/or producing or allowing new knowledge. Touch is, it is clear, an effective way to catalyse memory and in the process to glean information from the body. The hands are legitimate instruments in this process (though not the only ones),[16] since one of the skin's functions is as a 'perceptual system', providing 'a wide range of information about the surrounding environment' (Rodaway 1994: 43). Skin is 'a remarkably sensitive interface between our body and the environment and gives us a vast amount of vital information' (1994: 43). This seems commonsensical to us, given how natural touch's role as an authenticating sense (M. Smith 2007: 97) is in our times, unlike in earlier times, where, as noted above, the taking of a case history – even by letter – was considered not only sufficient but indeed superior to tactile examination (Porter 1993: 181–3). Touch was understood as distracting from the truth of the physician's *intellectual* engagement with the illness: 'The physician was a thinker not a toucher' (184–5).

But what if touching could *enable* thinking, bringing about preternatural possibilities for two-way *verbal* communication, in addition to the pathways of non-verbal communication for which it is so valued? In my experience, this is the case:

the structured, ritualized stillness that characterizes therapeutic settings undoubtedly enhances the hands' function as 'an outer brain of man' (Kant, qtd in Merleau-Ponty, 1962: 316). In therapeutic touch, the hands, to recall my earlier metaphor, act as both transmitters and receivers. They transmit heat, and in the case of reiki they are also understood to be transmitting a higher energy that does not come from the practitioner. In everyday life the hands are both touching and touched – they are doing and receiving. So when you switch off the doing, as in reiki, and just sit with them for a long period of time, perhaps their receptive capacities are enhanced.

But receptive to *what?* Bodywork, perhaps more literally than phenomenology, conceives of the body as 'the medium of both thoughts and things' (Young 2002: 28). So what kinds of truths do bodyworkers think can be picked up by sensitive and trained hands? When bodyworkers claim that 'truths are bone deep' (F.F. Smith 2005: 91) or that a craniosacral pulse is 'a signal from the soul' (Milne 1995a: 5), what do they mean? Where do such truths and signals come from? From the client's unconscious, or their stored bodily memories, or from 'spirit'? And to whom do they belong – to the practitioner, or the client, or are they generated only in interaction and hence 'belong' to both of them? And if they are 'true', what kind of truth is at stake? These are big questions indeed, which I cannot answer in either philosophical or physiological terms, but which I have explored in another register – that of experience and lay reflection. It is here that I need to turn to my own experiences of reiki.

Reiki is a difficult object for Cultural Studies to examine, except critically. The same fact that is used within the healing literature to give credence and value to the idea of reiki energy – the observation that the idea of a universal life force and healing energy pervades most cultures – is, within Cultural Studies, more likely to function as proof of its non-existence than its existence – evidence of a historically and culturally pervasive vitalism that modernity has not yet been fully able to stamp out. So it is with some trepidation that I attempt this bridging exercise.

I first did an introductory reiki course in the late 1980s, and it brought about significant questions and provocations. But these were nothing compared to the tumult precipitated by a higher level course I did one year later, which claimed not only to deepen the reiki experience but also to teach a method of absent healing and to open up expanded possibilities for intuitive receptivity. For many, such claims may well seem at best arcane, at worst risible, but for me, they are live issues. For when I did this upper-level reiki training course, the effect was instant and unmistakable. It was as if a tap had been turned on. I could pick up information – detailed, precise, not infrequently involving proper names – not only from people in the room but about people I had never met (who had given permission). One of my initial reactions, and one that has persisted, was amazement at how *technical* this was. I had undergone some mysterious physical process, granted, but I had also 'simply' been *taught* a protocol for connecting at this level – and it had worked. Where were the years of patient spiritual self-development? Where the apprenticeship in a communal context? No, I was the classic Western consumer: I had paid money to do a course, and suddenly I had found myself (seemingly) in possession of some hitherto unrealized ability.

The result was that, three days later, I found myself back in my suburban home wondering what to do with this new-found 'capacity'. I was not completely isolated. The teacher had asked us to commit to practising every day for thirty days after the course to lock the practice in, and I had diligently done this, and the reiki programme I had chosen also involved a degree of community, plugging one into a network of amateur exchange, if one wanted. I took the opportunity and joined a group. I discovered that not everyone had had the same depth or specificity of intuitive awakening that I had experienced. Many of the intellectual and ethical issues that arose I have therefore grappled with alone, though a network of intelligent interlocutors and willing reiki recipients – including many female academics – has allowed me some measure of the 'intersubjective confirmation' that helps distinguish perception from hallucination (Merleau-Ponty, discussed in Kruks 1981: 12).[17]

Now, by this stage, I may have lost some of my readers, who may indeed have already shut the book in disgust, and reached instead for their Richard Dawkins. But over twenty years of reiki practice I have participated in so many incidents of heightened or meaningful perception that it would actually be irrational of me simply to have ignored them. I have no interest in abandoning the call of reason. Rather, I have found myself having to live out Merleau-Ponty's exhortation that the task of the twentieth century is to re-envision what rationality might *be*, by 'attempt[ing] to explore the irrational and integrate it into an expanded reason' (*Sense and Non-Sense*, qtd in Kruks 1981: 12).[18] There have been so many instances of accurate and pointed intuitive perception that I hardly know where to start, nor am I sure how to recount them, having few genres to rely on except that unwelcome staple of the self-help genre, the testimony.[19] No doubt as we continue to rethink reason over the coming century, a task that involves neuroscience as much as it does esotericism, we will develop new genres, but in the meantime, I am stuck with whatever discursive resources are currently to hand. So, here I go, beginning with a list:

- I recall, many years ago, giving reiki to someone I had never met before and picking up that she was having trouble with a woman at her workplace called Margaret. She was.
- More recently, I gave reiki to a good friend of mine because he was in some distress and who wanted to know if I could pick up anything. I picked up that the issue at stake was too intimate for disclosure to me, but that if he wanted

an image for it that would speak meaningfully to him but remain opaque to me, then it would find it in the ornament in the shape of a budgerigar that was sitting on a bench nearby. He burst into tears and described, a little, what the budgerigar signified.

■ Once I was giving some reiki to a man I had only just met, at his request. It was a public setting and I sat next to him with my hands on his shoulder. I am very guarded about giving unbidden information, but the phrase 'You really do have to forgive yourself' insisted itself and I passed it on quietly. Without hesitating a moment he said to me quietly, 'I know, but I just can't let go of the guilt', and he explained a set of circumstances to me that I will not recount here.

■ Another time, I was giving reiki to a young friend when an odd little phrase came up. Always aware of the potential to feel a bit foolish, and always wondering what is worth mentioning or not, I said hesitantly, 'I don't know what this means but I'm picking up that "You really need to decide what you're going to do with that carrot".' He laughed. He had recently been given a barbeque apron decorated with a strategically placed carrot and two onions in unsubtle reference to the genital area. (He had come out, sexually, some time earlier.) This event occurred over a decade ago but the story has stuck with me, since I am attracted to the quirky humour with which something (his unconscious?) had communicated with me. After all, Freud saw jokes, puns and double entendres as the staple of the unconscious, so why should we expect deep intercorporeal experiences to be always earnest or pious? When I recently asked the person involved in this story for permission to recount it, he had no recollection of it at all, though he did recall other images I had picked up in the same session, which I had myself forgotten. He gave permission willingly: 'It's your experience as much as mine', he said.

I could go on, tumbling out story after story, but I fear that I myself am falling for the seductions of the party trick approach against which many spiritual traditions warn. It is an understandable pull: over the years, it is these types of story – involving seemingly verifiable 'facts' – to which I have become attached, as my bridge back to a traditionally conceived reason. And it is tempting to bulwark oneself against external criticism with a roll-call of names and facts. But perhaps the stories that matter most in the end are less these showy instances of neat coincidences than other forms of intelligence that may be equally particular but also more abstract. For example, I recently did reiki for someone I had met socially on a couple of occasions and who suffered from a chronic shoulder pain that had emerged somewhat mysteriously, having not been brought on by injury. She asked for my perceptions and what came through was something like this: 'You are very meticulous and your preferred way of processing information is to ponder it systematically and respond to it before moving on to the next problem. But your everyday life doesn't allow you to operate according to your preferred cognitive mode, and it is as though your mind is clogged up with an enormous backlog of material to process. It is as if your interactions are subject to a kind of time-lag. After many years of this mismatch between your preferred cognitive mode and the rhythms and temporalities of your everyday life, you feel as though your action in the world is blocked.' This, then, is a commentary pitched at that primordial layer of being of which phenomenologists speak, and one that resonated with the recipient. The advice that came through was equally abstract: 'You need to reorganize the network'. None of it, of course, can be proven true by reciting facts, let alone by the randomized trials required by evidence-based medicine, but it rang true for the recipient, and she found it enabling. What interests me is how this is quite abstract – to do with cognition, temporality, intention and agency – yet also very particular, unguessably so.

To a philosophical tradition that has characterized reason as producing facts that are generalizable, repeatable and that exclude context (Lloyd 1984: 50), this individual, contextual, unrepeatable intelligence – produced in its singularity and only available through interaction – is a feminized form of knowledge that falls short of reason as an attainment (Lloyd 1984: Ch. 3). There are, however, exciting scientific discussions opening up – for example, about intention, perception, neuroplasticity and epigenetics – that hint at future explanatory pathways. Simon Ings describes experiments in sensory perception that indicate that 'the mind is not overly fussy where it gets its sensory information from':

> What matters is what 'shape' the information takes. If visual information is received through the skin of your back [e.g. in experiments where cameras are strapped to a person's back], it only takes your brain a couple of hours to start seeing through your back. (2007: 19–20)

Even under these strange experimental conditions, says Ings, the brain is still capable of making discriminations, and doesn't process all the information coming from your back as a messy perceptual oneness: 'If your back starts itching, you won't mistake the itch for a flash of light. The "shape" of an itch is different to the "shape" of a face, and the brain knows how to deal with each' (2007: 20). New fields, like epigenetics and psychoneuroimmunology, and new fields of practice, like integrative medicine, seem at this historical moment full of promise. My highly trained osteopath (himself a neurology researcher) tells me that many of the phenomena I am describing here fall within the purview of cutting-edge neurology. We may not need mysticism at all. In future decades it may well be possible to see how much the new science of perception and intra-corporeal communication accords with the models and explanations that come from traditional esoteric anatomies like the subtle body schemas which, in their own way, provide an explanation for more-than-rational modes of knowing and communicating. In yoga, for example, two of the sheaths or subtle bodies are bodies of thought, which interact with all the other bodies, including the physical body. Conceiving of thought as thoroughly material and materiality itself as inherently energetic in nature, the emphasis in yoga and meditation is less on answering the question 'how is this so?' than on teaching and cultivating the methods of perception that enable practitioners to refine their perception. While I do not personally have the intellectual resources to bridge esotericism and the emerging science, I suspect that contemporary neuroscience and the newly emerging field of epigenetics might ultimately give us a scientific understanding for such phenomena and we may eventually be able to take seriously the question of the materiality of thought (just as the materiality of emotion is currently in view) and the role of intention and trained attention in affecting not only states of mind but also, potentially, our genes (Church 2007).

Meanwhile, the current cultural politics of such possibilities involves fierce battles about legitimation and authority, especially in the face of global concern about the rise of unreason (Barcan 2009a). In this conflicted political domain, how might we value testimony? In seeking to bridge academic and popular discourse, I have found myself with a limited concept bank to think with and precious few genres of writing on which to draw. While Anthropology provides Western academics with both data and genres that are relatively protected from ignominy, Cultural Studies and Sociology have provided me with few guiding stories, having currently few discursive resources for dealing with practices such as reiki. I have read three accounts of reiki coming from these disciplines, only one of which comes from the point of view of an academic who also practises reiki (Garrett 2005 [2001]). Of the other two patient narratives, the first is a decidedly unhappy one: Jackie Stacey's account of visiting a reiki practitioner after having been diagnosed with a form of ovarian cancer, and having had her condition interpreted for her metaphysically and in rigidly normative terms, as resulting from a rejection of her femininity. Stacey's response, understandably enough, is fury and resistance, followed by a biting and convincing feminist analysis. The second account of receiving reiki comes from Mark Paterson, who opens an essay on therapeutic touch and affect with a description of lying on a reiki table and being suddenly overcome by an unexpected cathartic reaction in the form of weeping. He uses this experience as a catalyst for thinking about reiki, and other forms of therapeutic touch, as affective experiences in which one body can catalyse another in what he describes, drawing on the feminist philosophical uptake of Spinoza and Deleuze, as 'the exchange of affective intensities' (2005: 167).

To someone who has been involved in reiki for many years, neither story surprises. The unwilled[20] emotional releases on the table are a familiar response to reiki; but so too, the naive will to interpret – especially in prescriptive, essentialist and normative terms – is also a familiar part of the landscape, especially given the fact that enthusiastic amateurs (like myself) make up the bulk of reiki 'practitioners'. In the face of Stacey's experience of gender essentialism, prescriptive metaphysics and the will to power (whereby all her resistance was understood as a further symptom), it is tempting, certainly, to decide that non-diagnostic touch – touch that 'invites rather than demands', and that is made 'without any intention to change' the other person (Geggus 2004: 67) – is certainly the ethical way to go.

But stories *invite* interpretations, at least in the intellectual heritage of which I am an heir.[21] And reiki throws up no end of stories, and hence no end of fascinating invitations and ethical dilemmas. Indeed, the body seems to have too *much* to say! It positively *hums* with language, to borrow Elizabeth Gilbert's lovely phrase (2006: 340). Its stories are not the universal metaphysical propositions beloved of the New Age, but individual, contextual, dynamic narratives whose abode is not the dictionary but the *encounter*. Perhaps because my original training was in literary criticism, or perhaps, simply, because I find the practice of prescriptive reading abhorrent, I have spent many long years wrestling about both the epistemology and the ethics of these telling stories.

So, for example, as I pick up something I wonder: is this literally true or a symbol? Is it my metaphor or hers? If it's true, is it true now, or in the future, or from a long time ago? And if it's true for her, then what part of her – her everyday self, her unconscious, or some higher self? How best should I think of my role? Conduit? Translator? Crystallizer? Catalyst? Perhaps, after hearing an eminent sceptic speak, I'll be less focused on questions interior to the practice and more prone to shame, and find myself wondering whether I am, rather, a fake, or deluded, or a horribly well-meaning fool. Perhaps, after all, I am making all this up; it might all be gibberish or just a cliché. After all, one could say 'You really need to forgive yourself' to anyone at all and they would have some meaningful response to it; guilt is hardly an unusual experience. On and on goes the mental wrestling: perhaps my inventions don't *need* to be true, as such; perhaps they can be useful, like the interpretations we make of our dreams. In any case, it's not all interpretations. Sometimes it's narration – stories, or pictures. But sometimes it's not that at all – it's *advice*. And not necessarily only about the person on the table. Sometimes, the information comes in chains – with my hand on one person, I pick up information about his/her mother, or brother, or *cat*! How could we meaningfully talk of giving permission when one body gives access to so many others? And if one were doing this professionally, what then? After all, informed consent is the cornerstone of medical ethics; in the UK, for example, 'medical' treatment without consent constitutes an assault (Bensouilah 2005: 138).

As someone who has allowed herself to flail about in this murky landscape, for me each experience begets yet more questions. Are there different levels of significance in what one can pick up? How can you tell what is good information and what isn't – what is accurate and what isn't, what matters and what doesn't, what should be spoken and what not? Perhaps some of the flow of information is really something like Freud's detritus of the day and other parts are more like the repressed or, even more mysteriously, some 'message' from elsewhere. If the hands *do* provide knowledge beyond that of physical sensations, then in the reiki context it is certainly not in the empirical, unreflective, unexamined way theorized from Kant on, as a 'direct, unreflected, physically proximate comprehension of the world' (qtd in M. Smith 2007: 100). Rather, it is inextricably caught up in the dilemmas, uncertainties and politics of interpretation.

Fortunately, and fittingly, not all this rumination takes place inside my head; rather, the reception and transmission of information has its own tactile dimensions. I 'pick up' (a metaphor both tactile and technological) lots of information when I do reiki, but I actually need to concentrate quite hard to do this, and in any case it comes to me most fluidly when I speak the information aloud. Although I can hold a perception silently for some time – usually while I am deciding whether I ought to speak it or not – the holding blocks any ongoing perception. Mostly, then, I need to speak in order to know; the information comes to me *in and as* a flow. In that sense, I am not really able to know very much at all, unless the recipient has given permission for me to start the flow by speaking. Moreover, there are different physical sensations associated with different types of information. In Chapter 5 I will describe a clairvoyant who told me that she gets unmistakable bodily sensations when her intuition, in her words, 'drops in':

> Everybody gets their intuition in lots of different ways. But the way it happens for me, it's like a touch. It's like your whole body becomes alive. I get a feeling going all the way down my back and it's like goose bumps and it gets so strong.

Sensation for her is itself a form of information. I have something similar: lots of different parts of my mind are active, but there are occasions where the flow just *streams out* and the whole sensation is quite distinctive. Then I 'know' (that is, I believe) that whatever is happening is something somehow stronger or truer or more significant. Since information flows through me in/as sensation, I need to remember that it flows through the recipient in the same way. In Chapter 2 I noted the intermeshing of eye and hand that characterizes much bodywork, but in these interactions in which I speak what I perceive, it is touch and *sound* that interweave. My interpretations are spoken as words that course through the body in its deeply relaxed state – not just ideas about the person but a sensory flow through his/her body. This makes the ethical questions even more serious, since whatever one says has the potential to move through the body of the person as one speaks it.

So, what are possibilities of an ethical practice of reading the body? I asked a masseur who offers a service she calls 'psychic massage' (in which she recounts what she picks up as she massages the body), 'What does a client's body know?' She replied: 'What can you pick up from them? Their body stores everything'. In the slippage between the two questions – 'what might a body know?' and 'what can be known from a body?' – lies a whole ethical drama, which I have spent two decades thinking about, without resolution. Here is a banal distillation of some of these threads of thought into a series of 'options'.

Option one. Don't do it at all. Leave narrativization, interpretation, and reading well alone. Stick to the body; stay with the body. There is considerable ethical merit to this. Many practitioners advocate non-diagnostic, non-ideational bodywork practice. (Smith, as we have seen, explicitly calls ZB non-diagnostic and says it should be performed with minimal talk (2005: 2)). This is especially understandable in the North American context, where talking therapies have such dominance. Critics of psychoanalysis or talk-based psychotherapy see it as yet another way of distancing oneself from the body and from emotion – interpolating a defensive bank of talk between the person and the experience of the body. Narration, interpretation, analysis are just yet more ways of evading stillness – interesting ways, certainly, but ultimately a form of defence and even interference. Thus Smith, in response to a client who recounts a dream, says:

> I'm not a dream analyst and I don't believe we or you need to figure out the dream. Just let things flow through you. Let things stay in motion. (2005: 23)

Many practitioners believe that 'the deep truth of clear touch' (Beaumont 2005: xi) will do its own work, without need for help from the analytical brain or the defensive ego. Professional bodyworkers in particular often believe that it is more ethical and more important (and, no doubt, more professionally feasible and sustainable) for the client to process this flow of 'information' below the level of consciousness and narrativization – for it to remain non-mental context. In a bodywork treatment

> the client often has a transformative experience – seeing for *himself*, at the level of his 'deepest presence', what really troubles him. This revelation to the self may have more power to it than would the same observation from the most skilled outsider. (Milne 1995a: 5, original emphasis)

(Foucauldians reading this will undoubtedly nod in frustrated agreement, for Foucault has taught us much about the power of self-constitution that imagines itself to be revelation. But at this point in the chapter, I have bade a temporary farewell to Foucault. After all, an insistently Foucauldian reading can, in its own way, potentially be as prescriptive or programmatic as any other intellectual framework, when mechanically applied (see Barcan 2008)).

Part of me agrees, utterly, with the idea that narration by the practitioner is an imposition and admires the restraint, discipline and patience involved in rejecting it as a therapeutic practice. But another part feels that this is to look a quite fascinating gift-(horse) in the mouth. If the body is capable of giving out such precise information – and another person capable of picking it up and, moreover, this technique can sometimes be quickly *learnt* or acquired – surely this is of such interest and import that it is quite perverse not to learn more about how this happens? It is possible – quite possible – that my curiosity is spiritual under-development and that those practitioners who adhere to a practice of non-interpretation are, quite simply, wiser and less ego-driven than I. After all, the aim of meditation is not only to still the mind but also to quieten down the body's language-hum. Should we learn to hush this hum or to *listen* to it, I wonder? It may well be the case that it is both more therapeutically effective and more ethically sound to avoid narration. If this appears to return the body to its all too familiar role as mute counterpart to the mind, perhaps it doesn't matter, and bodywork should, after all, be about catalysing and *using* bodily intelligence rather than translating the body into narrative. Perhaps the obsession with verbalization is simply a Western, ego-driven, analytical thing – at best unnecessary, at worst deluded, dangerous and counterproductive. So much for option one, then: dead-end.

Possibility two is to read the body, but recreationally, not therapeutically. That is, groups of interested friends might do it, but keep it divorced from situations of serious therapeutic or medical import. This, on the surface, seems a reasonable response – but the division into harmless recreation and humourless healing is untenable. Who can know in advance whether the question of what to do with one's carrot will cause grief or merriment? In any case, the healing energy itself and the intimate intercorporeal context have their own trajectories that cannot be willed or known in advance.

Possibility three is to do it but with care, explicit permission-asking and ongoing negotiation. This option situates us in the terrain of spiritual traditions, in which the imperative to self-cultivate is usually contextualized within a community and an ethic of caution and care. To this, my intellectual training asks me to add a special and serious caution about the formulaic metaphysics that so permeates New Age thought.

For there is no shortage of testimony about the potentially damaging impact of both normative interpretations and popular exhortations about how serious illness should be managed. Having experienced cancer, Jackie Stacey says that from the patient's point of view, 'It is impossible to have cancer and not be seduced by the power of [the] cultural narratives' (1997: 13) in which it is enmeshed – illness narratives of fortitude, will-power and the heroic triumph of good over evil. Despite this, she doesn't argue that we can or should do with narratives and metaphors per se – rather, that we need to be attentive to their politics and their effects. Likewise, when faced with bodies that throw up such wondrous stories, jokes and wisdom, neither can I, as an amateur practitioner, forgo the lure of narrativization. I cannot turn my back on the infinite possibilities of stories, symbols, puns and even prophecies that are generated, mysteriously, when hands meet bodies. But I only do it when people want such shared exploration, and even then, only cautiously. I am slower to speak these days, and since I only 'know' through speaking itself, I am also more modest in my 'knowing'. Over the years I have learnt to be more cautious, more discerning, more hesitant to convert sensations to words, in acting as the body's 'translator'.

But in any case the stories of the budgie and the carrot remind me that the practitioner is not always the one with the power to unlock the code, and that often the interpretive process can be one of dialogue not imposition, or indeed, of private contemplation, leaving the practitioner as an uncomprehending catalyst. In the case of the story about the budgie, the feeling that the recipient did not want or need to explain his story came through *as part of* the flow of information, and the recipient was able to process the image in private, sharing with me only those parts of the explanation that he wanted to.

But there is yet another complication. So far, most of my stories can be explained (away) via notions of a kind of intense but localized intercorporeality – bodies articulating, anticipating, responding, projecting, absorbing, blending and communicating with, into and for each other. But what if touch is not always direct or intimate – not a matter of fingers melting into the face of a partner but of connections made over distances? What if one can be trained to use other forms of connection – ritualized permissions, proxy objects, protected expressions – to make connections with strangers, dispersed in space, elsewhere in time? These, then, would be intercorporeal blendings less familiar, less visible, altogether less *reasonable*, than the intense but localized 'exchanges and mutual transfers between therapist and client' (Paterson 2005: 164–5) that are a recognizable part of therapeutic touch. Then, touch would no longer be the closest sense, as I claimed at the outset. Or rather, such possibilities would require us to rework our very notions of proximity and distance, presence and absence.

What, moreover, if the communicative possibilities I have just been discussing were also available at a distance, and what if such information could not plausibly be wished away as imagined, fantasized – what, for example, if it involved proper names, facts, times, places? What if you could produce verifiable facts – write them down, record the time of their arrival – for/with/about people you had never met? Surely, at that point, rationality would consist not in denying or evading such troublesome events, but in scrutinizing them. In contrast to what many might think, to *ignore* them might sometimes be to be run by emotion – to be anxious, defensive, embarrassed – rather than acting from some supposedly dispassionate reason. In these circumstances, seemingly strange, yet experienced by many, one could even argue that rationality consists of being unafraid to look them in the face and to wrestle with them and to wonder how they come about, and what they mean. This would require us to see new questions not as a threat but as a gift (Rubik 1995: 39).

Such an event occurred to me. It involved just such an irrefutable catalogue of proper names and events, recorded in writing some hours before the events actually occurred, involving some people I had never met, and picked up *in absentia*. It stands clear in my memory. For this was a threshold event, one that marked an irrevocable borderline between being someone who can shrug or dismiss or evade or scoff and someone who could no longer indulge in such luxuries. Crossing that line doesn't mean I know what happened. It means that, like it or not, I had been invited on an adventure, one which it would be ungrateful, ungenerous and, ultimately, anti-intellectual of me not to pursue.

So, I had crossed a line – not from ignorance to certainty, dogma or even belief – but into a space of possibility, conjecture, rumination and struggle. And of course, since I am a Humanities academic, being willing to countenance engagements with such possibilities – which are popular in an embarrassing, rather than a cool, way – inevitably brought me into a space of shame and vulnerability. For the human sciences, as Serres provocatively asserts, involve a constant struggle to find the place from which one cannot be attacked, a game which, for him, involves an element of duplicity (2008 [1985]: 43). The critical method, he asserts, is also hypocritical, involving 'the worst kinds of double dealing, whether from beneath the table or behind your back' (43). In a scathing condemnation that anticipates Sedgwick's later critique of 'paranoid' reading strategies (2003), Serres criticizes the staple Humanities argument structure that involves countering any claim with a critical 'yes, but':

> The hypocritical method consists in always placing oneself behind, and this immediately creates a queue. One must therefore get quickly behind the last person in the queue, stand behind the last one whose back can still be seen,

then hide one's own back for fear of being caught in turn by someone who has understood the game. (43)

In revealing my own implication in practices of scant academic respectability, I am saving the sceptical or annoyed reader the trouble of placing themselves in that line, for I present my open front to them, a posture both vulnerable and defiant. Like the bodywork client, I am prepared to front the dangerous world in the interests of openness to its possibilities. Being upright – one of the distinctive features of human embodiment – involves presenting an open front, at once receptive and vulnerable, to the world. This makes the front of the body a prime site for meanings and experiences of connection: 'The front of us is an extended surface of contact and connection. This is what we present to the world' (Keleman 1981: 23).

Still, I would rather interest you than defy you, and deciding how to write about this threshold event, where I picked up events, names and places, in writing, before they occurred, has inevitably called up dilemmas about one of the key themes of this chapter – the wisdom of revelation. On the one hand, perhaps a detailed recounting of this threshold event could convince you, as it did me, that these things are at least worth thinking about. And I would be in plentiful, if not exactly academically respectable, company, since my tale would be an example of what Arlie Russell Hochschild calls the 'magnified moment' – the exemplary moment from which, in the women's self-help genre, a moral hangs (2003: 16).

But I don't want to try too hard to prove anything to you, the reader, because I know I can't. After all, if I were you, I'd be wondering if I were lying, or misremembering, or deluded, or fulfilling unconscious desires, or caught up in a collectively generated fantasy. No big reveal – no final full emergence from the closet[22] – can counter those doubts. Even though it is hard to resist the showy proof, the big finish, the final unveiling, I cannot go on with the show. I am far too implicated in the politics and genres of revelation – and have thought far too much about nakedness (Barcan 2004)! – to believe that the striptease reveals the naked truth. The event convinced me, utterly, that something very interesting indeed was going on. Would telling all its details convince you, or would it just devalue my magnified moment? My story is precious to me, and like the man with the budgie, I don't want to share.

So, in the end, my show turns into a no-show. Having just stepped out of a closet, I have chosen to leave the details of my threshold story, my 'magnified moment', back there in the closet – which can function both as a sacred space to be kept free from prying eyes and as a cultural repository for that which is excessive or shameful, or threatens order. After all, my story would not have convinced anyone who didn't already believe that things might be a little bit more mysterious – a little bit more full of *possibility* – than a narrow understanding of reason would have us believe, and

I have learnt that one person's sacred moment is another person's nightmare, joke or cliché. The other participants and close bystanders in my threshold story have, I know for sure, forgotten the event. But my story won't be lonely back there; the closet is a good place to find lively companions.

5 THE SIXTH SENSE: INTUITION

[W]hat is socially peripheral is often symbolically central.

Stallybrass and White, *Politics and Poetics of Transgression*

I finished the last chapter at the door of the closet. In this final chapter, I walk inside it, via a study of two sacred healing techniques: spiritual healing and medical clairvoyance. The chapter focuses on perceptual questions (what practitioners claim to perceive); philosophical questions (the metaphysical underpinnings of the practices, and the concept of intuition on which they rely); and political questions (the gendered politics of intuition).

These therapies are organized around a putative 'sixth sense' – intuition – that is believed to be accessed via clairvoyance or some other form of sensitivity. Those who believe in the existence of this specialized form of intuition may see it in different ways: as a very particular gift (an aspect of the practitioner's own being that is fundamentally given rather than learnt); or an innate human potential more developed in some people than in others; or a capacity that can be enhanced through training, practice or experience.

Spiritual healing and medical clairvoyance have several things in common. The first is that they are sacred healing techniques: they involve interaction with spiritual forces in the form of spirit guides, angels or other otherworldly entities. A second thing in common is that they rely on specialized forms of perception or intuition – what might commonly be called clairvoyant or psychic abilities – for diagnosis and/or healing. The third feature they share is that they centralize the role of communication. The giving and receiving of information is not purely functional, but an active and central part of the 'therapy'. In this, these practices, though they are undoubtedly more socially marginal than many of the therapies discussed in this book, are conceptually quite central to alternative medicine. They represent a stark form of the metaphysics underpinning alternative medicine more broadly, which centralizes the body's expressive and communicative possibilities. In the techniques examined in this chapter, healing is understood as resulting from a complex communicative interplay between spiritual guides, the practitioner and the client. The practitioner's body is understood as a channel for 'higher energies', while that of the client functions as an expressive medium, one capable of giving up information not only in the form of sensations, reactions, movements and transformations, but also in the form of specific pieces of information.

As we have seen, in alternative metaphysics, the entire body, from the toenails to the scalp and beyond, is always in unseen communication with the rest of the body, with others and with the environment. In the therapeutic context, this potentially infinite flow of information, picked up, channelled or relayed between client, healer and the spirit world, is understood to have diagnostic, catalytic and even curative functions. Since information is conceived of as a form of energy, understood in more than conventionally physical ways (Rubik 1995: 38), these transactions are understood as simultaneously a kind of complex information relay and a movement or transfer of energy across a dispersed and mostly invisible energetic network. Energy and information flows are thus not two separate, parallel channels; rather, they are conceived of as completely intertwined. Intuitive healing modalities thus provide a good opportunity to consider Judith Fadlon's question of the relation between the metaphor of an immaterial body and current technological arrangements. 'The question to be addressed', she asks, 'is whether the narrative of CAM that focuses on the notion of a dematerialising body, defined by energy, *chakras*, auras, and the vital force, points to a new phase in the relationship between the body and society' (2004: 72).

Certainly, a study of intuitive medicine has much to suggest about the relationship between gender and knowledge. For medical intuition and spiritual healing are even more highly feminized than other forms of CAM. The vast majority of psychics and clairvoyants are women, as are their clients, and intuition itself is popularly understood as a feminine sense. The hidden nature of the sacred medical system makes it hard to formally confirm its client demographic, and the social class of the clientele would be especially hard to work out.[1] But the question of gender and age is quite clear-cut. Says the clairvoyant Mary:

> Well, I know the majority of [my clients] are women and they're usually from early twenties through to … mostly the twenties and the thirties … and sometimes I get people older than that – forties, fifties, sixties. But after about seventy, people aren't interested in seeking out this, although I have had some. But mostly they're in that younger – twenties, thirties, forties – age group, and then it sort of declines from that point on.

One of the commonly reported motivating factors for taking up alternative medicine – the failure of other options – appears to be true of Mary's clientele:

> I get a lot of people coming because they've tried the conventional medical routes and a lot of them have even done the alternative medical searches and they've not got themselves sorted out. So then finally they hear about me ... This is the end-of-the-line kind of thing for most people.

This hints at medical clairvoyance as the fringe of the fringe – located at the edge even of alternative medicine. This may be true in systemic terms, but not necessarily in the experience of individuals, for there may well be people for whom it is such a naturalized practice that it is their medicine of first resort. A study of marginal therapeutic techniques matters, therefore, not only because of the segment of the population who make use of spiritual healing or medical clairvoyance (whose numbers are hard to gauge), but also because it illuminates the fundamental process of world-making and 'paradigm surfing' (Barcan 2009a) that characterizes postmodern pluralist societies. Moreover, sacred intuitive healing techniques push to the limits the question discussed in Chapter 1 of how to model and regulate the relations between different medical systems.

While intuitive healing techniques may appear to be at the fringe of the CAM scene, a number of the pragmatic, philosophical, conceptual and political questions they provoke are similar to those posed by alternative therapies generally. Intuitive medicine shares, and pushes to the limit, many of the qualities of alternative medicine more broadly. As both the closet logic dramatized at the end of the previous chapter and the epigraph from Stallybrass and White (1996) suggest, practices that might not be highly visible can still operate as a conceptual or symbolic core. In the case of intuitive medicine, medical doctor and spiritual healer Daniel Benor considers that the holistic approach and underlying principles of spiritual healing are so fundamental to complementary therapies that, rather than constituting a fringe, they can be considered to offer 'a unifying theory and a unifying influence' in the field (1995: 237).

Although this book makes few explicit claims about the medical effectiveness of any of the therapies I discuss, I have made clear my general appreciation of them as bodily and therapeutic encounters. So in this chapter I need to begin by stating that I have visited one of the medical clairvoyants I interviewed in the role of client as well as in that of researcher. It would be an intellectual sham to pretend that I made these visits with a sense of curiosity, excitement, nervousness and hope that was confined to my identity as a researcher. On the contrary, and obviously, I brought many aspects of my being to these sessions and found them both interesting and beneficial. Given the 'feminist research imperative of attending to the relationship between the researched and the researcher' (Reger 2001: 606), it is important, ethically and intellectually, for me to declare that I now consider medical intuition – under certain circumstances and only with a particular practitioner – to be a part of my own personal repertoire of available medical techniques, one I use quite infrequently but have nonetheless found useful.

I have not, however, cast discernment to the winds. Rather, the intellectual interest and the medical-regulatory dilemma of these practices lie precisely in their particularity, fallibility and amenability to the worst kinds of deception and self-deception. One or two practitioners I would willingly place my trust in; some others, I would never dream of consulting. This is the practical problem posed by a commodified and medically pluralist landscape, in which the various types of medicine are based on different and often competing knowledge forms, and in which practitioners vary greatly in skill, knowledge, training, experience, maturity and professional ethics. Medical intuition makes starkly visible the very real regulatory dilemmas of a medically pluralist environment, since its underlying medical paradigm could not be more different from that of biomedicine, nor the case of practitioner training and regulation more difficult. So, while practitioners of *all* forms of medicine and therapy are marked by great differences in skill, training and sensitivity, the basis of the knowledge claims underpinning medical intuition – in an unverifiable, possibly unteachable, possibly imaginary, perceptual skill – makes it particularly unamenable to regulation.

This lack of amenability to scrutiny and regulation is undoubtedly a very real problem for those interested in the formal control of health care and for consumers wanting to move safely and effectively across different medical options. Nonetheless, from a social analyst's point of view, it is fascinating. How can a medical system based on a radically different 'curative cosmology' (M. Stacey 1986: 10, n. 2) from that of biomedicine function alongside it? Or, as the anthropologist Elizabeth Povinelli asks in relation to the anthropology of radical difference:

> How do incommensurate worlds emerge and how are they sustained in their incommensurability? In other words, how is the inconceivable conceived? (2001: 320)

I have explored these types of systemic questions about the coexistence of different medical worlds in depth elsewhere (Barcan 2009b) in an analysis of spiritual healing and medical clairvoyance as a quasi-clandestine yet publicly available network of sacred healing practices in complex relationship with mainstream medicine. These practices are both widespread and hidden, legal yet largely outside medical regulation, sacred, yet also recreational, consumerist and 'medical'. They are based on the antithesis of a number of core principles underpinning Western medicine, supplanting rationalism and empiricism with non-, extra- or supra-rational concepts like those of the 'gift', intuition and spiritual guidance. And yet they nonetheless operate in a relationship with orthodox medicine that is much more complex than simple oppositionality. The clairvoyant's consulting room can be considered a 'heterotopic' space (Foucault 1986) – that is, a place that is set aside somewhat from the rules of the outside world; that allows different times and spaces to coexist within it; and whose rules invert many of those of the outside world. Such spaces are not sealed off completely from the outside world – they are isolated but penetrable (1986: 26). As we will see, there are interesting hidden pathways between the clairvoyant or healer's rooms and the medical mainstream.

Exploring and bridging incommensurate worlds involves, in part, struggling to find a language in which to write the incommensurate – a language that is neither *of* the 'other' world, nor a purely external commentary on it. As a writer it has taken me a long time to find such a voice. It seemed to me at first that there were only two available discourses in which to write about these practices – a language *from* that world (e.g. a New Age discourse), or a sceptical, critical, and, if not derisory, then at least ironic, voice that keeps its writer safe. A third possibility – the expository language of anthropology – seemed, for complex reasons, less available for the analysis of middlebrow, culturally appropriated practices used especially by white middle-class women. Although I would now see a neutral analytic voice as an available option, it was one I ultimately decided not to take. I am not intellectually or ethically content to hide behind it. I took some inspiration (and indeed courage) from the anthropologist Paul Stoller's (2004) personal account of his experience of lymphoma, in which he describes matter-of-factly and analytically his use of some techniques of Songhay sorcery as a form of healing, solace and inspiration. Having, however, no anthropological training to tacitly legitimate my own interest in energetic and intuitive medicine, I still struggled to find a voice that was analytical without being 'neutralizing' (Reger 2001: 611), and that could allow space for different articulations of belief, scepticism and dissent, including my own often fractured and contradictory responses. This search is all the more important since the struggle to think and speak about stigmatized practices is, in fact, part of their very functioning.

For the relatively marginal practices described in this chapter may well be experienced with uncertainty and ambivalence by some clients. Certainly, in wider social debate they are bound up in particularly intense and volatile affective webs of suspicion, fear, doubt, anger, derision, shame, curiosity, joy or hope. The wide range of emotions these practices commonly arouse (sometimes within the one person!) points, in fact, to the cracks, fissures and unreconciled contradictions that always characterized the modern experience of reason and to the diversity of ways of being and thinking that characterize any late-modern society. Accordingly, in this chapter, as in the previous one, I have left visible some of the signs of my own intellectual struggles, writing what the Australian writer and critic Robert Dessaix (1998) calls an 'including' text. The including voice is, he says, 'more openly emotional and personal (emphasising vulnerability)' (1998: 124). It respects the reader by levelling with him or her, rather than trying to bluff. I didn't want to produce a polished, invulnerable account – a shiny surface that can rebuff all attacks. Rather, I want to *stage the struggle*, since it is of philosophical, political and indeed, in this context, medical importance. For as I noted in Chapter 1, almost all CAM clients use a variety of CAM forms and combine them with biomedicine. In doing so, they move between different practices, practitioners, medical systems, body models, concept bases and language forms. Some of these practices may be paradigmatically almost incommensurable with orthodox medicine and yet there are plenty of people – myself included – who move between them. How do both practitioners and clients negotiate radically different medical systems, often simultaneously, and the radically different conceptual bases of these systems (Barcan 2009b)? These paradigmatic tensions, negotiated privately, with close friends or within communities of practice, constitute the context in which spiritual healing and medical intuition operate as working medical practices. Moreover, they connect with broader social tensions. Are we seeing a growth in popularity of a system built on forms of knowledge traditionally associated with the feminine, and if so, how will these opposing epistemologies be operationalized as workable 'alternatives' or 'complements'? Is it realistic to imagine these secret sacred healing techniques becoming mainstream, and if so, how desirable might that be?

In this chapter, I draw again on my interviews with clairvoyants and healers to canvass some of the epistemological questions about perception and the nature of the knowledge produced in intuitive medicine. For example, what do medical psychics claim they actually *see*? Is it like a movie, or a photograph, or a dream? Do they see in black and white or in colour? When they hear voices, is it the same as hearing a real voice? Do spirits have accents? These questions about the perception of reality are tied in with broader systemic and political questions about how much credence and faith we place in accounts of non- or supra-rational perception. Since I am interested in contradictions, cracks and overlaps between systems, logics and practices, I have deliberately let stand certain linguistic disjunctions without attempting to regularize or resolve them. My decision, for example, to bring into unholy assembly sacred, professional, neoliberal and medical discourses ('healer', 'practitioner', 'therapy', 'client', 'patient') is a deliberate mobilization of the current cultural context into which ancient practices have been brought and reinvented – a context at once consumerist, bureaucratic, medical and sacred.

The central role these practices accord to the practitioner's own perceptual capacities makes her role particularly powerful, whatever her commitment to a model of client empowerment. In keeping with the alternative medical philosophy, these practitioners still typically consider themselves channels for healing rather than instruments of it, but the exclusiveness implied in the concept of a gift, and its unamenability to testing, means that questions of power, authority and ethics run especially deep. Is the medical clairvoyant to be thought of as a medical practitioner, a CAM therapist, a spiritual adviser, a guru, a special friend or a particular form of counsellor? Of course, to many people, she is none of these things – rather, she is a charlatan, fraud, self-deceiver or fool. Since the rational critique of clairvoyance is commonplace, I do not elaborate it directly; rather, I look at how it functions in relation to the practices it simultaneously excludes and constitutes. For the commonsensical debunking of clairvoyance inevitably underpins these practices, helping to structure, for example, the legal status of clairvoyant practice, its forms of professionalization, and clients' experiences, which may be marked by ambivalence, distrust or excitement. The taken-for-granted nature of the rational critique also means that I have not deemed it necessary to litter the text with caveats such as scare quotes or qualifiers ('so-called', 'allegedly', 'putative') but have largely described the practices using a language internal to their own logic and suppositions. This does not mean I tacitly agree with (all) the claims made; it means that a rational critique is self-evident. This is not the same thing, however, as arguing that reason is a singular, simple opposite to intuition. On the contrary, one of my interests in this chapter is precisely how clairvoyance does not simply oppose a monolithic idea of reason. Rather, in its more elaborated formulations, the New Age metaphysics espoused by my interviewees is often based on something more subtle and more complex than a simple valorization of intuition over reason, or even a model of complementarity, common though that is. Rather than seeing intuition in dualistic terms as the feminized and denigrated other to reason, the subtle body model that informs their practice imagines *all* forms of knowing (cognition, intuition, emotions) as inherently embodied and as located less in a simple hierarchy of value than in a complex matrix of ways of knowing. Cultivating intuition thus involves learning to discriminate intuition not just from rational thought but also from *all* elements of 'the mental world' (Shumsky 1996: 168) – beliefs, ideologies, subconscious fears, the 'ego-chatter of the surface mind' (168) – as well as from other-worldly communications, such as those coming from 'astral entities' (174). It is precisely such a vision of a manifold anatomy inextricably enmeshed in a complex mix of cognitive and perceptual faculties and situated in a wider cosmos that makes the cultivation of intuition in spiritual traditions as difficult and lifelong a task as the cultivation of intellect is in rationalist institutions such as the academy.

The chapter begins with some definitions and descriptions of spiritual healing and medical clairvoyance. I then consider the ethics and gender politics of marginalized (yet popular) knowledge practices, via a discussion of, in turn: information relay;

sensory perception; the understanding of intuition at the core of these practices, and its relation to reason; and the question of gendered knowledge. The chapter concludes with a consideration of how the relationship between these systems has been modelled, and the gendered politics of 'complementarity'.

INTUITIVE MEDICINE AND SPIRITUAL HEALING: DEFINITIONS AND DESCRIPTIONS

As I have already suggested, it is impossible to separate out intuitive/spiritual medicine as a discrete branch of alternative medicine: first, because it shares so many core precepts (e.g. body models) with other alternative therapies; second, because it shares healing mechanisms – intuition and the sacred – with many other therapies (Benor 1992: 44); and third, because, as we have repeatedly seen, alternative therapies are characterized by a high degree of combination, hybridization and customization by both practitioners and clients. In any case the semi-clandestine nature of these practices means that many of them are advertised euphemistically (e.g. 'intuitive counsellor') or are masked behind other, more recognized, disciplines in which a practitioner may have been trained (e.g. homeopathy or naturopathy). From the outside it can be hard to know just what is being performed under a particular name. So there can be no clear-cut taxonomy whereby spiritual healing, for example, might be separated distinctly from psychic healing, or from medical intuition, or even from seemingly more remote practices like kinesiology or reiki. Moreover, intuition may play a significant role in many other CAM modalities and indeed also within orthodox medicine. Many biomedical practitioners allow a role for intuition and/or the sacred in their work, whether it be the GP's hunch, the nurse's gut feeling or the physician who also prays for his or her patient.

From within this broad spectrum of intuitive or sacred practice in medical or therapeutic contexts, this chapter focuses on only a very small subset of sacred healing techniques, both of which are commodified forms of healing found in the mainstream of consumer culture. In industrialized societies, traditional healing practices of many kinds continue to be practised; in multicultural societies, indigenous and migrant communities often actively continue traditional medicine, usually in combination with the dominant medical system. But in this chapter, my focus is on commodified forms of spiritual and intuitive healing, which excludes many forms of sacred medicine and of communal religious practice, however widespread they may be in contemporary Western multicultural societies.[2] Even within this narrowed focus, some practices have been excluded for reasons of scope (e.g. I have not considered the New Age appropriation of shamanism). I have limited my study to medical intuition and spiritual healing (known by some as 'psychic healing').

Medical intuition is the use of clairvoyance for the purposes of diagnosis and/or healing. While all clairvoyants are regularly asked to give information about illnesses, not all specialize in health. Those who do may call themselves medical intuitives, medical clairvoyants or medical psychics, or other more euphemistic titles like intuitive counsellor. Medical intuitives give a clairvoyant reading of their clients' health, whether in general terms or focused on a particular issue. The client may be present in the room or the process may occur *in absentia* – for example, over the telephone or by email. Physical touch is not required. Medical intuitives carry out intuitive 'diagnosis', whether or not they use orthodox anatomical or medical labels. Some, though not all, also suggest treatment regimes (e.g. by 'prescribing' naturopathic remedies). Some see their central role as the passing on of medical information; others integrate information and healing, e.g. by the use of visualization, which is where it may overlap with spiritual healing.

Spiritual healing is a blanket term for a range of techniques. Daniel Benor, a medical doctor, psychiatrist and spiritual healer, defines spiritual healing as 'the intentional influence of one or more people upon one or more living systems without utilizing known physical means of intervention' (1995: 234). He breaks it down into two main approaches: techniques involving the physical laying on of hands (or hands held slightly above the body), and a hands-off approach using 'focused intent', such as meditation or prayer. Both approaches are often combined with visualizations (such as imagining a cloud of healing light surrounding the patient), and the two approaches (hands-on and -off) may be used in the same session (234). Many spiritual healers work actively with entities from a spiritual realm – guides, spirits, deceased relatives and so on. As with medical intuition, some practitioners may also prescribe naturopathic, homeopathic or essence remedies, especially if they are also formally trained in these fields. In such cases, guidance about what to prescribe may arise spiritually or psychically and/or it may derive from their formal training.

Some practitioners differentiate between psychic and spiritual healing. For those who do, psychic healing involves 'work[ing] with energy in a very deliberate and conscious manner, with awareness of where and how the energy is moved' (MacDonald 1997: 58). Examples might include *chakra* balancing and the channelling of universal energy into the client (MacDonald 1997: 58; Litchfield 1996: 40). Not all practitioners make this distinction. One spiritual healer I interviewed, Regina, didn't see much difference between spiritual, psychic or clairvoyant healing: 'Psychic healing and spiritual healing are really not very separate because you are getting information and you are picking up from the body what's wrong and you are getting guided by spiritual realms to work on different areas.' This definition involves three things: the invocation or intervention of a spiritual realm; some form of diagnosis (in a broad rather than strictly medical sense); and some pointer towards treatment or healing.

Some practitioners call their work simply 'healing' (rather than spiritual healing), perhaps in order to sidestep or de-emphasize the role of the spiritual in their practice. Daniel Benor, for example, argues that healing has 'been confused with ritual, religious and magical practices, as it is often given within these contexts' (1992: 45). Though he calls himself a spiritual healer, at least in some contexts, much of his writing, published in journals such as *Complementary Therapies in Medicine*, is couched in social-scientific language rather than in spiritual discourse. Spiritual entities or guides, for example, are not mentioned, even while studies exploring the effectiveness of distant healing, prayer or intuitive diagnosis are cited. This seeming omission – talking about spiritual healing without talking about spirits – is made possible by the fact that the spiritual and intuitive healing practices in question are underpinned by the energetic conception of the body and thus they might equally well be characterized as forms of energy medicine (like reiki or kinesiology) as spiritual medicine. Benor's particular bent is on understanding energy medicine as an essentially scientific medicine, one whose acceptance has been limited by cultural bias and the lack of a conventional theory to explain it (1992: 44). His research output includes meta-studies of research into spiritual healing and energy medicine, in which previously published claims are held up to scrutiny and subjected to the rigours of social scientific assessment. (See, for example, his four-volume meta-study *Healing Research: Holistic Energy Medicine and Spirituality* (1993).) His long-term project is to critique and query the biomedical traditionalism that has resulted in the medical community 'taking a more tentative position than the evidence necessitates' (Dreher, in Benor 1992: 45). Thus, whether or not Benor is personally comfortable with a spiritual discourse, he argues that in any case:

> The impressive body of research which demonstrates significant effects on enzymes, tissue cell cultures, bacteria, yeasts, plants and animals shows that healing is a natural process which need not be dependent upon faith or religious belief for its effects. (1992: 45)

For many, the energy paradigm means that the distinction between spirits and energy is meaningless. Spirits are understood, precisely, *as* energies in a hierarchically organized cosmos.

In this, the subtle body model is crucial. Benor uses it as a challenge to scientific rationality to expand its concepts of energy, arguing that Western society commonly rejects as unreal or immaterial that which cannot be measured with mechanical, electromagnetic or particle physics instruments, rather than accepting it as 'representing a different class of phenomena for which the measuring instruments of the reductionist, material world are inappropriate' (1995: 235). Like so many writers on the energetic body, Benor sees quantum physics as pointing the way to a scientific understanding of the workings of energy medicine, intentionality and absent heal-ing (1992: 46). As noted in Chapter 3, the paradigm shift from Newtonian to quan-tum physics is almost ritually cited by writers in the field as providing the missing link between traditional energetic concepts of the body and modern science and as mandating a new or revived concept of the body as an energy system (see also Barcan 2011, forthcoming). In many writers, the ritual invocation of quantum physics is less than convincing. This is hardly surprising, given the specialization needed to understand it in any depth.[3] The intellectual difficulty involved in making convinc-ing bridges between esotericism and contemporary science lies less, it seems to me, in the intrinsic plausibility or otherwise of the connection than in the degree and number of specializations required to make such connections convincingly, as well as in the question of an appropriate language in which to write and think them. At this point in the trajectory of energy medicine in the modern West, then, the dominant popular discourse is still one of spirit, with a passing nod to quantum physics and, more recently, to psychoneuroimmunology, neuroscience and epigenetics. While it is not impossible to imagine a distant future in which these currently marginal techniques are medically mainstreamed, and while it may be that spirituality might eventually disappear as a metaphor for the understanding of currently inexplicable phenomena, at this historical juncture, intuitive medicine clearly functions as a form of sacred medicine, in which the practitioner is understood as a mediator between different worlds.

MEDIATING INFORMATION

In Chapter 2, I noted Jackie Stacey's analysis of the impact of the rise of 'information cultures' on our curiosity about ourselves (1997: 3–4). I argued that this insight enables us to understand medical intuition, based as it is on the relay of hidden information about the self, as a modern articulation of traditional sacred practices to fit contemporary desires. In this section, I explore what type of information medical intuitives and healers claim to pick up.

The reason many people go to a medical clairvoyant is that they want to find out what is ailing them when conventional medicine cannot tell them. Medical psychics pass on what one might consider 'diagnostic' information, even though, like most CAM practitioners, they know not to use the term for legal reasons. As the medical psychic Glen Margaret explained:

> You never diagnose and you never give advice. What you do is say, 'Let's just work with removing whatever comes up.' They're happy, you're happy, and you're within the legal system. You can never promise a cure.

Some healers will give medical names for conditions; others will sidestep the issue of diagnosis in favour of a description of what they are seeing. As I described in Chapter 2, this may be a visual image of something wrong; a symbolic representation of an illness; or it may be something distinctive in the aura. Despite practitioners' cautions about diagnosis, it is indubitable that many clients *want* the clairvoyant to tell them everything they see. Moreover, as I discussed in relation to iridology, they usually don't want to assist the process by contributing much information. They often seek a one-way information relay (from spirit to clairvoyant to client), and their faith in the process may be secured by giving the clairvoyant as little information as possible. Though a medical intuitive trained in any form of CAM would be committed to the partnership model of practitioner-client relationships, the client's desire to test and/ or be thrilled by the clairvoyant's abilities introduces a particular nexus of desire and power that adds to the interpersonal complexity of the encounter.

In addition to diagnostic information, clients will often be interested in the question of causation. Knowing the cause of an illness is an important cosmological component of alternative medicine. It fits in with the sacred character of this medicine, whereby nothing is meaningless. Illness is not generally perceived as random; it has a 'meaning', perhaps even a purpose. In medical cosmologies that foreground the emotional, the psychological, the spiritual or the social, knowing 'why' is an important part of living with a disease and/or effecting healing. In a biomedical setting, we might be equally curious about the cause of an illness, but biomedicine is essentially pragmatic, solutions-driven and disease-centred rather than person-centred. Thus, causation is important on a broad scale (in aetiology and epidemiology, for example) but at the level of the individual it is not always crucial to treatment. There are exceptions of course. (For example, it is important to know the cause of digestive disorders or allergic reactions in order to eliminate ongoing triggers.) But in the case of an individual suffering from an illness such as cancer, influenza, a cold, or a frozen shoulder, treatment does not rely on a theory about 'why' someone has contracted the disease or condition. Ultimately, the 'why?' question is often outstripped by the question of what to *do* about the problem. But for metaphysical branches of alternative medicine the question of causation lies at the heart of the ability to heal and to learn from illness. Take, for example, the following lines from the physician, neuroscientist and medical intuitive Mona Lisa Schulz, author of a popular book on intuition. Her chapter on the metaphysical meanings of health and disease begins:

> 'Why me?'
>
>   It's the first question we ask when illness strikes. At a loss to understand what's happening to us, we let the questions fly. Why did this happen to me? Why now? Why can't I get better? Who can help me? Illness seems random, inexplicable, and the answers of science still limiting and unsatisfying.

In truth, however, these questions *can* be answered. In many cases, the situations that set the scene for an illness can be traced and understood. (1998: 113)

This metaphysical view of illness differs not just from biomedicine, but also from the more fully social conceptions of illness that typify traditional world-views – in which the import of illness may extend beyond the sick person. As de Rosny describes in the context of Cameroon:

[The patient] is essentially the member of a family. In the sick bay, this is not just an isolated individual, visibly spread out on a mat; in reality the whole family is sick. The patient is the living sign of an ill which affects this family of which he or she is an integral part, to the degree that the invalid identifies with the family and the family recognizes itself in the invalid. (1998: 10–11)

This social conception of illness is shared by some in alternative medicine. For example, Jobst et al.'s conception of modern illness as 'diseases of meaning' is broad enough to encompass community violence, genocide and environmental devastation as 'illnesses' (1999: 495), but more commonly, the New Age influence on alternative health means that the meaning of an illness is construed as an *individual* psychological or emotional drama, even though it may affect the rest of the family.

A third type of information commonly sought or given is suggestions about treatment. Given the holism that typifies CAM modalities, treatment suggestions may range from practical suggestions (clean up your office), to naturopathic or essence remedies, relationships advice, emotional clearing techniques, spiritual guidance, or conventional medicine. Some medical intuitives receive and pass on quite precise information about naturopathic or other remedies, including dosage and required length of treatment. If the intuitive is a trained naturopath, she may have her own dispensary, and might combine intuitive work with a naturopathic case history. If not, she may 'prescribe' psychically and the client will go to a health shop or another practitioner to get the remedies. The prescription is not always for 'natural' remedies. Sometimes the information may be that the client needs to get an X-ray, or to see a GP to get prescription medicine or even to have surgery. The patient may well take back a diagnosis to his/her GP and ask to have it formally confirmed. This is where systemic questions (and their medico-legal implications) become interesting (see Barcan 2009b).

Occasionally, information is given precognitively, with clairvoyants claiming to intuit, see or predict illness to come. This may be spiritually given information and/ or a particular form of visual perception, such as the interpretation of a visual symbol or the reading of an aura. In this latter case, telling a client about potential future illnesses may not always be understood as clairvoyant precognition or prediction so much as a more acute form of vision – based on an expanded model of the body and the cultivation of an amplified form of vision.

This, then, leads me back to the question of what clairvoyants claim to perceive. In Chapter 2 I described what the clairvoyants I interviewed claimed to see. But which other senses do they use, and how do the 'standard' senses relate to the over-arching idea of a sixth sense?

SENSORY PERCEPTION AND INTUITION

One way of making clairvoyance conceivable is by expanding the category not only of perception but also of the perceptible. This double expansion underpins the Theosophist Leadbeater's list of three types of clairvoyance: simple clairvoyance (the ability to see whatever astral or etheric entities happen to be around the person, but not to see anything from other times or places); clairvoyance in space (the capacity to see scenes or events either distant or normally concealed) and clairvoyance in time (the power of looking into the past or future) (1918: 27–8). Many intuitives also consider mediumship (the ability to communicate between the living and the dead) to be a discrete ability within the clairvoyant spectrum.

Leadbeater sought to normalize clairvoyance by seeing it as an extension of the perception processes of everyday life. We live, he said, 'surrounded by a vast sea of mingled air and ether' and our sense organs respond to only a small percentage of these vibrations (1918: 8). The human retina responds to only a very small percent-age of all the 'exceedingly rapid vibrations which affect the ether' (8); likewise, the human tympanum responds to a very small range of comparatively slow vibrations – those slow enough to affect the air around us (8). These perceptive ranges constitute only a small segment of all that which is potentially perceptible in the universe:

> In both cases it is a matter perfectly well known to science that there are large numbers of vibrations both above and below these two sections, and that consequently there is much light that we cannot see, and there are many sounds to which our ears are deaf. (9)

Among the welter of vibrations 'of every conceivable degree of rapidity' (9), humans can perceive only a small fraction:

> So we begin to understand that the vibrations by which we see and hear are only like two tiny groups of a few strings selected from an enormous harp of practically infinite extent, and when we think how much we have been able to learn and infer from the user of those minute fragments, we see vaguely what possibilities might lie before us if we were enabled to utilize the vast and wonderful whole. (10)

There are names for the seeing, hearing and feeling of these vibrations – clairvoyance, clairaudience and clairsentience respectively – but these terms, which date from the mid-nineteenth century, do not capture the full variety of ways in which clairvoyants and healers claim to receive information. Benor lists common ways in which healers reported an intuitive awareness of their patients' problems:

> [Understanding] may come to them as sensations in their hands during laying-on of hands treatments (heat, cold, stickiness, prickliness and the like); as words appearing in their minds (including in rare cases technical diagnoses which they themselves do not comprehend but which doctors later confirm to be accurate); as body sensations (especially pains) which mirror patients' symptoms; as smells; as visual images of organ dysfunctions; or simply as an 'inner knowing'. (1992: 43)

I asked the intuitives I interviewed which senses were most active when they did a reading. They reported the types of sensations listed by Benor, all claiming to receive information in a variety of ways. Glen Margaret, for example, said:

> I hear the subconscious of the person talk to me. I have X-ray vision of the person's body, so I can see all of their organs and what's happening with them. I feel energies and I'm a medium and have spirits come in and give me information as well.

The spiritual healer Regina described how she knows spirits are in the room:

> I can feel them and I can smell. Sometimes I can smell. I have very, very perceptive smells, and sometimes with my patients I might say, 'Does coconut biscuits mean anything to you?' and they'll say 'Oh my God! That's my great aunt.' So I'll smell something which might trigger something in them which will unfold with what the problem is. It won't just be about Great Aunt Fanny; it will be that this coconut smell is bringing up an issue around this time and around this person that is connected to what's happening to them.

Her perception of spirit presence is very tangible:

> When I was working on someone the other day I was jammed up there – and this might sound a bit strange – but I could hardly move because I had all of these people behind me and I'm thinking, 'Give us a bit of room here, you know!' 'Cos you can feel them you know. You can absolutely feel them.

In addition to this sensory input, the practitioner is managing a lot of other information simultaneously: her own bodily feelings (e.g. pain, shivers), the bodily cues given off by the client; his or her tone of voice; even overly insistent spirits which, my interviewees said, can sometimes be very keen to butt in! They are also trying to relay or 'channel' a stream of information and at the same time manage the type of question-and-answer dialogue that typifies a counselling session. How, then, can they tell what is what – where sensations, ideas or information come from, and what belongs to whom?

For some practitioners, the information comes through in symbolic ways, raising the question of who has generated the symbol, how, and to whom it belongs. In Regina's description above, the smell of coconut biscuits is perceptible but not meaningful to the healer, and, imperceptible but literally and/or symbolically meaningful to the client. Some practitioners understand the information to be given by the client, as in Glen Margaret's observation quoted in Chapter 2 that clients show you the information in the way *they* want to show it. Others conceive of the visions as something shown to them by the spirit guides:

> They [i.e. the spirit guides] will show me things really clearly – like a snapshot. I can describe at times what they were wearing or what the people around them are wearing, or it's like a TV screen. Sometimes it is like a bit of a movie, or sometimes it's like really quick, still shots – all in one go. (Suzie)

How about the client's unconscious, I wondered. Is the clairvoyant perhaps 'simply' the master of a highly nuanced empathy? I asked Mary whether at least some of the information came from the client – whether she is perhaps mirroring something that the client unconsciously knows, or whether she sees herself strictly as channelling from another realm:

> Yes, that's how I see myself. I don't see that I'm reading the client's subconscious mind or whatever. I feel the information is given externally from the universal energies and so that's how I deliver it.

Her word 'deliver' is quite significant, because Mary sees herself as relatively uninvolved in the process – as a conduit:

> I, Mary, don't give this advice. It comes through me. But that would be very hard to argue in law, of course it would. That's my understanding of it – it's not me. So if I'm delivering, I'm the messenger.

While Mary conceives of the process as a more or less straightforward communication of a message, for others it involves a greater degree of entanglement. For Suzie, the 'psychic masseuse', the knowledge is contextual and processual: it is known only from moment to moment in a dynamic process. When she massages a body, she passes on to the client information that relates to that particular bodily area, material she believes to be stored in bodily memory. She picks this information up with the help of spiritual guides, using a variety of senses. Her particular ethics is to pass this information on, seeing it as part of her 'duty of care'. Moreover, she believes that passing the information on also keeps her from taking on board anything that belongs to the client:

Anything I get, any feeling, you know, any physical feeling, emotional – anything I see, anything I hear – I'll relate it to them. One, because I like to know that I'm on the right track; I don't want to assume anything … So quite often I'll just ask for yes and no answers … It's better for me. I can be more objective if I don't get caught up in it; it's just like a clean slate. And the other reason I tell them everything is because as soon as I speak it out it leaves my body, whatever it is.

This sounds to me like a double process of disentanglement. First, receiving brief verification that she's on the right track disentangles her intuitive and reasoning capacities, freeing up her intuitive mind to keep working free of rational doubt. (Her reasonable, doubting mind paradoxically prevents her from being 'objective'.) And second, passing on information allows her not to become too intercorporeally entangled with the client, allowing the information to pass through her rather than becoming lodged in her own body.

In contrast to Mary's 'package' that she 'delivers' to the client, Suzie's practice sounds as though it involves something a bit more intermingled. In the following explanation, she begins by talking about what the spirit guides tell her, which then shades into the sensations she picks up more directly from the client's body and feels sympathetically in her own body. In a language that echoes the intercorporeality of her practice, in the following description self, other and spirits flow into one another:

They [the spirit guides] will tell me stuff really clearly and so I'll hear it. When I say I hear it, it is in my head but at the same time it's as if someone is speaking to me. I guess it is that loud now. It never used to be, but it sort of is now, but I can differentiate between whether it's someone standing beside me or them, so it's a bit more of an internal thing, or feelings. I'll either feel their [the client's] physical sensations or their emotional sensations, and that's why it can be quite accurate in some ways. You know, sometimes I could go 'Oh, I feel like crying' and I will feel like crying but I won't actually cry [laughs]. How inappropriate that would be?! Oh my God! [laughs]. But I actually do feel like that and I'll say 'I'm on the verge of tears' and it'll be totally relevant to what the client is releasing in their life.

Similarly, the clairvoyant Darlene spoke of the intersubjective entanglements, blockages and projections that can occur between practitioner and client. Darlene understands the process as involving both a special intuitive gift and a heightened professional expertise at reading body language, voice and so on, developed through experience. Her description of a complicated intersubjective encounter sounds very different from Mary's experience of clairvoyance:

> You are tuning into the energetic as well as gauging their reactions to some of the answers that they're given. [With some lines of questioning] you already know intuitively what you are trying to get at. You haven't actually got the strong message yet, but you know that you are being guided towards this particular area that is very, very sensitive for them, purely by their reactions to the different questions that you ask – not only their physical reactions but their senses as well. You know, they may frown or they may tense because intuitively *they* already know where you are going. And they may quite often put up a smoke screen and try to steer it in other ways. So you *are* doing a lot behind the scenes as well as actually trying to get out of them what's really going on.

Darlene, in fact, finds reading easier by phone rather than in person, since it reduces the amount of communication to be managed, leaving her to deal only with verbal cues.

The degree of inter-implication between practitioner, client and context clearly differs between practitioners. But in all cases, this sixth, 'highest', sense is believed to involve knowledge that isn't arrived at merely via the collection of sensory data (as in simplistic accounts of perception), nor by transcending or ignoring the senses and the body (as in, for example, the Cartesian conception of reason). Rather, it involves bodily perception without being reducible to it. And though this sixth sense functions complexly and differently for each practitioner, all insisted that it couldn't be reduced to the sum of its parts, and many believed it cannot really be enhanced by training or experience:

Ruth: Does that integrated knowing become stronger with experience? Or is it a distinct part of clairvoyance?

Mary: It is – it's a separate component.

Separate or otherwise, it is clearly something that permeates to greater or lesser degree many other, much more mainstream, forms of alternative medicine. For it is not just clairvoyants who believe in the centrality of intuition. The naturopath and iridologist Nancy whom I quoted in Chapter 2 made it clear that she understands there to be an intuitive element in her practice. The following exchange, in which we discuss the advantages of the close physical proximity involved in iridological diagnosis (where the practitioner looks closely in the client's eye), makes it clear not only that intuition is a valued component of *many* alternative therapies (but also that she understands it to be something over and above the tacit, component professional decoding of a range of bodily signs:

Ruth: When you approach someone there must be a whole lot of bodily signs. I assume you must be able to see the skin close up and feel it and smell the breath and a whole lot of other signs.

Nancy: You can, you can, and I also think that when you come close to somebody there's all sorts of intangible things you pick up. If you are quite tuned into receiving those, that information, it does tell you stuff.

Ruth: So is there an intuitive component to the reading of the body?

Nancy: Oh, totally there is. There is definitely one you develop.

This sense that calls on, synthesizes yet transcends the information known through other sensory channels is, finally, an overarching 'knowing'. In contrast to the way that reason has traditionally been understood, as operating via compartmentalization or the breaking down of a problem into its component parts, intuition is understood as a holistic sense. This is, however, no simple inversion. For despite a commonsensical framing of reason and intuition as *opposites*, the body model that underpins intuitive medicine, as we have seen, understands the self as an organized assemblage of interpenetrating layers rather than a binary between mind and body. This opens the way for a more complicated picture of both knowledge and gender.

GENDERED KNOWLEDGE: THE PROBLEM OF COMPLEMENTARITY

The New Age concept of intuition clearly owes a debt to Romanticism, which pinned its faith on imagination as the divine capacity that transcends rational knowing. It is, in part, a descendant of the 'intuitive, spiritual faculty' that the Romantics celebrated as superior to the Enlightenment's 'critical analytic intellect' (Berlin, qtd in Hanegraaff 1998: 415). Although Romanticism retained some ambivalent attachment to Enlightenment rationality (Hanegraaff 1998: 415),[4] its legacy of a challenge to the supremacy of reason flies in the face of the aspiration 'to a Reason common to all, transcending the contingent historical circumstances which differentiate minds from one another' (Lloyd 1984: ix). This ideal of reason, has, as philosopher Genevieve Lloyd argued in detail, historically excluded and indeed constituted the category of 'woman' (1984: 106).

In alternative/New Age thought, the place of intuition in relation to this traditional dualism is complex, since intuition fits on neither side of a neat binary, being neither reason (rationality, logic, analytical capacity) nor emotion. Rather, it represents the pinnacle of perceptive capacities, but one that needs to work in conjunction with other modes of knowing.

I have considered relations between intuition and reason in alternative thought elsewhere (Barcan 2009a). Here, I want to use the persistent, though complex, historical gendering of emotions, unreason and intuition as feminine as a way of returning to the vexed theme of complementarity and the gendered politics of alternative medicine.

In Chapter 1, I spelled out some of the difficulties – philosophical, political and pragmatic – that plague attempts to conceive the relation between different medical practices and systems. Such difficulties are particularly acute when it comes to the relationship between practices founded on seemingly incommensurate cosmologies, such as those explored in this chapter. Yet movement – indeed *co-operation* – does occur between systems. Elsewhere (Barcan 2009b), I have described some of the largely invisible back-and-forth between spiritual healing/medical intuition and biomedicine, as when healers refer patients to GPs and, less frequently, the reverse occurs and GPs refer patients to a healer or intuitive and even visit one themselves.

Since sacred medical practices usually occur beneath the biomedical radar, most Western physicians are able to ignore their esoteric 'alternatives'.[5] Not so the healers and clairvoyants themselves. The nature of the Western medical landscape means that all professional medical clairvoyants have had to actively consider, negotiate and operationalize their relations to orthodox medicine and to the rationality on which it reposes (Barcan 2009b). Their modes of doing this vary, but the practitioners I found most fascinating were those who actively (if largely invisibly) worked across both systems. The clairvoyant Glen Margaret, for example, works in private practice, sometimes in conjunction with orthodox medical practitioners. She has worked in nursing homes and hospitals, where doctors and surgeons have called her in to help with intractable or puzzling cases. This mode of work involves finding sympathetic doctors who are open to the unorthodox and are professionally secure enough to act on this. It relies on a network of doctors with whom she enjoys a professional relationship, albeit one with a degree of secrecy involved: 'Generally they don't let too many people know they've called in a medical psychic.' So how are such doctors to be found?

> Some have heard of me and just ring and just say I'm absolutely stuck on this. Some of them have patients who have said 'Look, I've just been to see this lady and she says it's this and this, could it be?' and they've sort of explored that and found, yes, that's right, and therefore have been happy with my work.

The clairvoyant Mary thought that it was best to think of medical intuition and orthodox medicine as different areas of competence rather than as directly in competition. She has a number of medical specialists who consult her regularly, mostly for their own ailments but occasionally in relation to their patients. Many other mainstream medicos would no doubt find this absolutely horrifying – to me it's both intellectually and medically fascinating, despite the host of ethical, intellectual and political problems it so obviously invites. Mary's vision of an ideal medical system is one in which we could 'have the best of both worlds', and in which the advantages and limitations of different medical paradigms could be recognized and accommodated:

Mary: You've got to work with the strictly scientific medical arena as well. I think so.

Ruth: So you think that medical psychics should belong in a separate sphere, as it were, like separating consulting rooms?

Mary: Yes, but possibly working in harmony with each other. Like if I break my leg I'm not going to rush off to a psychic for healing. I'm going to go to a doctor; I want it set. That sort of thing. So there are areas. I think psychics can work well with emotions as long as they're the right psychics. I think they can do a lot of healing with the emotional body and the mental body and I also think that for lots of illnesses psychics can diagnose. I had a client … who had a son who was very ill so he rang me and asked me what could I see was the cause of the boy's problem. And I tuned in and I said, look he's got glandular fever. So he went and asked for a test for glandular fever and it showed up that's what he had. So it can be something which can be very useful in speeding up the process of diagnosing.

What we see here is the renunciation neither of orthodox biomedicine nor of the scientific rationality on which it is founded, but rather a professional practice based on the active negotiation of different modes of knowing and different institutional contexts.

The task of operationalizing new relations between reason, emotion and intuition in a working medical practice is intertwined with the broader intellectual and cultural project of attempting to forge or discover plausible biological or scientific equivalents, explanations or correlates for intuitive knowledge. In recent decades the popularization of the idea of the complementary functions of the two hemispheres of the brain has provided one avenue for such cultural translation. It's an interesting example for a study in the gendered politics of knowledge, since it illustrates the ongoing currency of the gendered politics of difference and complementarity, lodging such principles within the body itself.

According to Susan Leigh Star, studies of the 'asymmetry' of the bicameral human brain began with Roger Sperry in the early 1960s (1991: 239–40). Right from the outset, she says, there was stereotyping: the left brain became known as the 'major lobe', despite the fact that the two lobes are of the same size and function equivalently in both sexes (240). This set the stage for the subsequent gendering of the two halves of the brain, based on cultural stereotypes associated with the functions they control. Star's essay critiques from a feminist point of view the popularization of what was at that time a relatively new field of science. She argues that it drew on existing gender stereotypes and further entrenched them by extending their use into '"scientific" research' (237). Her essay was first published in 1979, and at that time her major target was the current interpretation of the right ('feminine') side as controlling faculties deemed less valuable than those associated with the left brain: that is, intuition as opposed to rationality and linear thought. It was, she argued, a 'classic case of sexist language, sexist interpretation of biological findings, and an interesting reflection of male-centred valuation' (241).

Some decades on, the discourse of brain hemisphere asymmetry is still gendered, but somewhat differently. Now the discourse is much more one of complementarity than of an implied superiority. The elaboration of a distinct feminized mode of thinking and a model of complementarity is, according to Lloyd, relatively recent in the Western philosophical tradition, beginning around the middle of the eighteenth century (1984: 75). Early philosophers saw femininity as an inferior version of masculinity rather than as distinct and complementary (75). But the themes of an internal struggle for dominance hark back to Plato. Today, complementarity is such a mainstay of our thinking about gender as to be commonsensical, permeating many forms of popular gender discourse, from self-help genres to chick flicks. No surprise, then, that it is a staple of New Age thought. As Hanegraaff points out, there is 'a rather pronounced tendency in New Age thinking' to conceive of holism as 'a dynamic harmony of opposites' (1998: 152). Harmony, whether individual, ecological or cosmic, is understood to result from 'a creative tension between both poles, which hold each other in balance' (153).

For co-operative endeavours to occur between intuitive medicine and biomedicine there must be people willing to engage in scientific and practical 'translation' by actively straddling or cutting across seemingly incommensurate paradigms and medical worlds. I want to explore these adventures in paradigm crossing by focusing on two examples, both from the US. Both are examples of boundary crossing occurring in the public eye rather than clandestinely. The first is someone who herself straddles two intellectual and practical worlds.

Mona Lisa Schulz, as noted earlier, is a medical doctor with a PhD in neuroanatomy and behavioural neuroscience who also practises as a medical intuitive and who has written a number of books on developing intuition. Schulz uses her scientific background in brain research to bridge these worlds, and she makes use of the picture of complementarity described above to do so. In *Awakening Intuition* (1998), she outlines the by now conventional theory of the different functions of the left and right hemispheres of the brain, but refuses either the traditional rational hierarchy in which reason (the left brain) is seen as superior to the right brain or the reversalist position that valorizes intuition (right brain) over rationality. Instead, she elaborates a theory of complementarity in which not only is each hemisphere seen as distinct and valuable, but rationality is actually seen as crucial to the optimum functioning of intuition, since intuition can only be interpreted and communicated through logic and reason:

> The two hemispheres complement each other. The right brain provides the intuition while the left gives it expression and communicates the intuition to the individual and to others. Without input from the left brain, the right brain's messages to you can be gibberish. (1998: 61)

The left brain grounds intuition in the world, without which it would be useless (62). Schulz's version of holism is a classic vision of complementarity as the working together of two equal halves:

> [W]hen it comes to understanding what intuition has to tell us, one brain is as essential as the other. Just as the brain needs both its halves to function with maximum efficiency, you need both your right brain and your left brain, indeed, your whole brain and all of its parts, to tap into your intuition most effectively. (58)
>
> You get the best value out of intuition only when the two halves of your brain (and indeed the entire brain) 'work together' (59).

This division of brain labour is explicitly and conventionally gendered: Schulz supports the commonsensical idea that women have better access to the right brain than men (1998: 58). Similarly, the right brain is more 'emotional' than the left, which is 'fact-based' (65). In this, she is not atypical: Hanegraaff claims that the gendering of 'polarity-holism' is 'particularly strong in the minds of New Age adherents' (1998: 153). This gendered conception implicitly maps the social body in the individual body. Thus, in Schulz's model, developing one's intuition represents a model both of gender complementarity and of social harmony:

> Ideally the two hemispheres should work in tandem, but they usually don't. The left brain tends to lord it over the right, like the president or Congress, running things and making laws. The right hemisphere acts like the electorate, which is there to be governed. (1998: 63)

This picture of habitual brain activity as an ongoing battle of the sexes naturalizes gender inequality even while it hopes for change, especially as Schulz grounds this gendered distinction in biology, arguing that it is more than cultural bias and may well proceed from a biological basis (63). Familiar gender claims underlie this model of a brain divided into two different but complementary halves, one of which is, by nature as well as culture, 'more submissive and receptive' than the other (65). Despite the familiarity of this gendered cluster – femininity, intuition, submission, receptivity – it is not essential to a model of complementarity. Hanegraaff notes that not all New Agers subscribe to the 'patriarchal' interpretation of complementarity as the interactions of a masculine principle conceived of as active and a feminine principle understood as passive (1998: 152).

In any case, complementarity is only one of the ways we might imagine the relations between intuition and reason. Jonas Salk, for example, recognizes their interaction and mutual dependency, as Schulz does, but does not envisage them as complements. Rather, he inverts the classic hierarchy of intuition and reason via a metaphor of the wise master and respectful servant:

> The intuitive and reasoning realms operate separately and together. It is necessary to educate and to cultivate each separately, and both together. I suspect that if appropriately cultivated, the two would work best together if the intuition were liberated from bondage and constraints, and put in charge of a respectful intellect. If a respectful intellect becomes conscious of intuition and reflects upon what it observes, a self-correcting, self-modifying and self-improving process is established. (1983: 79–80)

But Schulz rejects a hierarchical model. As noted above, she claims that it is counterproductive to think in terms of either separateness or superiority (1998: 26). It is clear that she wants to break out of the left-right dichotomy. At moments throughout the book – indeed, in its very sub-title – she prefers the metaphor of the network, speaking of the 'mind-body network' and the 'intuition network'. Though she still uses the language of difference ('one brain', 'the other brain'), she seems to be on the cusp of breaking out of a conventionally gendered dualist conception of complementarity. While she describes our mental processing as an ongoing tug-of-war between two 'opposing yet equally indispensable minds' (57), she also calls for the tug-of-war to be called off and for both brains to be integrated with all the other parts of the brain. But ultimately, this new metaphor of the network, which was only beginning to gain currency at the time her book was published, remains somewhat in tension with the dualism of the two brains model. This is hardly surprising, given the popular pervasiveness of gender dualism and essentialism at the time she was writing; the 1990s were, after all, the decade in which women were deemed to come from Venus and men from Mars (Gray 1992).

Schulz was not alone, of course, in arguing for the interdependency of different modes of knowing. In the late 1980s, the philosopher Ronald de Sousa made a similar argument about the indispensability of emotions to the functioning of reason. In his book *The Rationality of Emotion* (1987), he argued that emotions help the reasoning faculties to recognize *what matters*:

> [E]motions are among the mechanisms that control the crucial factor of *salience* among what would otherwise be an unmanageable plethora of objects of

attention, interpretations, and strategies of inference and conduct. (xv, original emphasis)

Like both Salk and Schulz, he was making an argument about the mutual dependency and the functional interactions between various modes of thought, an argument that involved some rhetorical inversions. (Emotions, for once, are seen as *controlling* the otherwise unmanageable world, rather than a prime instance *of* unmanageability!) The old tug-of-war between reason and emotion was, he claimed, outdated: 'Despite a common prejudice, reason and emotion are not natural antagonists' (1987: xv). De Sousa argues this as a philosopher of emotions and of mind. From a different disciplinary base, the neurologist Antonio Damasio (2000 [1994]) has made a similar argument about the relations between reason and emotion. He argues that feelings are crucial to reasoning processes. Arguing against 'Descartes' error' – the disembodying of mind – he demonstrates that feeling and reasoning cannot help but be processes of the brain, and that there is a biology of reasoning and of feeling:

> Feelings do seem to depend on a dedicated multi-component system that is indissociable from biological regulation. Reason does seem to depend on specific brain systems, some of which happen to process feelings. Thus there may be a connecting trail, in anatomical and functional terms, from reason to feelings to body. (2000 [1994]: 245)

As this view of both feeling and reasoning as underpinned by a 'complex biological and socio-cultural machinery' (246) develops and popularizes, it will be interesting to see if the gendering of intuition and emotion remains intact!

To close this chapter I want to turn to a second US boundary-crossing example: the collaboration, since 1985, of the medical intuitive Caroline Myss and the Harvard-trained physician and neurosurgeon Norman Shealy.[6] It is possible to read Myss and Shealy as embodying complementarity, and its traditional gendering. Perhaps their model of co-operation splits the reason/intuition binary by personifying each and operationalizing them as mutually respectful and co-operative. Like Schulz's, their practice connects different medical worlds; it is, in their words, 'bridge work' (1993: 7). Again like Schulz's, their vision is ultimately integrative; they seek a 'SYNTHESIZED paradigm of health' (18, original emphasis). Thus, Shealy's history of intuitive diagnosis in a book he co-wrote with Myss entwines the history of intuitive diagnosis with that of orthodox medicine, beginning with the commonly imagined starting point of Western medicine:

> The use of intuitive diagnosis is probably as old as medicine, and it almost certainly goes back to the days of Hippocrates. Many famous physicians throughout the history of the world seem to have been involved in things that today we would

call parapsychology, and many of them were probably outstanding intuitives. Paracelsus is one example of such an individual ... (1993: 63)

Shealy continues by discussing the study of intuitive diagnosis made by the British physician John Elliotson, who 'introduced to England the stethoscope, the use of narcotics and a variety of other medical techniques' (64). Linking the history of intuitive diagnosis with two icons of Western biomedicine – drugs and the stethoscope – is obviously intended to intertwine the two systems. Indeed, the subtitle of the first edition of this book is '*Merging* Traditional Medicine with Intuitive Diagnosis' (my emphasis).

As discussed in Chapter 1, in the current biomedical context, 'merging' involves submitting medical intuition to some form of evidentiary test. The problem of how to test and evaluate radically different healing practices is a familiar one in the CAM literature generally, and especially in relation to spiritual healing, energy medicine and intuitive medicine. The key themes and problems of this debate include how to assess the efficacy of spiritual healing, energy medicine and other forms of spiritual medicine, such as prayer-for-health (see, for example, Astin et al. 2000; Dossey 1993; Brown 2000). Core problems include the difficulty of accounting for intention methodologically (Brown 2000: 171); the incompatibility of goals, whereby healing is not the same thing as cure (Brown 2000: 171; Barcan and Johnston 2011); particular problems with controls and placebos (Brown 2000: 173) and with defining outcomes (2000: 173). Despite these difficulties, some healers believe that the way to further the cause of intuitive medicine is by having it meet the criteria of the dominant system. (Indeed, one of the often repeated stories about the origin of Myss and Shealy's collaboration is that Shealy tested Myss's intuitive diagnoses and found she was 93 per cent accurate (1993: 72) – in contrast with what he estimated to be the average biomedical accuracy rate of around 80 per cent (1993: 59)!) Daniel Benor, as I have noted, has made a research career founded on the systematic scientific evaluation of spiritual healing. Methodological discussions are growing, including books published in the Health Sciences on the science and research methods appropriate to healing and energy medicine (e.g. Jonas and Crawford 2003).

Beverly Rubik, the scientist of energy medicine cited in Chapter 2, claims that the accumulation of anomalous data is never enough to effect a shift in the scientific paradigm (1995: 34). What is needed, rather, is conceptual work that can contribute to new explanatory theories (34). So the legitimization of spiritual healing and medical intuition as therapeutic practices has become intertwined with attempts to push the knowledge base itself. Myss and Shealy attempt to make currently inexplicable phenomena intellectually legible in terms of the new science: they have put out a CD set called *The Science of Medical Intuition* (2002). In the US there are a variety of frames in which such attempts occur: research into the medical efficacy of prayer, for example, constitutes a recognized medical sub-field (e.g. Dossey 1993; McCaffrey et al. 2004) and there are many projects on energy medicine taking place under the rubric of integrative medicine. Mainstream institutions such as the National Center for Complementary and Alternative Medicine (NCCAM), for example, fund studies on reiki and energy or aura medicine under the rubric of 'biofield therapeutics' (Baruch 2002: 43).

The process of legitimization is not without its risks. Some believe that different evaluation criteria are needed. Medical doctor Karen Lawson, for example, argues that medical science needs to recognize the inappropriateness of traditional criteria in judging healing systems that are fundamentally inimical to it:

> The greatest challenge is to develop good research designs that do not obviate the very processes we seek to maximize, such as the placebo effect, mind-body interactions, self-healing, or the power of intention. Forcing other philosophies of healing to fit into our mechanistic model will decrease the potential of these other approaches. For example, we require proof of a biochemical/mechanical mechanism for energetic systems such as Reiki because we do not know of any other way to measure or understand them. (2002: 17)

According to this logic, not only is medical science an inappropriate vehicle, its methodological foundations, based as they are on a set of separations – intention from practice, personnel from contexts, desire from action – actually work against the foundational mechanisms of alternative healing techniques, which are based on intermingling (of mind and body, healer and patient, intention and practice, person and context). This chapter returns us then to arguments raised in Chapter 1 about the complications involved in understanding, modelling and practising disparate therapies. For Myss and Shealy, though, the future is clear: 'The two paradigms of health that now co-exist in this world are here to stay' (1993: 39).

I said at the outset of this chapter that these sacred intuitive practices are important as they represent a stark form of the more general CAM phenomenon. As we have seen, they centralize a number of assumptions, properties and logics common to most alternative medicine – the expressive potential of the body; the communication between bodies and between different parts of the self; the role of the sacred; and the centralizing of intuition. They also raise in the starkest form the issues of safety and medical regulation common to the whole CAM landscape: questions of training, regulation, evidence and integration. I have also argued (Barcan 2009a) that intuitive medicine is best understood not as an overthrow of reason but as its relativization and its revisioning as one tool among many. This prospect understandably frightens those who fear that the West is succumbing to an assault on reason, but it certainly tallies with the relativism, pluralism and customization that typify postmodern knowledge practices.

As a footnote to this excursion beyond the boundaries of 'legitimate' medicine and 'legitimate' academic work, I need to say that one thing I have learnt through the process of writing this book is the truth of the insight, found in different ways in many disciplines and philosophies, from anthropology to deconstruction to psychoanalysis, that we are formed in part through what we exclude. I found that almost everyone I have interviewed, no matter what their healing modality, needed to identify an outside, a fringe – someone or some practice that was less professional or more 'kooky' than they were. Almost all the clairvoyants I interviewed, for example, described performing 'corrective readings', in which they remedied the errors of other, less accurate, less professional, or less ethical, clairvoyants. Perhaps I, too, in describing my own reiki experiences, needed to perform my own ambivalence (Carter and Hooker 2010) to stabilize my own sense of reasonable identity. How congruent do I consider my practice of reiki with the practices described in this chapter? Do I want to consider myself part of this spectrum? I hardly know.

6 CONCLUSION

In his book *The Politics of Life Itself*, the Foucauldian scholar Nikolas Rose argues that in contemporary Western societies, human beings have come increasingly to 'understand themselves in somatic terms' (2007: 254). Bodily life, he claims, has become one of the most important sites for ethical judgements and techniques (254). Rose argues that where once the management of health and vitality might have been derided as 'obsessive or narcissistic self-absorption', it has now achieved 'unparalleled ethical salience' in the lives of many (258). His focus is on biomedicine, whose successes have, he notes, extended the possibility and responsibility for 'choice' right down 'to the very fabric of vital existence' (254): 'Our biological life itself has entered the domain of decision and choice' (254). This biopolitical regime is so significant as to constitute a new mode of citizenship – 'biological citizenship' (132) – with its own sets of bodily techniques and its own new arenas of decision, debate and uncertainty. He terms this new practical and ethical terrain 'somatic ethics' (254). Somatic ethics is not made up only of the self-evidently ethical issues surrounding biomedical research and practice; it is far more pervasive than that. Rose argues that it constitutes a new set of relations to the body, in which the fashioning, transformation, restoration and augmentation of the body are not only the province of exceptional medical interventions but also constitute the terrain of everyday bodily life. Though Rose mentions alternative medicine only in passing,[1] it is clear that his argument extends across the broad spectrum of contemporary health practices. Certainly, the therapeutic practices explored in this book are examples par excellence of this contemporary extensive medicalization, in which the body is a site of action not just for external interventions and internalized strictures but also for consumer pleasures, and where the boundaries between medicine, pleasure, recreation, asceticism, consumerism and spirituality are not clear-cut.

Clearly, this is significant both socially and medically. My analysis has deliberately skirted the question of the medical effectiveness of CAM therapies. Nonetheless, since I have stated from the outset that I am a 'fan' of alternative medicine, and since its medical success and its social significance cannot help but be intertwined, it is important for me to acknowledge in this Conclusion their potential to assist, relieve or cure, which I have experienced first-hand and witnessed in others. It ought, I hope, to be self-evident that my enthusiasm is not a blanket endorsement. The diversity of CAM modalities, the variation in practitioner skills, and the free market context all mean that a productive negotiation of these therapies as medical phenomena requires skill, social and economic capital and also, importantly, luck. Luck is of course a feature of any medical system, since all forms of health practice are characterized by unevenness of practitioner skill and therapeutic effectiveness, and there is always an element of mystery, intractability and unpredictability to physical suffering. I am definitely not among those who believe that if only you try long enough and hard enough you will inevitably find physical relief or cure – whether that be through biomedicine or CAM. In this, I reject the absolutism of New Age thought, which holds that any medical therapy 'will work if you desire and believe it will' (Gawain 1978: 61).

My sidestepping of specifically medical questions in a book about alternative therapies does not undercut my claim that they are highly significant as bodily practices. For while the social and medical fortunes of alternative therapies are inevitably tangled together (in that it is hard to imagine them thriving as social practices if there were not at least some degree of therapeutic effectiveness to them), they address the body in ways that surpass or lie outside the question of their medical effectiveness. My arguments for the significance of CAM as a bodily phenomenon do not hinge on its medical successes. For, whatever one thinks of the medical claims, effects and significance of alternative therapies (and given the extraordinary diversity of alternative modalities and practitioners, this is not a question that can be addressed through generalities), their impact on the conception and experience of the body at a cultural level is indisputable.

I have argued, then, that alternative medicine is not only a medical phenomenon, but also a new popular form of conceptual practice. Whatever else they are, the new body practices of alternative medicine are invitations to rethink the body. Its singularity is opened out by the multiplicity of the subtle body model; its materiality by the concept of matter as energy; and its boundedness by the profound forms of intercorporeality promised in its practices. The body is a repository for life history and for memory and its dynamization in therapeutic practice allows us access to different corporeal temporalities, not as time-locked capsules but as an 'alluvial' flow, to recall Yehuda Tagar's beautiful metaphor. This body extends across space – where does it end? – and is conceived of as affecting and affected by the bodies of others, themselves dispersed across time and space. In some of the more esoteric therapeutic practices, objects can be made to serve as proxies for bodies, or one part of the body may be invited to act as a proxy for another body part.[2] This body couldn't be more different from the sealed-off, individual body of the high-modern cliché, and, as Jay Johnston (2008) has argued, it implies not only a radically different ontology but also, potentially, an ethics founded on intersubjectivity. And yet, in the current cultural context, this open body-self is all too often urged to fulfil its own individual desires, and the collectivity is imagined as a crowd of individuals.

Alternative therapies have not only expanded our ways of thinking about the body, they are also invitations to new forms of bodily *experience*, and this book has used the senses as a way of demonstrating the experiential richness of these bodily encounters. Alternative therapies can deepen the experience of particular senses through focused attention (e.g. touch in massage; smell in aromatherapy). But they also enrich and complicate sensory experience by creating cross-, inter- or synaesthetic sensory experiences: they may allow us to feel colours, to intuit through touch, to enjoy aromatic caresses or bathe ourselves in sound. This, then, is the hedonic aspect of alternative medicine, which provides pleasure, solace and comfort and also makes CAM so amenable to the market.

What, then, are we to make of this intertwining of medicine, pleasure and consumption? Should we celebrate it as the re-humanizing of a mechanistic modern medicine? After all, we could follow the arguments of the utopian philosopher Charles Fourier, who claimed that 'societies could be judged according to how well they gratified and developed the senses of their members' (Howes 2005a: 282), a claim that influenced Marx's analysis of capitalism as an alienation of the body (282). Or should we critique is as a selfish indulgence? Or see it not as the opening out of a new vision of the body but as yet one more manifestation of biological citizenship?

In wrestling with this question it is important to note that alternative medicine does not construe pleasure simply as an end in itself, even while it values it. Sensory experience is conceived of as a pathway to self-knowledge, and the senses frequently operate as 'ways into' different aspects of the body and emotional life, opening up new ways of knowing the body. Practitioners see with their hands, feel with their eyes, listen with their intuition. But the process is not only one-way, for the practitioner's touch may spark memories, associations or insights; the scent of the aromatherapy oil may trigger changes in physical, emotional and cognitive states; or meditation on a particular colour may bring about alterations in heart-rate, cognition or the depth and frequency of breathing. How are such rich sensory experiences to be valued? For some, these new modes of perception are less about self-indulgence than about the hope for a broader social shift in which constraining forms of rationality and sociality may be broken through. In Chapter 4 I described the MFR practitioner Thomas Myers's argument that kinaesthetic intelligence had social ramifications, enabling us to live more attentively to the world around us – to become, finally, more humane. Merleau-Ponty would have agreed. He claimed that 'synaesthetic perception is the rule, and we are unaware of it only because scientific knowledge shifts the centre of gravity of experience, so that we have unlearned how to see, hear, and generally speaking, feel, in order to deduce, from our bodily organization and the world as the physicist conceives it, what we are to see, hear and feel' (1962: 229).[3]

For others, though, CAM would have to be seen as congruent with a host of biomedical and lifestyle 'enhancement technologies' (Elliott 2003), which construe pleasure as part of one's 'right' to self-fulfilment (Rose 1999: xxiv). For such critics, the ideal of happiness-as-individual-optimization is not only self-defeating (being, it is argued, more likely to make us miserable (Elliott 2004)), it is also ethically impoverished. This is the position taken by Nikolas Rose who, although he makes little mention of CAM, has been an insightful and trenchant critic of the

> ethical paucity of the contemporary obligation to fulfil ourselves through the
> mundane achievements of our everyday lives, and to evaluate all aspects of our
> livers in terms of the extent to which they do or do not contribute to such
> an inexorable trajectory of self-improvement and personal happiness through
> career enhancement and lifestyle maximization. (1999: xxiv)

This ethics is, he claims, matched by the 'poverty of the therapeutic ethic' that goes with it (xxiv–xxv).

I respect the critical task of pointing out the psychological and social dangers of making therapy the only game in town. And it is true to some extent that the individualized tenor of the contemporary quest for pleasure and self-actualization has left in its wake a lost realm of other ways of relating to ourselves and each other. Rose, for one, laments the loss of 'dependency, mutuality, fraternity, self-sacrifice, commitment to others' (1999: xxiv). But if there is one type of human experience that can bring us inexorably back to the importance of such values, surely it is illness itself – which can make us see, sometimes in an instant, the poverty of the neoliberal ideal of autonomous self-reliance, even while it might make us pine to re-establish our place back in the everyday social practices founded on such conceptions of the self. For, despite the various forms of individualism in which alternative medicine is enmeshed – the individualism implicit in the contemporary injunction to optimize one's capacities; extolled in New Age ideology; and structurally underpinning commodity relations – it is also true that as social *practices*, alternative therapies are bound up in webs of reciprocity and care. Those forms of interaction and inter-reliance whose erosion Rose notes have not absented themselves from the field of everyday action, though it is indubitable that neoliberal consumer societies are no longer structured around them. I share Rose's dismay at the rise of a narrowly conceived individualism, but I do take some comfort that the new forms of somatic ethics brought into being in biological citizenship are not *solely* individualist. After all, the alternative health movement arose from the interventions of the feminist health movement and from the hippie counter-culture. Even the notorious individualism of the New Age as a system of thought is cut across somewhat by one of its favoured metaphors and organizational structures – that of the network (Hanegraaff 1998: 107). Perhaps more pertinent, though, is the tenacity of care in everyday practice. For on the level of the everyday, even the most fervent adherents of New Age individualism (those utterly committed to the 'we are each 100% responsible for all of our experiences' philosophy (Hay 1987: 5)) are in my experience nonetheless still likely to be galvanized by the illness of others – dropping off bottles of homeopathic medicines, coming around and doing reiki, giving someone a foot massage or driving him/her to appointments.

This informal ethics of care, seemingly countermanded by New Age, neoliberal and consumerist ideologies, is, perhaps, a valuable political and ethical legacy of the ongoing feminization of CAM. It signals, moreover, the ongoing importance of alternative medicine to feminism – not only because currently most clients and practitioners of CAM are still women, but also because however much it has been mainstreamed, domesticated or co-opted by hegemonic medicine, at this stage many forms of CAM still represent a feminized rebellion against both the power and the knowledge base of a still subtly masculinist biomedicine. As Beverly Rubik says, 'Alternative medicine remains alternative because it poses serious challenges to the mainstream biomedical paradigm of mechanical reductionism and because it requires a new framework' (1995: 34). In its valuing of emotion, expressivity and intuition, and its suspicion of overly reductionist forms of reason, alternative medicine continues to provide an important challenge. Naturopath Judy Singer suggests that the type of (feminized) care practised in alternative settings occurs in no other Western therapeutic encounter (2008: 200). In caring, respectful CAM settings, which she calls a 'meeting place', home, she claims, can be (re)created; past connected with present; 'female' knowledge respected; deep care practised; and the unspeakable voiced through the body (197–8, 205).

There is, perhaps, no agreement to be reached between those who see a progressive future as lying in the extension of the sensory pleasures of CAM to all members of society and those for whom such a prospect is a nightmare. Wherever one sits on such a continuum, it is important, I believe, to recognize the role of ideological and political values in determining which body practices are available to whom. This is what the critical Humanities and Social Sciences allow us to do. They also allow us to remain alert to contradictions, paradoxes and cracks – for example the fact that, as noted in Chapter 1, the logic of neoliberalism has been able to support the extension and sometimes centralization of alternative health practices to marginalized or disadvantaged groups, through indigenous health programmes, alternative therapy programmes for HIV/AIDS patients, refugee health programmes and so on. The contingency of economic rationalism (which values, in the end, cost-effectiveness over particular biomedical truth claims) means that although when purchased through private means alternative therapies produce pleasure for the happy few, the recipients of their care are not solely 'the articulate, health-aware and information-rich middle-classes' (Greenhalgh and Wessely 2004: 197). Moreover, as noted in Chapter 1, the paradoxical agnosticism of evidence-based medicine – in which the *fact* of a therapy's effectiveness is ultimately more significant than the reasons behind it (Willis and White 2004: 54) – can give some CAM practices unexpected purchase in mainstream health care systems. Such paradoxes are part of the complex picture of contemporary medicine as it struggles its way towards something more integrative.

TOWARDS INTEGRATION

In the Introduction to this book I noted that my personal hope is for the emergence of a form of integrative medicine that would not flatten out alternative medicine's useful points of difference. This dream requires us to think multiply: to be aware of the congruencies of biomedicine and alternative medicine as well as their differences; to keep alternative medicine's challenge to biomedicine alive; to enrich CAM's scientific and conceptual base; and to hold both biomedicine and CAM politically, socially and intellectually accountable. Clearly, this complex set of tasks requires input from many disciplines.

The rich somatic potential of alternative therapies and their larger social context are not always able to be reconciled or held in one view. The transdisciplinary approach of this book has not been an attempt to attain a position of mastery whereby we could see alternative medicine from above, in all its complexity and contradiction. Rather, it represents an attempt to bring into proximity many different perspectives, and to make the meetings, merging and collisions as rich and productive as I can.

In particular, I have tried in this book to be a mediator or bridge between two big bodies of knowledge: my home discipline of Cultural Studies and some of the popular and professional discourses of CAM. I have argued that though they will not ultimately agree on all things, each has something useful to learn from the other. CAM has an exciting and evolving new science base, which it has been impossible for me to do anything but gesture towards, but which must contribute to our future understanding of the body. Alternative medicine can also offer Cultural Studies a working model of non-dualism, and a potential mechanism for thinking about non- or extra-rational phenomena – or, perhaps, for helping us to reconceptualize reason itself. Moreover, the materiality of CAM's engagement with the senses, in which sounds, colours and smells are understood to *do* things as well as *mean* things, provides an ongoing corrective to those currents in Cultural Studies that might still bring an overly textualist perspective to bear on the body.

Cultural Studies, meanwhile, can bring important conceptual subtlety and a political sensibility to bear on those streams in CAM where critical thought and conception remain underdeveloped. In particular, it can offer an understanding of the limitations of simplistic ideas of nature that still plague some of the CAM literature; a much more historically and socially aware view of the body and body practices; an acute sensitivity to cross-cultural perspectives and a wariness of universal claims; and a trenchant political critique of neoliberalism, individualism and the politics of cross-cultural appropriation. My aim in this book, therefore, has not been to undercut critiques of therapeutic culture but to enrich and complicate them.

The intellectual and practical project of integrative medicine requires specialization – not only in medicine and CAM science but also in the Humanities and Social Sciences. But it also requires people willing and able to combine or traverse several disciplines or fields of practice. This need for enrichment and translation explains, in part, my excitement at the existence of crossover figures who work between or across different intellectual paradigms and/or medical worlds. Throughout the book I have mentioned people like the molecular biologist-physiotherapist-yoga teacher Simon Borg-Olivier; or the surgeon-psychotherapist-hypnotherapist René Mateos; or the neuroscientist-physician-medical intuitive Mona Lisa Schulz. Such people are, for me, among the most exciting and challenging drivers of the ongoing project of integrative medicine.

It does not require especially subtle perception to notice that the themes of bridging, paradigmatic pluralism and boundary crossing might also attract me because they speak to my own personal experiences. I have used the feminist emphasis on experience as an intellectual resource – aware, however, of the cautions about using it as an unexamined byword for authenticity (Scott 1991). Perhaps my use of personal experience is not to the taste of some readers, but it springs from two interlinked ethical drives. First, I have drawn on my own experience as a way not only of deepening my analysis but also of *implicating* myself in it, to avoid a sense of detachment from the material that is unethical insofar as it is both untrue and lacking in moral courage. Second, in aiming to write a book that is open rather than closed – that makes manifest my own uncertainties, doubts and desires – I have aimed to write a book that ultimately pays respect to the reader.[4]

This book has been trying to write itself for over twenty years but has benefited incalculably from the wait. Two decades of ripening have broadened my personal experiences with alternative therapies, put me in the way of truly gifted and intellectually exciting practitioners, and also, I hope, dulled or curbed some of the mawkishness of my early enthusiasms. Twenty years from now and it would no doubt have been a better book still. For one thing, I suspect that I would no longer have had to devote so much time to engaging the somewhat programmatic thematics of a sceptical Cultural Studies and been able to take for granted an approach to the body in which the biological and the cultural are more fully integrated. But I write at a bridging moment, and my book bears the traces of this.

It also, inevitably, bears the traces of my own living attempt at an integrative process. Rose argues that the era of somatic ethics obliges modern citizens to answer for themselves in new ways the three questions famously posed by Kant at the end of his *Critique of Pure Reason*: What can I know? What ought I to do? What may I hope? (Rose 2007: 257). I am one of these new types of citizen. My own twenty-year journey along the parallel train tracks of post-structuralism and alternative medicine has certainly brought these questions to the fore – both as intellectual issues and as lived dilemmas, occasionally agonizing ones. My accounts in this book of my own experience render this process of questioning very visible and make evident its implication, as per Rose's concept of somatic ethics, in the deepest aspects of life – whether it be childbirth, back pain or knowing the boundaries of reason and reasonableness itself.

Now, however, I no longer have one foot in each parallel. I'm more in the thick of things – at a place of multiplicity and possibility. At this meeting point, many different ways of knowing rub shoulders with each other – sometimes jostling for space, at other times opening up to a wary embrace. In this place of possibility, I look around me, sniffing the air, feeling my way.

NOTES

Chapter 1

1. I am interested, by way of contrast, in the conclusion drawn by the eminent scholar of the New Age, Wouter J. Hanegraaff, about the artistic (rather than sensory) merits of New Age culture. He concludes that it is 'conspicuously lacking in artistic sensitivity' (1998: vii) – by which he means its music, art and literature do not match the great themes and beauty of the mainstream Western tradition.

2. Surveys and interviews were carried out as part of two studies funded by the School of Philosophical and Historical Inquiry and the Faculty of Arts at the University of Sydney, Australia. I would like to thank all participants for their time, generosity and insight. Practitioners were given the option of using a pseudonym, which they often chose themselves. Real names have been used only where permission was given.

3. I am referring here to the appropriation and commodification of indigenous knowledges and practices, and the invocation of 'the East' in much alternative and New Age discourse (see Stacey, 2000). Not all uses of the term 'traditional' in alternative medicine refer to non-European others, however. 'Traditional' can also refer to traditions in European herbalism, for example, or to English folk medicine. Adding to the confusion, sometimes the term 'traditional medicine' is used to refer to biomedicine.

4. This is not to say that what homeopaths call the Law of Similars has never had any place in Western medicine. Indeed, homeopath Ian Howden seeks to reclaim this principle as one of the fundamental underpinnings of Western medicine. The principle that 'like cures like' is, he notes, first found in Hippocrates and has 'often re-emerged' during the development of Western medicine. His examples of this, however – Galen (AD 129–200), Paracelsus (sixteenth century) and Samuel Hahnemann, the founder of homeopathy (late eighteenth century) – make it evident that it is not a dominant biomedical principle (2003: 213–14).

5. The original source is 'China Gives Limited Approval to Western Medicine' from a summary reported by Sin Hua, China News Agency, 1 April 2001. To what extent this is a neutral medical summing up or a subtle and targeted political irony I am unable to say, since I have obtained this quotation indirectly.

6. The term 'allied' has a longer history, having been used by the American Medical Association as early as 1926 in relation to 'allied sciences', like physiology, pharmacology and biochemistry (Donini-Lenhoff 2008: 47). Donini-Lenhoff dates the first usage of the term 'allied health' in the US at 1969, reporting that in 1970 the AMA officially replaced the terms 'ancillary' and 'paramedical' with 'allied'.

7. 'CAM' is, for example, the term used by the World Health Organization.

8. The pragmatic movement across medical systems need not necessarily be a feature of privilege; it also characterizes the attitudes and practices of most non-First-World people, including indigenous peoples and refugees (see, for example, Singer 2008: 188; Macintyre 2003: 45–7).

9. For an atlas depicting biomedical uptake around the world, see Bodeker et al. (2005).

10. Throughout this book I use the term General Practitioner (or GP) to refer to what is usually known in the US as the 'family doctor'.

11. Thanks to Sam McCarthy and Anita Bressan for conversations about osteopathy, and to the aromatherapist Salvatore Battaglia, who made this observation in an interview with the author.

12. On the American Academy of Medical Acupuncture website, for example, the 'classical Chinese explanation' for how acupuncture works is followed by 'the modern scientific explanation', in which energy channels (meridians) are re-explained as the effects of nervous system stimulation on biochemistry. Even so, this site does recommend acupuncture for a broad range of physical conditions, and not just for classic Westernized uses like pain relief. http://www.medicalacupuncture. org/

13. On the other hand, the editorial to a 2000 issue of the journal *Complementary Therapies in Medicine* argued that CAM should *not* be exempt from the biomedical standard of the placebo-controlled study (White 2000: 225).

14. 'Physiotherapist' is the term preferred in the UK, Australia and Canada for what is known in the US as 'physical therapy'. I use the term 'physiotherapist' throughout this book, except when I am referring specifically to a US practitioner.

15. For a careful empirical consideration of whether there is, indeed, a spiritual revolution in the UK and the US, see Heelas et al. (2005).

16. The House of Lords Select Committee cited above found that in the UK anyone, with or without training, has the right to treat a sick person provided informed consent is given, but they may not use various protected terms (like 'doctor') or prescribe registered drugs (Bensouilah 2005: 138). They may even claim to cure some diseases, but not particular diseases listed in the law (138). Similarly, in most Australian states it is an offence for a CAM practitioner to provide medical services and/or to offer 'medical advice' (Weir 2003: 303). Clearly, the question of what constitutes a 'medical' service is a core issue. Grace et al. (2006: 695) note that in Australia CAM practitioners have increasingly come to use many of the simpler Western diagnostic techniques (such as the taking of blood pressure or a case history) to augment their own assessment procedures. In another study they also found that many CAM practitioners lacked confidence in performing such techniques, even though they had training in them (Grace et al. 2008: 44).

17. Wouter J. Hanegraaff identifies four fundamental types of holism in New Age thought, not all of them necessarily philosophically compatible with each other, though they nonetheless may often be found in combination (1998: 120).

18. *Chakras* is the yogic term for the energy centres in the body, which mediate between physical and subtle energies (Dale 2009: 235). The idea of a system of subtle energy centres is found in many traditional healing systems around the world, with the number of *chakras* varying from system to system. The yoga guru B.K.S. Iyengar names six principal *chakras* (1991: 130), but the Hindu system alone has 'dozens of variations within it' (Dale 2009: 236).

19. See, for example, *The Journal of Religion and Health*. This line of research is particularly strong in the US. For an overview of the literature on religion and health, see Sutherland et al. (2003: 316–17).

20. Holmes was active in the first decade of the twentieth century. He founded the Institute of Religious Science and Philosophy in 1927. Affiliated groups sprang up and slowly began calling themselves churches (Albanese 2007: 429).

21. For a detailed discussion of how New Age thought is both similar to and different from Freudian ideas of repression see Stacey (1997: 112–21). For a detailed lineage of New Age thought in the context of American religious history see Albanese (2007).

22. Hay's book *You Can Heal Your Life* (1987) was on the *New York Times* bestseller list for thirteen consecutive weeks and has sold more than 35 million copies. *Heal Your Body* (1988) has been translated into twenty-five languages. (Figures sourced from http://www.hayhouse.com; accessed October 2009).

23. John Harrison's *Love Your Disease: It's Keeping you Healthy* (1984) is a psychological version of the idea of disease as a useful lesson. Harrison argues for the psychological basis of disease and its unconscious psychosocial payoffs.

24. Seth is an entity channelled by Jane Roberts, in *Seth Speaks*.

25. An important exception is the widespread opposition to vaccination found in homeopathy.

26. Hanegraaff argues that the New Age is 'a far broader *religious* movement, which happens to include approaches to healing as an important part of its ideology' (1998: 243, original emphasis).

27. In an article on medical doctors' and CAM practitioners' legal obligations, Michael Weir notes that in Australia the National Health and Medical Research Council's guidelines stipulate that a full discussion of treatment options is required, and that similar requirements exist in other countries (e.g. Canada). While this has mostly been taken to refer to information about material risks associated with particular biomedical interventions, the question arises as to whether doctors could be understood to be required by law to extend their advice to CAM options (2003: 298).

28. This comes from *Time Magazine*, who selected Chopra in 1999 as one of their Top 100 Icons and Heroes of the Century.

29. There exists, in fact, a 'physical immortality' strain of New Age thought, which holds that ageing and death result from a deeply engrained unconscious belief in the inevitability of mortality. The repudiation of ageing and death is a striking example of the desire for mastery noted by Stacey (1997: 238), and an interesting reversal of the desirability of all things 'natural' (since, presumably, animals don't share this death-wish, and yet they die).

30. More detailed engagement with these ideas can be found in Barcan (2008) and Barcan and Johnston (2011).

31. For critiques of Cultural Studies' Romantic attachment to the spectacular and the subversive, see Bennett (1998) and Couldry (2000). Cultural Studies' relation to religious/spiritual discourse is discussed in greater length in Barcan and Johnston (2005).

32. For an exploration of the attractiveness and cultural plausibility of the energetic or subtle model of the body, see Barcan 2011, forthcoming.

33. Nutton (1993) reports that the taste of sweat was believed to provide useful information in Galenic medicine (2003: 11); Bylebyl notes that the tasting of various excretions, including urine, was one component of Renaissance diagnosis (2003: 46–7).

34. Thanks to David Howes for bringing this text to my awareness.

35. Traditional Chinese Medicine incorporates a schema of five phases or elements – wood, fire, earth, metal and water – each of which has a related set of associations, or 'correspondences', including colours, emotions, seasons, climates, body organs, tastes, smells and sounds (Patching van der Sluijs and Bensoussan 2003: 71). These correspondences are an important component of diagnosis.

36. Ayurveda is the traditional medicine of India. Nutrition is an important component of this medical system. Its herbology takes account not only of the effects of herbs, but also of their qualities (e.g. their moistness, heaviness, lightness) and their taste. The six tastes are sweet, sour, salty, pungent, bitter and astringent. In this taxonomy, taste *itself* is understood to have effects on the body (Matthews 2003: 29).

Chapter 2

1. Anatomy was not of course the only medical discipline of this time. Lisa Cartwright's (1995) study of the visual culture of modern medicine, while it makes use of Foucault's *Birth of the Clinic*, also makes it evident that physiology gave a quite different picture of the body, and that post-revolutionary French laboratory medicine evinced a strong fascination with the body in movement, not just with the inanimate corpse (11). Foucault himself notes that the anatomic gaze was a dominant but not the only medical gaze.

2. To take one example, there have been many analyses of the effects of medical imaging on pregnant women's attitudes and relation to the foetus (e.g. Van Dijk 2005: Ch. 6).

3. I was once having an ultrasound and, ever curious, I asked the ultrasonographer what the distinctive white ring I could see was. It turned out I was, somehow, looking up (or was it down?) my own anus.

4. While I agree with Stacey's argument about the centrality of fantasies of control to biomedicine and alternative medicine, we also need to remember the power of the discourse of 'healing' to alternative medicine, whose techniques – at once legally restrained and spiritually invested – speak less of cure than of transformation and reconciliation (Barcan and Johnston, 2011).

5. Nowadays all Australian bodywork training courses incorporate anatomy and physiology, and the depth and subtlety of a bodyworker's observational powers are undoubtedly enhanced by the kind of detailed anatomical knowledge provided by biomedicine.

6. I am indebted to Margaret Mayhew's (2010) study of life drawing and art education for bringing Nicolaides's work to my attention.

7. Crary argues that in the seventeenth and eighteenth centuries touch was an 'integral part' (1990: 19) of theories of vision, but receded in the nineteenth. The philosopher Immanuel Kant considered sight the 'noblest' of the senses as it was 'furthest removed from the sense of touch', which he considered 'the most limited condition of perception' (2006: 48).

8. This is an assertion based on my conversations with alternative practitioners over many years. Clearly, it is a generalization, but I have found that many CAM practitioners scoff at Freud (though not necessarily at Jung), unaware of the degree to which his theories have permeated contemporary popular thought and culture.

9. Among them: Freud and Breuer's insistence on multi-causality, on specificity and on the possibility of organic disorders whose origins are not psychosomatic, including hereditary ones (Stacey 1997: 120). Stacey cites a number of instances where Freud specifically insisted that symptoms cannot and should not be interpreted 'as direct tropes of the mind' (120).

10. In its turn, 'soul' came to be replaced in modern medical discourse with 'psyche' and eventually 'personality' (Stacey 1997: 125), and in New Age/alternative medical discourse 'emotions' tends to predominate and/or act as a catch-all for all feeling and mental states.

11. The 1990s were designated such by the US Congress. See Rose (2007: 187) and Mitchell (2000).

12. I would like to acknowledge the work of Lisa Zipkis, an Honours student in the Department of Gender and Cultural Studies at the University of Sydney, Australia, whose thesis *Beyond the Binary: Wilhelm Reich: Somatic Theories of Embodiment* (2006) brought Reich's work to the forefront of my attention.

13. I once shared a house with several people, one of whom was a bodyworker. In one of those moments of frustration that characterize shared living, the bodyworker once exclaimed to me in exasperation about the controlling tendencies of another flatmate: 'I swore I'd never move in again with someone who held her pelvis like that!'

14. 'Unwinding' is a term used by bodyworkers to describe sequences of involuntary release of tension in the muscles and fascia that might be catalysed by a bodywork treatment. These often take a quite

visible form, as when, for example, an arm may start lifting up, a shoulder moving back, the neck turning, or the chest arching up from the table. To an onlooker, these may well look willed, forced or faked, but from personal experience I know that they are often not. This doesn't mean, however, that they are immune to the subtle influences of desire and intention.

15. In this instance, I am happy to use the feminine gender to resolve the grammatical awkwardness of 'himself/herself'. As I argue in detail in Chapter 5, clairvoyance is an empirically and metaphorically feminized practice.

16. There are, it appears, professional associations (the Spiritual Healers' Association, the Australian Association of Psychics) but how useful or representative they are is unclear. Certainly, none of my interviewees had had any involvement with them and didn't see them as a potential source of ethical training.

17. By mid-2007, the hardback edition of the book had sold 3.8 million copies in the US alone (McGee 2007: n.p.)

18. For the intersections of yoga and modern science, see Borg-Olivier and Machliss (2003).

19. Epigenetics is the branch of science devoted to the study of the effects of environmental factors on the genes and the expression of genetic material.

20. The practice is now widely known as 'Calmbirth'.

21. René explained to me that his practice has developed out of a number of fields: humanistic psychology (in particular Abraham Maslow, Virginia Satir and Fritz Perls, the developer of Gestalt Therapy); transpersonal psychotherapy (in particular Carl Jung and Roberto Assagioli, the founder of 'psychosynthesis'); and a number of strands of hypnotherapy: medical, clinical and analytical.

22. It is possible for me to make use of it sporadically because the groundwork was laid many years back when I visited this practitioner for a series of sessions. The ability of the body to recognize, remember and rapidly respond to a known and trusted practitioner is discussed in Chapter 4, in relation to bodywork.

Chapter 3

1. Schmidt links Ong's and McLuhan's lament for the 'living presence' of the Word (2003: 47) to their Christianity. McLuhan was a Catholic convert; Ong, a Jesuit priest. Schmidt detects a 'deeply Pauline' conviction underpinning Ong's faith in hearing (45).

2. To take another example, Roland Barthes considers 'the intentional reproduction of a rhythm' to distinguish the human from the animal (1985: 248).

3. In sound and music therapy, toning is a form of chanting, often of a vowel sound, that involves voicing a single note. When performed in a group, it usually promotes the phenomenon of entrainment – whereby vibrations in proximity gradually begin to synchronize. Some therapists combine it with intention, breath and visualization to turn it into a cathartic as well as energizing procedure (Tokalon n.d.). Some music therapists consider yawning, screaming, sighing, moaning and crying to be spontaneous forms of toning: http://www.peacefulmind.com/music_therapy.htm

4. Gioia notes that the human body finds it hard to adjust to different time zones and interruptions to its natural rhythms, such as shift work (2006: 1). 'The body fights back', he says, in the form of accidents, errors, mishaps and health problems (2).

5. This axiom is frequently cited but, after considerable searching, I have not been able to find the original source, nor that of the other quotations from Novalis in this chapter.

6. Throughout this chapter, as elsewhere, unsourced quotations come from interviews carried out for this book. Where I have drawn on published material written by interviewees I have referenced it in the References.

7. For an account of the developmental significance of the decline of the cradle in the West (from the 1890s onwards in the US), see Montagu (1986: 147–62).

8. A 'sonic bath' is not a formal sound therapy but a technique used in sound workshops. An Australian called Peter Gleeson, for example, runs spontaneous vocal/singing events known as the Spontaneous Choir. Gleeson's sonic bath technique involves a volunteer lying on the ground while a crowd of people direct sounds over his/her body in what is to all intents and purposes a vibro-acoustic massage. Gleeson directs the crowd in what sounds to make: perhaps 'sshhhh' or 'mmmmmm' or, if the volunteer is willing, softly intoning his/her name. I have experienced a sonic bath and, depending on the sounds used, it is like being gently rained on, or tapped, or caressed. The body responds – for example with shivers or goose bumps. Such techniques can have therapeutic applications.

9. Sound therapist Chris Tokalon, for example, offers 'playshops and sound journeys' that include a variety of activities, including singing your name to yourself with a loving intention and having a group singing your name back to you 'as you are silently absorbing a sonic bath of loving energy, thrilling to your being' (Tokalon n.d.).

10. 'Nature uses maths' is the subtitle of a website of Hindu philosophy (Gould-King n.d.).

11. Royal Raymond Rife was a US inventor who developed a theory that electrical currents could be used to kill pathogens, and could be useful in curing cancer. Interest in Rife's work waned in the 1950s but revived in the 1980s following the publication of a book by Barry Lynes: *The Cancer Cure that Worked: Fifty Years of Suppression* (1987), which accused the American Medical Association of a cover-up. Mainstream medical scientists accuse Lynes of conspiratorial thought and consider Rife machines to be quackery and pseudoscience (see, for example, a review of Lynes's book published on the Australian Council against Health Fraud website http://www.acahf.org.au/books/reviews/bl_rife.htm

12. Given exactly the right conditions (extreme purity of tone, correct resonant frequency, intensity of volume, and a lucky assemblage of fault-lines in the glass), the soprano can indeed shatter glass (Schrock 2007).

13. For example: 'Mantras are Sanskrit-invocations of the Supreme Being. Reinforced and propelled by japa meditation, they pass from the verbal level through the mental and telepathic states, and on to pure thought energy. Of all languages, Sanskrit most closely approaches telepathic language because of its affinity to the fifty primeval sounds. It is the most direct way to approach the transcendental state' ('Bija Mantras' n.d.).

14. Fifer and Moon, for example, discuss the effects of vibro-acoustic stimulation, especially at low frequencies, on foetal development (1995: 357).

15. Jacques Lacan was a twentieth-century French psychoanalyst who influenced post-structuralism. The core of his theory is the belief that identity is founded on lack. The search for the 'whole self' is in his schema an impossible quest to regain the infant's sense of oneness that preceded the development of individuality.

16. For a longer discussion of the phenomenology of breathing in relation to intersubjectivity, see Barcan 2000.

17. The *bija* mantras are known in the Sufi and Sikh traditions. Gaynor gives the following, but there are many variants: LAM is assigned to the root *chakra*; VAM to the belly; RAM to the solar plexus; YAM to the heart; HAM to the throat; OM to the third eye and ALL SOUND to the crown *chakra* (1999: 14).

18. In fact, the vibratory effects are believed to be more subtle than this schematic summary suggests: A – emerges from the throat, originating in the region of the navel; U – rolls over the tongue; M – ends on the lips; A – waking, U – dreaming, M – sleeping … It is the primordial fundamental

sound symbolic of the Universal Absolute. In fact, when correctly pronounced, or rather, rendered, the 'A' can be felt as a vibration that manifests itself near the navel or abdomen; the 'U' can be felt vibrating the chest, and the 'M' vibrates the cranium or the head. The abdominal vibration symbolizes Creation; it is interesting that the 'creative' or reproductive organs are also located in the lower abdomen. The vibration of the chest represents Preservation, which is also where the lungs are situated (the lungs sustain or preserve the body through breath). The vibration of the head is associated with Destruction or sacrifice, since all that one gives up or destroys is first destroyed mentally. Hence, the entire cycle of the universe and all it contains is said to be symbolized in AUM ('Pronunciation of Om' n.d., some punctuation amended).

19. As proof of this, in this chapter I and my interviewees still occasionally use semiotically inspired words like 'code' and 'encryption'.

20. Freud wrote that the analyst's own unconscious had to become like a kind of receiver 'able to reconstruct the patient's unconscious' (qtd in Barthes 1985: 252). He advised a particular form of listening that he described as an '"evenly hovering" attention' in which the analyst tries not to select or judge what is important – a form of attention that is the counterpart to the demand on the patient to recount everything that occurs to him/her without judgement or selection (qtd in Barthes 1985: 253). This attentiveness without judgement whose aim is to prevent the replication of that which is already known (qtd in Barthes 1985: 253) is not dissimilar from the forms of meditative perception advocated by bodyworkers, which will be described in the next chapter.

21. Equally routinely, we construe onomatopoeia as a notable exception to this rule.

22. These are not exact equivalents, of course. For a critique of 'energy' as a translation of *chi*, see Mayor (2009).

Chapter 4

1. David Chidester's essay on tactility in Christianity paints a complex picture of the role of touch and sight in faith. He begins with the story of the disciple Thomas, who said he could not believe in the resurrection of Christ until he could put his fingers into the stigmata and his hand into the wound in Christ's side. When Christ appears before him, and offers his body up to Thomas's touch, the conclusion is a complex interchange between seeing, touching, truth and belief: 'Jesus saith unto him, Thomas, because thou hast seen me, thou hast believed: blessed are they that have not seen, and yet have believed' (John 20: 29). For his role in this complex drama, Chidester wryly calls Thomas 'the patron saint of Christian tactility' (2005: 72), noting the ongoing centrality of touching (and not-touching) to Christianity (2005: 72–3).

2. Benthien (2002) is summarizing the views of the phenomenologist Etienne Bonnot de Condillac.

3. Tactile reciprocity begins at the very beginning of life. Montagu (1986) emphasizes the reciprocal physiological benefits of close physical contact between mother and child immediately after birth and in the early months of life.

4. One of the medical contexts for their increasing popularity is the increasingly sedentary nature of modern work, and the resultant rise in chronic back problems. The most conservative forms of biomedicine tend to offer treatments that are either palliative or risky (pharmaceutical painkillers or surgery).

5. Grimm claims that scientific interest in the fascia has recently begun to emerge, claiming that it has 'spiked' since 2004 (2007: 1234).

6. This understanding of reiki as non-directive does not accord with the explanation of reiki received by Jackie Stacey, who experienced reiki with someone who appears to have understood it as 'the redirection of the energy field surrounding [one's] body' (1997: 38). In the teaching I received, we

were continually reminded that we were *not* healing another person, nor in fact *doing* anything at all ourselves. Rather, we were to conceive of ourselves as channels or conduits for an energy that had its own mysterious trajectories and agency and that worked in concert with the patient's own conscious or unconscious will and the body's own intelligence. Our job was to contribute time rather than skill, and to strive in the interests of our own spiritual development and the wellbeing of the patient to keep our own ego as much out of the picture as possible.

7. Touch for Health is a form of Applied Kinesiology developed specifically for amateurs to use safely at home. It was founded by Dr John Thie in the early 1970s (La Tourelle 1997: 16).

8. This comparison was passed on to me by the MFR trainer Barbara.

9. On the Imperial scale, this range is equivalent to 0.001574 to 0.059055 inches.

10. Milne uses the example of the disturbance caused to patients by variations in dental crowns, which dentists assess and correct using carbonated paper as thin as three microns (1995a: 5).

11. The concept of EQ has a long genealogy, but was popularized in Daniel Goleman's 1995 book *Emotional Intelligence*.

12. Traditionally, Rolfing, one of the precursors of MFR, has involved the direct use of force to relieve tension in the fascia, but there is some emerging scientific evidence that the force is unlikely to produce results (Grimm 2007: 1235), and that the effectiveness of Rolfing may be due to other elements in the procedure.

13. Of course, the devotees of alternative medicine are likely to hold contradictory views about modernity and individualism. I doubt that many would like to give up the freedoms and choices associated with modern individualism in favour of the more constraining structures of pre-modern societies!

14. For the sociologist Pierre Bourdieu, *habitus* is 'an acquired system of generative schemes' (1990: 55) – that is, a set of body structures and habits that are culturally learned, but nonetheless allow for agency. The body thus conceived is both constrained and free. Its habits and patterns are generated within a particular sociocultural context, but within those limits it is free to act and be acted upon.

15. Carol Davis notes that some people believe the fascia 'acts as the "copper wire" – the conduction mechanism to transmit bioenergy – the ch'i of our body/minds, the flow that is responsible, in part, for homeostasis, for self-regulation, for our ability to stay in remarkable balance, to heal ourselves and maintain our healing state as our natural state' (2009: 12).

16. Though not the only possible ones. Barbara believes that any part of the body could, theoretically, be trained to be a subtle instrument; she talks about the use of feet by shiatsu practitioners, including blind ones. Cf. Ings (2007: 19–20) on the body's ability to adapt and receive sensory information from a variety of sources.

17. Merleau-Ponty believed that we can make a distinction, though not an absolute one, between valid or true perception and hallucination (1962: 334–5). Typically, he saw the intersubjective nature of perception as the guarantor: 'Since all perception is subjective it cannot be its subjective character that distinguishes hallucination from true perception. But true perception, although subjective, is not purely subjective and receives objective confirmation: it opens on to and confirms itself in the world. It is when I act on the basis of my perception that I can confirm its truth; or when I share it with others my perception receives an intersubjective confirmation, if it is true. A hallucinatory perception does not have these qualities …' (Kruks 1981: 12, summarizing Merleau-Ponty 1962: 339).

18. The philosopher Emmanuel Chukwudi Eze notes the paradox whereby critiques of reason may repose on a tacit claim to their own higher reason. He considers that calls to think through 'reason's essential multiplicities' are, in fact, advocating more pragmatic forms of reason (247). I do not

attempt to evade or break through this irony; rather, I hope to dramatize what it is like to live through and with these contradictions.

19. The testimony has more valued contexts, e.g. in Holocaust studies. It has also been a staple genre of feminist and queer studies, where it is, as here, an obviously gendered genre that is ambiguously valued: it is linked to the perceived authenticity of experience and the strategic deployment thereof, but it always threatens to shame the testifier. I would like to thank Anna Gibbs for conversations about this, and other, matters.

20. The question of when and how 'unwilled' might mean the same thing as 'unwilling' is at the heart of what I discuss next.

21. I am speaking in a broad sense of the post-Enlightenment Western analytical tradition. Speaking personally, I have inherited it in various guises, including through a Protestant upbringing and through university education in literary criticism.

22. The closet is a paradoxical space – hidden yet central. As Eve Sedgwick has demonstrated, it reminds us of what is important to any society – what it simultaneously values, repugns, fears and desires. Its space is 'curious', both 'internal and marginal to the culture: centrally representative of its motivating passions and contradictions, even while marginalized by its orthodoxies' (2008 [1990]: 56).

Chapter 5

1. One might expect clients of medical clairvoyants to come from the economically privileged, since medical clairvoyance is unlikely to be recognized by either national health care schemes or private health insurers, but this is only one factor among many. I suspect that clients come from right across the social spectrum and that participation in these practices is governed by dispositional and belief structures more than economic ones.

2. A 1998 study of over two thousand English-speaking households in the US, made up largely of whites and almost exclusively of Christians, found that 35 per cent of respondents used prayer-for-health, while only 11 per cent disclosed this to their doctor. See McCaffrey et al. (2004).

3. There are a few individuals, however, in whose accounts it is tantalizingly more convincing. The medical intuitive Barbara Brennan, for example, is a former researcher for NASA, with a Masters degree in atmospheric physics (1988: 10). The New Age end of the alternative health literature is populated with a few such cross-over figures: Norman Shealy, the MD who works with the medical intuitive Carolyn Myss, whose collaboration is described later in this chapter; Deepak Chopra, an endocrinologist and Ayurvedic physician who specializes in mind-body medicine; Mona Lisa Schulz, the physical and neuroscientist turned medical intuitive. These writers, naturally enough, gain some muscle from their scientific and/or medical training, but it doesn't indemnify them from criticism. For a critique of both Myss and Chopra, for example, see Stacey (2000: 126–8).

4. He notes, for example, that one of the various names by which Romanticism's higher faculty went was, in fact, 'reason' — in a sense reminiscent of Platonic conceptions of 'higher reason', a 'pure intellectual vision' quite discrete from 'a merely analytical Enlightenment rationality' (1998: 416).

5. Again, I want to emphasize that I am speaking of the popular, often commodified forms of sacred medicine, such as those that characterize the New Age. The use of sacred healing techniques among indigenous people or migrants may perhaps have a higher degree of official visibility or recognition, though it is beyond the scope of this study to know in what circumstances this is true.

6. I haven't heard of a similarly high-profile example in my home country of Australia, though I do know of a medical intuitive who works one day a week for a GP. Perhaps the public nature of religiosity in the US makes combining esoteric spirituality and mainstream medicine a more thinkable proposition, at least in some states.

Conclusion

1. He notes that CAM to a large extent continues the logic of this biomedical phenomenon (2007: 28) and is bound up in a shift from understanding sick people as patients to health consumers (23).
2. I refer here to certain absent healing techniques, and also muscle testing techniques in kinesiology.
3. Thanks to Drew Leder for bringing this quotation to my attention.
4. I concur with Ann Game and Andrew Metcalfe, who associate honest writing not only with lack of bluff but also with a lack of condescension (1996: 33).

REFERENCES

Abrams, R.M., Gerhardt, K.J. and Peters, A.J.M. (1995), 'Transmission of Sound and Vibration to the Fetus', in J.-P. Lecanuet, W.P. Fifer, N.A. Krasnegor and W.P. Smotherman (eds), *Fetal Development: A Psychobiological Perspective*, Hillsdale, NJ: Lawrence Erlbaum Associates, pp. 315–30.

Ackerman, D. (1990), *A Natural History of the Senses*, New York: Random House.

Adorno, T.W. and Horkheimer, M. (1979 [1947]), 'The Culture Industry: Enlightenment as Mass Deception', in *The Dialectic of Enlightenment*, London: Verso, pp. 120–67.

Albanese, C.L. (2007), *A Republic of Mind and Spirit: A Cultural History of American Metaphysical Religion*, New Haven, CT: Yale University Press.

Alcoff, L. (2006), *Visible Identities: Race, Gender, and the Self*, New York: Oxford University Press.

American Academy of Medical Acupuncture (n.d.), viewed 3 August 2007, http://www.medicalacupuncture.org

Angell, M. and Kassirer, J.P. (1998), 'Alternative Medicine: The Risks of Untested and Unregulated Remedies', *New England Journal of Medicine*, 339(12): 839–41.

Appadurai, A. (1996), *Modernity at Large: Cultural Dimensions of Globalization*, Minneapolis, MN: University of Minnesota Press.

Aristotle (1906), *De Sensu and De Memoria*, trans. and introd. G.R.T. Ross, Cambridge: Cambridge University Press.

Aristotle (1960 [350 BCE]), *Metaphysics*, trans. R. Hope, Ann Arbor, MI: Michigan University Press.

Armstrong, D. (1986), 'The Problem of the Whole-Person in Holistic Medicine', *Holistic Medicine*, 1: 27–36.

Armstrong, D. (1995), 'The Rise of Surveillance Medicine', *Sociology of Health and Illness*, 17(3): 393–404.

Astin, J.A., Harkness, E. and Ernst, E. (2000), 'The Efficacy of "Distant Healing": A Systematic Review of Randomized Trials', *Annals of Internal Medicine*, 132(11): 903–10.

Augustine (1964 [387–395]), *On Free Choice of the Will*, trans. A.S. Benjamin and L.H. Hackstaff, Indianapolis: Bobbs-Merrill Co.

Australian Traditional-Medicine Society (2006), *Code of Conduct*, viewed 8 November 2009, http://www.atms.com.au/PDFS/ATMS%20Code%20of%20Conduct%20website.pdf

Baer, H.A. (2004), *Toward an Integrative Medicine: Merging Alternative Therapies with Biomedicine*, Walnut Creek: Altamira Press.

Baker, J. (2001), *The Bowen Technique*, Fishbourne, Chichester: Corpus Publishing.

Barcan, R. (2000), 'Breathing Space', *UTS Review*, 6(1): 130–49.

Barcan, R. (2004), *Nudity: A Cultural Anatomy*, Oxford: Berg Publishers.

Barcan, R. (2008), 'Alternative Therapies as Disciplinary Practices: The Uses and Limitations of a Foucauldian Approach', in N. Anderson and K. Schlunke (eds), *Cultural Theory in Everyday Practice*, South Melbourne: Oxford University Press, pp. 14–27.

Barcan, R. (2009a), 'Intuition and Reason in the New Age: A Cultural Study of Medical Clairvoyance', in D. Howes (ed.), *The Sixth Sense Reader*, Oxford: Berg Publishers, pp. 209–32.

Barcan, R. (2009b), 'Spiritual Boundary Work: How Spiritual Healers and Medical Clairvoyants Negotiate the Sacred', in E.B. Coleman and K. White (eds), *Medicine, Religion and the Body*, Leiden: Brill, pp. 129–46.

Barcan, R. (2011, forthcoming), 'Invisible, Dispersed and Connected: The Cultural Plausibility and Attractiveness of Subtle Body Models in the Contemporary West', in G. Samuel and J. Johnston (eds), *Religion and the Subtle Body in Asia and the West: Between Mind and Body*, London: Routledge.

Barcan, R. and Johnston, J. (2005), 'The Haunting: Cultural Studies, Religion and Alternative Therapies', *Iowa Journal of Cultural Studies*, 7: 63–81.

Barcan, R. and Johnston, J. (2011), 'Fixing the Self: Alternative Therapies and Spiritual Logics', in M. Bailey and G. Redden (eds), *Mediating Faiths: Religion and Socio-Cultural Change in the Twenty-First Century*, Farnham, UK: Ashgate Publishing, pp. 75–87.

Barthes, R. (1985), 'Listening', in *The Responsibility of Forms: Critical Essays on Music, Art, and Representation*, trans. R. Howard, New York: Hill and Wang, pp. 245–60.

Baruch, E. (2002), 'Biofield and Energy Therapies', in M.A. Herring and M. Manning Roberts (eds), *Blackwell Complementary and Alternative Medicine: Fast Facts for Medical Practice*, Malden, MA: Blackwell Science, pp. 41–6.

Basil, R. (ed.) (1988), *Not Necessarily the New Age: Critical Essays*, Buffalo, NY: Prometheus.

Beaumont, R. (2005), 'Foreword' to F.F. Smith, *The Alchemy of Touch: Moving Towards Mastery*, Taos, NM: Complementary Medicine Press, pp. ix–xii.

Bennett, J. (2005), *Empathic Vision: Affect, Trauma, and Contemporary Art*, Stanford, CA: Stanford University Press.

Bennett, T. (1998), *Culture: A Reformer's Science*, St Leonards: Allen & Unwin.

Benor, D.J. (1992), 'Intuitive Diagnosis', *Subtle Energies*, 3(2): 41–64.

Benor, D.J. (1993), *Healing Research: Holistic Energy Medicine and Spirituality*, Munich: Helix verlag GmbH.

Benor, D.J. (1995), 'Spiritual Healing: A Unifying Influence in Complementary Therapies', *Complementary Therapies in Medicine*, 3: 234–8.

Bensouilah, J. (2005), 'The History and Development of Modern-British Aromatherapy', *The International Journal of Aromatherapy*, 15: 134–40.

Benthien, C. (2002), *Skin: On the Cultural Border Between Self and World*, New York: Columbia University Press.

Berger, J. (1972), *Ways of Seeing*, London: BBC and Harmondsworth: Penguin.

Bess, F.H. and Humes, L.E. (2003), *Audiology: The Fundamentals*, 3rd edn, Baltimore, MD: Lippincott Williams & Wilkins.

Bharati, Swami Jnaneshvara (n.d.), 'Yoga Nidra: Yogic Conscious Deep Sleep', viewed 21 August 2009, http://www.swamij.com/yoga-nidra.htm

'Bija Mantras' (n.d.), Rudra Centre website, viewed 20 May, 2010, http://www.rudraksha-ratna.com/bija_mantra.php

Birke, L. (1999), *Feminism and the Biological Body*, Edinburgh: Edinburgh University Press.

Block, K.I. (2006), 'Why Integrative Therapies?' editorial, *Integrative Cancer Therapies*, 5(1): 3–6.

Blumenberg, H. (1993), 'Light as a Metaphor for Truth: At the Preliminary Stage of Philosophical Concept Formation', in D.M. Levin (ed.), *Modernity and the Hegemony of Vision*, Berkeley, CA: University of California Press, pp. 30–62.

Bodeker, G. (2000), 'Complementary Medicine and Evidence', *Annals, Academy of Medicine* [Singapore], 29(1): 3–6.

Bodeker, G. (2001), 'Lessons on Integration from the Developing World's Experience', *British Medical Journal*, 322: 161–7.

Bodeker, G. Ong, C.K., Grundy, C., Burford, G. and Shein, K. (eds) (2005), *World Health Organisation Global Atlas of Traditional, Complementary and Alternative Medicine*, Kobe: World Health Organisation Centre for Health Development.

Borg-Olivier, S. and Machliss, B. (2003), 'Yoga and Meditation', in T. Robson (ed.), *An Introduction to Complementary Medicine*, Crows Nest: Allen & Unwin, pp. 276–95.

Bourdieu, P. (1990), *The Logic of Practice*, Stanford, CA: Stanford University Press.

Bradford, N. (ed.) (1996), *The Hamlyn Encyclopedia of Complementary Health*, London: Hamlyn.

Brennan, B.A. (1988), *Hands of Light: A Guide to Healing Through the Human Energy Field: A New Paradigm for the Human Being in Health, Relationship, and Disease*, Toronto: Bantam Books.

Brennan, T. and Jay, M.(eds) (1996), *Vision in Context: Historical and Contemporary Perspectives on Sight*, New York: Routledge.

Brown, C.K. (2000), 'Methodological Problems of Clinical Research into Spiritual Healing: The Healer's Perspective', *Journal of Alternative and Complementary Medicine*, 6(2): 171–6.

Bull, M. and Back, L. (2003), 'Introduction: Into Sound', in M. Bull and L. Back (eds), *The Auditory Culture Reader*, Oxford: Berg Publishers, pp. 1–18.

Bury, M. (1982), 'Chronic Illness as Biographical Disruption', *Sociology of Health and Illness*, 4(2): 167–82.

Bylebyl, J. (2003), 'The Manifest and the Hidden in the Renaissance Clinic', in W.F. Bynum and R. Porter (eds), *Medicine and the Five Senses*, Cambridge: Cambridge University Press, pp. 40–60.

Byrne, R. (2006), *The Secret*, New York: Atria Books.

Cage, J. (1961), *Silence*, Middletown, CT: Wesleyan University Press.

Canaway, R. (2007), 'A Study of the Naturopathic Profession in Melbourne', Master's thesis, University of Melbourne.

Carlyle, T. (1846), *Critical and Miscellaneous Essays*, Philadelphia: Carey and Hart.

Carrette, J. and King, R. (2005), *Selling Spirituality: The Silent Takeover of Religion*, Abingdon: Routledge.

Carter, S. and Hooker, C. (2010), 'Exploring How Lay People Think about Cancer Risk', workshop presented at the Cancer Council of NSW, June 18.

Cartwright, L. (1995), *Screening the Body: Tracing Medicine's Visual Culture*, Minneapolis, MN: University of Minnesota Press.

Caspi, O., Sechrest, L., Pitluk, H.C., Marshall, C.L., Bell, I.R. and Nichter, M. (2003), 'On the Definition of Complementary, Alternative, and Integrative Medicine: Societal Mega-Stereotypes vs. the Patients' Perspectives', *Alternative Therapies in Health and Medicine*, 9(6): 58–62.

Chaitow, L. (2001), 'Foreword', in T.W. Myers, *Anatomy Trains: Myofascial Meridians for Manual and Movement Therapists*, Edinburgh: Churchill Livingstone, pp. ix–xii.

Chant and be Happy: The Power of Mantra Meditation (1982), Based on the Teachings of His Divine Grace A.C. Bhaktivedanta Swami Prabhupēda, Los Angeles, CA: Bhaktivedanta Book Trust.

Chidester, D. (2005), *Authentic Fakes: Religion and American Popular Culture*, Berkeley, CA: University of California Press.

Chopra, D. (2001), *Perfect Health: The Complete Mind Body Guide*, revised edn, Sydney: Bantam Books.

Church, D. (2007), *The Genie in Your Genes: Epigenetic Medicine and the New Biology of Intention*, Santa Rosa, CA: Elite Books.

Clapham, J. Saraswati, prod. (2006), *Shanti: Indian Chants and Music to Calm the Mind*, Bangor, North Wales: Life Foundation School of Therapeutics (UK).

Classen, C. (1993), *Worlds of Sense: Exploring the Senses in History and Across Cultures*, London: Routledge.

Classen, C. (1998), *The Color of Angels: Cosmology, Gender and the Aesthetic Imagination*, London: Routledge.

Classen, C. (ed.) (2005), *The Book of Touch*, Oxford: Berg Publishers.

Classen, C., Howes, D. and Synnott, A. (1994), *Aroma: The Cultural History of Smell*, London: Routledge.

Clennell, B. (1997), 'The Cosmic Body Map', *Yoga Vaani*, 13(4) (51) [*sic*]: 12–14.

Connor, S. (1999), 'Michel Serres's Five Senses', viewed 19 August 2009, http://www.bbk.ac.uk/english/skc/5senses.htm

Cope, S. (1999), *Yoga and the Quest for the True Self*, New York: Bantam Books.

Couldry, N. (2000), *Inside Culture: Re-Imagining the Method of Cultural Studies*, London: Sage Publications.

Coward, R. (1989), *The Whole Truth: The Myth of Alternative Health*, London: Faber & Faber.

Crary, J. (1990), *Techniques of the Observer: On Vision and Modernity in the Nineteenth Century*, Cambridge, MA: MIT Press.

Crawford, R. (1985), 'A Cultural Account of "Health": Control, Release and the Social Body', in J. McKinlay (ed.), *Issues in the Political Economy of Health Care*, London: Tavistock, pp. 60–103.

Crossley, N. (1995), 'Body Techniques, Agency and Intercorporeality: On Goffman's *Relations in Public*', *Sociology*, 29(1): 133–49.

Crossley, N. (1996), *Intersubjectivity: The Fabric of Social Becoming*, London: Sage.

Cunningham, A. and Andrews, B. (eds) (1997), *Western Medicine as Contested Knowledge*, New York: Manchester University Press.

Currivan, J. (2005), *The Wave: A Life Changing Journey into the Heart and Mind of the Cosmos*, Winchester: O Books.

Dale, C. (2009), *The Subtle Body: An Encyclopedia of Your Energetic Anatomy*, Boulder, CO: Sounds True, Inc.

Damasio, A. (2000 [1994]), *Descartes' Error: Emotion, Reason, and the Human Brain*, New York: Quill.

Daruna, J.H. (2004), *Introduction to Psychoneuroimmunology*, Amsterdam: Elsevier Academic Press.

Davis, C. (2009), 'Energy Techniques as a Way of Returning Healing to Health Care', in C. Davis (ed.), *Contemporary Therapies in Rehabilitation: Evidence for Efficacy in Therapy, Prevention, and Wellness*, 3rd edn, Thorofare, NJ: Slack Inc., pp. 7–14.

De Michelis, E. (2004), *A History of Modern Yoga: Patañjai and Western Esotericism*, London: Continuum.

De Rosny, E. (1998), 'The Longevity of the Practice of Traditional Care', in L.-M. Chauvet and M. Tomka (eds), *Illness and Healing*, London: SCM Press, pp. 8–14.

De Sousa, R. (1987), *The Rationality of Emotion*, Cambridge, MA: MIT Press.

Demby, C. (n.d.), 'Sanctum Sanctuorum', viewed 24 August 2007, http://www.constancedemby.com/sanctum_f.html

Derrida, J. (1997), *Of Grammatology*, trans. G.C. Spivak, Baltimore, MD: Johns Hopkins University Press.

Dessaix, R. (1998), 'Showing your Colours', in *(and so forth)*, Sydney: Pan Macmillan/Picador, pp. 121–33.

Dethlefsen, T. and Dahlke, R. (1992), *The Healing Power of Illness: The Meaning of Symptoms and how to Interpret Them*, Shaftesbury, England: Element Books.

Doidge, N. (2008), *The Brain That Changes Itself: Stories of Personal Triumph from the Frontiers of Brain Science*, Carlton North, Vic.: Scribe Publications.

Dolar, M. (2006), *A Voice and Nothing More*, Cambridge, MA, MIT Press.

Donini-Lenhoff, F.G. (2008), 'Coming Together, Moving Apart: A History of the Term *Allied Health* in Education, Accreditation, and Practice', *Journal of Allied Health*, 37(1): 45–52.

Dossey, L. (1993), *Healing Words: The Power of Prayer and the Practice of Medicine*, New York: HarperSanfrancisco.

Dovey, J. (2000), *Freakshow: First Person Media and Factual Television*, London: Pluto Press.

Doyle, B. (2006), letter to the editor, *Sydney Morning Herald*, 14 March: 10.

Easthope, G. (1993), 'The Response of Orthodox Medicine to the Challenge of Alternative Medicine in Australia', *The Australian and New Zealand Journal of Sociology*, 29(3): 289–301.

Eisenberg, D.M., Kessler, R.C., Foster, C., Norlock, F.E., Calkins, D.R. and Delbanco, T.L. (1993), 'Unconventional Medicine in the United States: Prevalence, Costs, and Patterns of Use', *New England Journal of Medicine*, 328(4): 246–52.

Eisenberg, D.M., Kessler, R.C., Van Rompay, M.I., Kaptchuk, T.J., Wilkey, S.A., Appel, S. and Davis, R.B. (2001), 'Perceptions About Complementary Therapies Relative to Conventional Therapies among Adults Who Use Both: Results from a National Survey', *Annals of Internal Medicine*, 135(5): 344–51.

Elliott, C. (2003), *Better Than Well: American Medicine Meets the American Dream*, New York: W.W. Norton.

Elliott, C. (2004), 'The Identity Clinic: Happiness has Become the Goal of Medicine – And it will make us Miserable', *The Guardian*, 27 March.

Eze, E.C. (2008), *On Reason: Rationality in a World of Cultural Conflict and Racism*, Durham, NC: Duke University Press.

Fadlon, J. (2004), 'Meridians, Chakras and Psycho-Neuro-Immunology: The Dematerializing Body and the Domestication of Alternative Medicine', *Body & Society*, 10(4): 69–86.

Farquhar, J. (2002), *Appetites: Food and Sex in Post-Socialist China*, Durham, NC: Duke University Press.

Ficino, M. (1980 [1489]), *The Book of Life*, trans. C. Boer, Irving, TX: Spring Publications.

Fifer, W.P. and Moon, C.M. (1995), 'The Effects of Fetal Experience with Sound', in J.-P. Lecanuet, W.P. Fifer, N.A. Krasnegor and W.P. Smotherman (eds), *Fetal Development: A Psychobiological Perspective*, Hillsdale, NJ: Lawrence Erlbaum Associates, pp. 351–68.

Filmer, P. (2003) 'Songtime: Sound Culture, Rhythm and Sociality', in M. Bull and L. Back (eds), *The Auditory Culture Reader*, Oxford: Berg Publishers, pp. 91–112.

Finnegan, R. (2005), 'Tactile Communication', in C. Classen (ed.), *The Book of Touch*, Oxford: Berg Publishers, pp. 18–25.

Foucault, M. (1979), *The History of Sexuality: An Introduction*, trans. R. Hurley, Harmondsworth: Peregrine.

Foucault, M. (1986), 'Of Other Spaces', *Diacritics*, 16(1): 22–7.

Foucault, M. (2003), *The Birth of the Clinic: An Archaeology of Medical Perception*, trans. A.M. Sheridan, London: Routledge.

Freud, S. (1973), *Civilization and its Discontents*, trans. J. Riviere, London: The Hogarth Press and the Institute of Psycho-Analysis.

Frow, J. (1998), 'Is Elvis a God? Cult, Culture, Questions of Method', *International Journal of Cultural Studies*, 1(2): 197–210.

Fulder, S. (1996), *The Handbook of Alternative and Complementary Medicine*, 3rd edn, Oxford: Oxford University Press.

Gabriel, Y. and Lang, T. (1995), *The Unmanageable Consumer: Contemporary Consumption and its Fragmentation*, London: Sage.

Game, A. and Metcalfe, A. (1996), *Passionate Sociology*, London: Sage Publications.

Garcia, E.E. (2009), 'Alexander Scriabin's *Mysterium* and the Transcendence of Music: Psychoanalytic Notes on Genius, Mysticism and Art', *The Psychoanalytic Review*, 96(3): 461–83.

Garrett, C. (2005 [2001]), *Gut Feelings: Chronic Illness and the Search for Healing*, Amsterdam: Rodopi.

Gawain, S. (1978), *Creative Visualization*, New York: Bantam Books.

Gaynor, M.L. (1999), *Sounds of Healing: A Physician Reveals the Therapeutic Power of Sound, Voice, and Music*, New York: Broadway Books.

Geggus, P. (2004), 'Introduction to the Concepts of Zero Balancing', *Journal of Bodywork and Movement Therapies*, 8(1): 58–71.

Gell, A. (1977), 'Magic, Perfume, Dream …' in I. Lewis (ed.), *Symbols and Sentiments: Cross-Cultural Studies in Symbolism*, London: Academic Press, pp. 25–38.

Giaquinto-Wahl, D.A. (2009), 'Craniosacral Therapy', in C. Davis (ed.), *Contemporary Therapies in Rehabilitation: Evidence for Efficacy in Therapy, Prevention, and Wellness*, 3rd edn, Thorofare, NJ: Slack Inc., pp. 75–87.

Gibbs, A. (2002), 'Disaffected', *Continuum: Journal of Media and Cultural Studies*, 16(3): 335–41.

Giddens, A. (2003), 'An Interview with Anthony Giddens', *Journal of Consumer Culture*, 3(3): 387–99.

Gilbert, E. (2006), *Eat Pray Love: One Woman's Search for Everything*, London: Bloomsbury.

Gioia, T. (2006), *Healing Songs*, Durham, NC: Duke University Press.

Gilman, S. (1993), 'Touch, Sexuality and Disease', in W.F. Bynum and R. Porter (eds), *Medicine and the Five Senses*, Cambridge: Cambridge University Press, pp. 198–224.

Goel, A. (n.d.), 'Understanding Deep Relaxation through Yoga Nidra', viewed 2 September 2009, at http://www.healthandyoga.com/HTML/news/nidrafollowup.html

Goldner, M. (2004), 'Consumption as Activism: An Examination of CAM as Part of the Consumer Movement in Health', in P. Tovey, G. Easthope and J. Adams (eds), *The Mainstreaming of Complementary and Alternative Medicine: Studies in Social Context*, London: Routledge, pp. 11–24.

Goldstein, M.S. (2004), 'The Persistence and Resurgence of Medical Pluralism', *Journal of Health Politics, Policy and Law*, 29(4–5): 925–45.

Goleman, D. (1995), *Emotional Intelligence*, New York: Bantam Books.

Gombrich, E.H. (1972), 'The Visual Image: Its Place in Communication', *Scientific American*, 272: 82–96.

Gordon, D. (n.d.), 'A-U-M-Silence: The Ancient Sound of 'OM'', viewed 2 September 2007 at http://www.spiritsound.com/aum.html

Gould-King, R. (n.d.), 'Anahata Nada: Uncreated Sound', viewed 14 September 2007, http://www.hinduism.co.za/anahata.htm

Govindan, S.V. (2005), 'Ayurvedic Medicine and the History of Massage', in C. Classen (ed.), *The Book of Touch*, Oxford: Berg Publishers, pp. 365–68.

Grace, S., Vemulpad, S. and Beirman, R. (2006), 'Training in and Use of Diagnostic Techniques among CAM Practitioners: An Australian Study', *Journal of Alternative and Complementary Medicine*, 12(7): 695–700.

Grace, S., Vemulpad, S., Reid, A. and Beirman, R. (2008), 'CAM Practitioners in Integrative Practice in New South Wales, Australia: A Descriptive Study', *Complementary Therapies in Medicine*, 16(1): 42–6.

Gray, J. (1992), *Men Are From Mars, Women Are From Venus: The Classic Guide To Under-standing The Opposite Sex*, New York: J.G. Productions Inc.

Greenhalgh, T. and Wessely, S. (2004), '"Health for Me": A Sociocultural Analysis of Healthism in the Middle Classes', *British Medical Bulletin*, 69: 197–213.

Grimm, D. (2007), 'Cell Biology meets Rolfing', *Science*, 318, 23 November: 1234–5.

Grosz, E. (2008), *Chaos, Territory, Art: Deleuze and the Framing of the Earth*, New York: Columbia University Press.

'Hand Development' (n.d.), Parent Information leaflet W41, Kew, Vic: Toddler Kindy GymbaROO.

Hanegraaff, W.J. (1998), *New Age Religion and Western Culture: Esotericism in the Mirror of Secular Thought*, Albany, NY: State University of New York Press.

Hankey, A. (2005), 'CAM Modalities Can Stimulate Advances in Theoretical Biology', *Evidence-based Complementary and Alternative Medicine*, 2(1): 5–12.

Hanna, T. (1977), 'The Somatic Healers and the Somatic Educators', *Somatics*, 1(3), viewed 16 January 2009, http://somatics.org/library/htl-somatichealed.html

Haraway, D.J. (1991), *Simians, Cyborgs, and Women: The Reinvention of Nature*, New York: Routledge.

Harrison, J. (1984), *Love your Disease: It's Keeping you Healthy*, London: Angus and Robertson.

Hay, L.L. (1987), *You Can Heal Your Life*, Concord, NSW: Specialist Publications.

Hay, L.L. (1988), *Heal Your Body: The Mental Causes for Physical Illness and the Metaphysical Way to Overcome Them*, Concord, NSW: Specialist Publications.

Heelas, P. (1996), *The New Age Movement: The Celebration of the Self and the Sacralization of Modernity*, Oxford: Blackwell.

Heelas, P., Woodhead, L., Seel, B., Szerszynski, B. And Tusting, K. (2005), *The Spiritual Revolution: Why Religion is Giving Way to Spirituality*, Malden, MA: Blackwell.

Hochschild, A.R. (2003), *The Commercialization of Intimate Life: Notes from Home and Work*, Berkeley, CA: University of California Press.

Hodge, B. (1995), 'Monstrous Knowledge: Doing PhDs in the New Humanities', *Australian Universities' Review*, 2: 35–9.

Horden, P. (2000), 'Musical Solutions: Past and Present in Music Therapy', in P. Horden (ed.), *Music as Medicine: The History of Music Therapy since Antiquity*, Aldershot: Ashgate, pp. 4–40.

Howden, I. (2003), 'Homœopathy', in T. Robson (ed.), *An Introduction to Complementary Medicine*, Crows Nest: Allen & Unwin, pp. 213–18.

Howes, D. (1991), 'Olfaction and Transition', in D. Howes (ed.), *The Varieties of Sensory Experience: A Sourcebook in the Anthropology of the Senses*, Toronto: University of Toronto Press, pp. 128–47.

Howes, D. (2005a), 'Hyperesthesia, or, The Sensual Logic of Late Capitalism', in D. Howes (ed.), *Empire of the Senses: The Sensual Culture Reader*, Oxford: Berg Publishers, pp. 281–303.

Howes, D. (2005b), 'Introduction: Empires of the Senses', in D. Howes (ed.), *Empire of the Senses: The Sensual Culture Reader*, Oxford: Berg Publishers, pp. 1–17.

Howes, D. (2006), 'Charting the Sensorial Revolution', *Senses and Society*, 1(1): 113–28.

Howes, D. (2009), 'Introduction: The Revolving Sensorium', in D. Howes (ed.), *The Sixth Sense Reader*, Oxford: Berg Publishers, pp. 1–52.

Hughes-Gibb, E. (1928), *The Life-Force in the Plant World Or Creative Nature*, London: George Routledge and Sons.

Huyssen, A. (1986), 'Mass Culture as Woman: Modernism's Other', in T. Modleski (ed.), *Studies in Entertainment: Critical Approaches to Mass Culture*, Bloomington, IN: Indiana University Press, pp. 188–207.

Ihde, D. (2003), 'Auditory Imagination', in M. Bull and L. Back (eds), *The Auditory Culture Reader*, Oxford: Berg Publishers, pp. 61–6.

Illich, I. (1976), *Medical Nemesis*, London: Calder and Boyars.

Ings, S. (2007), *The Eye: A Natural History*, London: Bloomsbury Publishing.

Institute of Medicine of the National Academies (2005), *Complementary and Alternative Medicine in the United States*, Washington: National Academies Press.

'Is Integrative Medicine the Medicine of the Future? A Debate between Arnold S. Relman, MD, and Andrew Weil, MD' (1999), *Archives of Internal Medicine*, 159, 11 October: 2122–6.

Iyengar, B.K.S. (1991), *Light on Yoga*, London: Aquarian/Thorsons.

Jackson-Main, P. (2004), *Practical Iridology*, South Melbourne: Lothian Books.

Jameson, F. (1990), *Signatures of the Visible*, New York: Routledge.

Jay, M. (1993), *Downcast Eyes: The Denigration of Vision in Twentieth-Century French Thought*, Berkeley, CA: University of California Press.

Jensen, B. and Bodeen, D.V. (1992), *Visions of Health: Understanding Iridology*, Garden City Park, NY: Avery Pub. Group.

Jobst, K.A., Shostak, D. and Whitehouse, P.J. (1999), 'Diseases of Meaning, Manifestations of Health, and Metaphor', *Journal of Alternative and Complementary Medicine*, 5(6): 495–502.

Johnston, J. (2008), *Angels of Desire: Esoteric Bodies, Aesthetics and Ethics*, London: Equinox.

Johnston, J. and Barcan, R. (2006), 'Subtle Transformations: Imagining the Body in Alternative Health Practices', *International Journal of Cultural Studies*, 9(1): 25–44.

Jonas, W.B. and Crawford, C. (2003), *Healing, Intention and Energy Medicine: Science, Research Methods and Clinical Implications*, Edinburgh: Churchill Livingstone.

Joudry, P. and Joudry, R. (1999), *Sound Therapy: Music to Recharge your Brain*, Sydney: Sound Therapy Australia.

Jung, C. (1997), *Jung on Active Imagination*, ed. and intro. J. Chodorow, Princeton, NJ: Princeton University Press.

Kant, I. (2006), *Anthropology from a Pragmatic Point of View*, trans. and ed. R.B. Louden, Cambridge: Cambridge University Press.

Kaptchuk, T.J. (2001), 'History of Vitalism', in M.S. Micozzi (ed.), *Fundamentals of Complementary and Alternative Medicine*, 2nd edn, Philadelphia, PA: Churchill Livingstone, pp. 43–56.

Keleman, S. (1981), *Your Body Speaks its Mind*, Berkeley, CA: Center Press.

Keleman, S. (1985), *Emotional Anatomy: The Structure of Experience*, Berkeley, CA: Center Press.

Keller, C. (2008), 'Sight Unseen: Picturing the Invisible', in C. Keller (ed.), *Brought to Light: Photography and the Invisible 1840–1900*, New Haven, CT: Yale University Press, in association with the San Francisco Museum of Modern Art.

Kramer, C. (2000), 'Music as Cause and Cure of Illness in Nineteenth-Century Europe', in P. Horden (ed.), *Music as Medicine: The History of Music Therapy since Antiquity*, Aldershot: Ashgate, pp. 338–52.

Kruks, S. (1981), *The Political Philosophy of Merleau-Ponty*, Brighton, Sussex: Harvester Press.

La Tourelle, M., with Courtenay, A. (1997), *Kinesiology: Touch for Health*, London: Thorsons.

Lawson, K. (2002), 'Political and Economic Issues in CAM', in M.A. Herring and M.M. Roberts (eds), *Blackwell Complementary and Alternative Medicine: Fast Facts for Medical Practice*, Malden, MA: Blackwell Science, Inc, pp. 14–19.

Leadbeater, C.W. (1918), *Clairvoyance*, 4th edn, London: Theosophical Publishing House.

Leder, D. (1990), *The Absent Body*, Chicago: University of Chicago Press.

Leder, D. and Krucoff, M.W. (2008), 'The Touch that Heals', *The Journal of Alternative and Complementary Medicine*, 14(3): 321–27.

Leslie, C. and Young, A. (eds) (1992), *Paths to Asian Medical Knowledge*, Berkeley, CA: University of California Press.

Litchfield, B. (1996), *On Wings Unfolded: A Journey Towards the Light*, Sydney: Angus and Robertson/HarperCollins.

Lloyd, G. (1984), *The Man of Reason: 'Male' and 'Female' in Western Philosophy*, London: Methuen.

Lynes, B. (1987), *The Cancer Cure that Worked: Fifty Years of Suppression*, Minneapolis, MN: CompCare Publications.

Lynxwiler, J. and Gay, D. (2000), 'Moral Boundaries and Deviant Music: Public Attitudes toward Heavy Metal and Rap', *Deviant Behavior*, 21(1): 63–85.

MacDonald, K. (1997), 'Healing', in F. Toy (ed.), *Directions: The Directory of Holistic Health and Creative Living*, Rozelle, NSW: Fiona Toy Trading.

Macintyre, M. (2003), 'Indigenous Healing', in T. Robson (ed.), *An Introduction to Complementary Medicine*, Crows Nest: Allen & Unwin, pp. 33–47.

MacLennan, A.H., Wilson, D.H. and Taylor, A.W. (2002), 'The Escalating Cost and Prevalence of Alternative Medicine', *Preventive Medicine*, 35(2): 166–73.

Marx, K. (1999), *Capital: A New Abridgement*, Oxford: Oxford University Press.

Massey, A. (1998), '"The Way we do Things Around Here": The Culture of Ethnography', Paper presented at the Ethnography and Education Conference, Oxford University Department of Educational Studies (OUDES), 7–8 September, viewed 29 April, 2005, http://www.geocities.com/Tokyo/2961/waywedo.htm

Matthews, S. (2003), 'Ayurveda', in T. Robson (ed.), *An Introduction to Complementary Medicine*, Crows Nest: Allen & Unwin, pp. 15–32.

Mayhew, M. (2010), 'Modelling Subjectivities: Life Drawing, Popular Culture and Contemporary Art Education', PhD thesis, University of Sydney.

Mayor, D. (2009), 'Reinterpreting *Qi* in the 21st Century', *The European Journal of Oriental Medicine*, 6(2): 12–20.

McCaffrey, A.M., Eisenberg, D.M., Legedza, A.T.R., Davis, R.B. and Phillips, R.S. (2004), 'Prayer for Health Concerns: Results of a National Survey on Prevalence and Patterns of Use', *Archives of Internal Medicine*, 164, April 26: 858–62.

McClure, T. (n.d.), 'Depression and Panic', interview with Stanley Keleman, viewed 19 June 2009, http://www.centerpress.com/html/iview.html

McDonald, R., Mead, N., Cheraghi-Sohi, Bower, P., Whalley, D. and Roland, M. (2007), 'Governing the Ethical Consumer: Identity, Choice and the Primary Care Medical Encounter', *Sociology of Health and Illness*, 29(3): 430–56.

McGee, M. (2007), 'The Secret's Success', 17 May, viewed 2 September 2009, http://www.thenation.com/doc/20070604/mcgee, hard copy version in *The Nation*, 4 June 2007.

McKee, A. (2002), 'What Cultural Studies Needs Is More Theory', *Continuum: Journal of Media and Cultural Studies*, 16(3): 311–16.

McLuhan, M. (1962), *The Gutenberg Galaxy: The Making of Typographic Man*, Toronto: University of Toronto Press.

McNeill, W.H. (1995), *Keeping Together in Time: Dance and Drill in Human History*, Cambridge, MA: Harvard University Press.

Meadows, A. (2002), 'Distinctions Between the Bonny Method of Guided Imagery and Music (BMGIM), and Other Imagery Techniques', in K.E. Bruscia and D.E. Grocke (eds), *Guided Imagery and Music: The Bonny Method and Beyond*, Gilsum, NH: Barcelona Publishers, pp. 63–83.

Melton, J.G. (1988), 'A History of the New Age Movement,' in R. Basil (ed.), *Not Necessarily the New Age: Critical Essays*, Buffalo, NY: Prometheus, pp. 35–53.

Melville, S. (1996), 'Division of the Gaze, or, Remarks on the Color and Tenor of Contemporary "Theory"', in T. Brennan and M. Jay (eds), *Vision in Context: Historical and Contemporary Perspectives on Sight*, New York: Routledge, pp. 103–16.

Menuhin, Y. (1999), 'Foreword to the First Edition', in P. Joudry and R. Joudry, *Sound Therapy: Music to Recharge your Brain*, Sydney: Sound Therapy Australia, pp. xi–xii.

Merleau-Ponty, M. (1962), *The Phenomenology of Perception*, trans. C. Smith, London: Routledge.

Merleau-Ponty, M. (1968), *The Visible and the Invisible*, trans. A. Lingis, Evanston, IL: Northwestern University Press.

Metz, C. (1982), *The Imaginary Signifier: Psychoanalysis and the Cinema*, Bloomington, IN: Indiana University Press.

Mick, D.G., Broniarczyk, S.M. and Haidt, J. (2004), 'Choose, Choose, Choose, Choose, Choose, Choose: Emerging and Prospective Research on the Deleterious Effects of Living in Consumer Hyperchoice', *Journal of Business Ethics*, 52(2): 207–11.

Milne, H. (1995a), *The Heart of Listening: A Visionary Approach to Craniosacral Work*, Vol. 1: *Origins, Destination Points, Unfoldment*, Berkeley, CA: North Atlantic Books.

Milne, H. (1995b), *The Heart of Listening: A Visionary Approach to Craniosacral Work*, Vol. 2: *Anatomy, Technique, Transcendence*, Berkeley, CA: North Atlantic Books.

Mitchell, E. (2000), 'Speak, Memory', *Time Magazine*, 28 February.

Mongan, M.F. (1998), *HypnoBirthing®: A Celebration of Life*, Concord, NH: Rivertree Publishing.

Montagu, A. (1986 [1971]), *Touching: The Human Significance of the Skin*, 3rd edn, New York: Harper and Row.

Montiel, I., Bardasano, J.L. and Ramos, J.L. (2005), 'Biophysical Device for the Treatment of Neurodegenerative Diseases', in A. Méndez-Vilas (ed.), *Recent Advances in Multidisciplinary Applied Physics*, Oxford: Elsevier, pp. 63–9.

Mulvey, L. (1975), 'Visual Pleasure and Narrative Cinema', *Screen*, 16(3): 6–18.

Myers, T.W. (2001), *Anatomy Trains: Myofascial Meridians for Manual and Movement Therapists*, Edinburgh: Churchill Livingstone.

Myss, C. and Shealy, C.N. (1993 [1988]), *The Creation of Health: The Emotional, Psychological, and Spiritual Responses that Promote Health and Healing*, New York: Three Rivers Press.

Myss, C. and Shealy, N. (2002), *The Science of Medical Intuition: Self-Diagnosis and Healing with Your Body's Energy Systems*, 12 CD set, Sounds True.

Nicolaides, K. (1941), *The Natural Way to Draw*, Boston, MA: Houghton Mifflin.

Noontil, A. (1994), *The Body is the Barometer of the Soul*, [Kilsyth South, Vic]: Brumby Books.

Nudd, P. (2006), 'The Hornsby Spine', Newsletter of the Hornsby Spine Centre, June.

Nutton, V. (1993), 'Galen at the Bedside: The Methods of a Medical Detective', in W.F. Bynum and R. Porter (eds), *Medicine and the Five Senses*, Cambridge: Cambridge University Press, pp. 7–16.

Olivelle, P. (1998), *The Early Upaniṣads: Annotated Text and Translation*, New York: Oxford University Press.

Oliver, K. (2001), 'The Look of Love', *Hypatia*, 16(3): 56–78.

Ong, W.J. (1967), *The Presence of the Word: Some Prolegomena for Cultural and Religious History*, New Haven, CT: Yale University Press.

Ong, W.J. 1988 [1982], *Orality and Literacy: The Technologizing of the Word*, London: Routledge.

Oppenheimer, M. (2008), 'The Queen of the New Age', *New York Times*, 4 May, viewed 4 March 2010, www.nytimes.com

Parsons, T. (1951), *The Social System*, London: Routledge & Kegan Paul.

Patching van der Sluijs, C.G. and Bensoussan, A. (2003), 'Traditional Chinese Medicine', in T. Robson (ed.), *An Introduction to Complementary Medicine*, Crows Nest: Allen & Unwin, pp. 67–85.

Paterson, M. (2005), 'Affecting Touch: Towards a "Felt" Phenomenology of Therapeutic Touch', in J. Davidson, L. Bondi, and M. Smith (eds), *Emotional Geographies*, Aldershot: Ashgate, pp. 161–73.

Philo, C. (2000), '*The Birth of the Clinic*: An Unknown Work of Medical Geography', *Area*, 32(1): 11–19.

Porter, R. (1993), 'The Rise of Physical Examination', in W.F. Bynum and R. Porter (eds), *Medicine and the Five Senses*, Cambridge: Cambridge University Press, pp. 179–97.

Povinelli, E.A. (2001), 'Radical Worlds: The Anthropology of Incommensurability and Inconceivability', *Annual Review of Anthropology*, 30: 319–34.

Prattis, J.I. (1997), *Anthropology at the Edge: Essays on Culture, Symbol, and Consciousness*, Lanham, MD: University Press of America.

Pringle, R. (1998), *Sex and Medicine: Gender, Power and Authority in the Medical Profession*, Cambridge: Cambridge University Press.

Probyn, E. (1990), 'New Traditionalism and Post-Feminism: TV Does the Home', *Screen*, 31(2): 147–59.

Probyn, E. (2000), *Carnal Appetites: Foodsexidentities*, London: Routledge.

'Pronunciation of Om' (n.d.), *The Hindu Life*, viewed 23 July 2010, http://www.thehindulife.com/mantra/pronunciation-of-om.html

Ramachandran, A. (2007), 'Diagnosis by Internet Wastes Time, say GPs', *Sydney Morning Herald*, 14–15 July: 12.

Reger, J. (2001), 'Emotions, Objectivity and Voice: An Analysis of a "Failed" Participant Observation', *Women's Studies International Forum*, 24(5): 605–16.

Reich, W. 1969 [1933], *Character Analysis*, 3rd edn, trans. T.P. Wolfe, London: Vision Press.

Rhodes, R. (1995), *The New Age Movement*, Grand Rapids, MI: Zondervan.

Rimke, H.M. (2000), 'Governing Citizens through Self-Help Literature', *Cultural Studies*, 14(1): 61–78.

Robertson-Gillam, K. (2004), 'Spirited Living Creates a New Vision: Using Meditation, Music and Choir Work for Elderly People with Depression and Dementia', unpublished paper.

Rodaway, P. (1994), *Sensuous Geographies: Body, Sense and Place*, London: Routledge.

Ronca, A.E. and Alberts, J.R. (1995), 'Maternal Contributions to Perinatal Experience', in J.-P. Lecanuet, W.P. Fifer, N.A. Krasnegor and W.P. Smotherman (eds), *Fetal Development: A Psychobiological Perspective*, Hillsdale, NJ: Lawrence Erlbaum Associates, pp. 331–50.

Root, D. (1996), *Cannibal Culture: Art, Appropriation, and the Commodification of Difference*, Boulder, CO: Westview Press.

Rose, N.S. (1996), *Inventing Ourselves: Psychology, Power, and Personhood*, Cambridge: Cambridge University Press.

Rose, N.S. (1999), *Governing the Soul: The Shaping of the Private Self*, 2nd edn, London: Free Association Books.

Rose, N. (2007), *The Politics of Life Itself: Biomedicine, Power and Subjectivity in the Twenty-First Century*, Princeton, NJ: Princeton University Press.

Rose, T. (1991), '"Fear of a Black Planet": Rap Music and Black Cultural Politics in the 1990s', *Journal of Negro Education*, 60(3): 276–90.

Ross, A. (1991), 'New Age: A Kinder, Gentler Science?', in *Strange Weather: Culture, Science and Technology in the Age of Limits*, London: Verso, pp. 15–74.

Rubik, B. (1995), 'Energy Medicine and the Unifying Concept of Information', *Alternative Therapies in Health and Medicine*, 1(1): 34–9.

Ruggie, M. (2004), *Marginal to Mainstream: Alternative Medicine in America*, Cambridge: Cambridge University Press.

Ruggie, M. (2005), 'Mainstreaming Complementary Therapies: New Directions in Health Care', *Health Affairs*, 24(4): 980–90.

Saks, M. (2003), *Orthodox and Alternative Medicine: Politics, Professionalization and Health Care*, London: Continuum.

Salk, J. (1983), *Anatomy of Reality: Merging of Intuition and Reason*, New York: Columbia University Press.

Schafer, M. (2003), in M. Bull and L. Back (eds), *The Auditory Culture Reader*, Oxford: Berg Publishers, pp. 25–39.

Schmidt, L.E. (1998), 'From Demon Possession to Magic Show: Ventriloquism, Religion, and the Enlightenment', *Church History*, 67(2): 274–304.

Schmidt, L.E. (2003), 'Hearing Loss', in M. Bull and L. Back (eds), *The Auditory Culture Reader*, Oxford: Berg Publishers, pp. 41–59.

Schmidt, L.E. (n.d.), 'Hearing Things: The Mystic's Ear and the Voices of Reason', Website of the Material History of American Religion Project, viewed 24 August 2007, http://www.materialreligion.org/participants/schmidt.html

Schrock, K. (2007), 'Fact or Fiction? An Opera Singer's Piercing Voice can Shatter Glass', *Scientific American*, 23 August, viewed 6 November 2010, http://www.scientificamerican.com/article.cfm?id=fact-or-fiction-opera-singer-can-shatter-glass

Schulz, M.L. (1998), *Awakening Intuition: Using your Mind-Body Network for Insight and Healing*, New York: Harmony Books.

Schwartz, B. (2004), *The Paradox of Choice: Why More Is Less*, New York: Ecco/HarperCollins Publishers.

Schwartz, L.R. (1969), 'The Hierarchy of Resort in Curative Practices: The Admiralty Islands, Melanesia', *Journal of Health and Social Behavior*, 10(3): 201–09.

Scott, A.L. (1998), 'The Symbolizing Body and the Metaphysics of Alternative Medicine', *Body & Society*, 4(3): 21–37.

Scott, J.W. (1991), 'The Evidence of Experience', *Critical Inquiry*, 17(4): 773–97.

Sedgwick, E.K. (2008 [1990]), *Epistemology of the Closet*, Berkeley, CA: University of California Press.

Sedgwick, E.K. (2003), 'Paranoid Reading and Reparative Reading, Or, You're so Paranoid, You Probably Think This Essay is About You', in *Touching Feeling: Affect, Pedagogy, Performativity*, Durham, NC: Duke University Press, pp. 123–51.

Sedgwick, E.K. and Frank, A. (1995), 'Shame in the Cybernetic Fold: Reading Silvan Tomkins', in E.K. Sedgwick and A. Frank (eds), *Shame and its Sisters: A Silvan Tomkins Reader*, Durham, NC, Duke University Press, pp. 1–28.

Serres, M. (2008 [1985]), *The Five Senses: A Philosophy of Mingled Bodies*, trans. M. Sankey and P. Cowley, London: Continuum.

Shannahoff-Khalsa, D. (1996), 'Sounds for Transcendence: Yogic Techniques for Opening the Tenth Gate', in R.R. Pratt and R. Spintge (eds), *MusicMedicine: Volume 2*, Selected papers from the International Society for Music in Medicine V, St Louis, MO: International Society for Music in Medicine, pp. 351–60.

Shumsky, S.G. (1996), *Divine Revelation*, New York: Simon & Schuster.

Sim, S. (2007), *Manifesto for Silence: Confronting the Politics and Culture of Noise*, Edinburgh: Edinburgh University Press.

Singer, J.B. (2008), 'Listening to Refugee Bodies: The Naturopathic Encounter as a Cross-Cultural meeting Place', PhD thesis, Southern Cross University, Lismore, NSW.

Singg, S. (2009), 'Reiki: An Alternative and Complementary Healing Therapy', in C. Davis (ed.), *Contemporary Therapies in Rehabilitation: Evidence for Efficacy in Therapy, Prevention, and Wellness*, 3rd edn, Thorofare, NJ: Slack Inc, pp. 261–77.

Skeggs, B. (1995), 'Theorising, Ethics and Representation in Feminist Ethnography', in B. Skeggs (ed.), *Feminist Cultural Theory: Process and Production*, Manchester: Manchester University Press, pp. 190–206.

Smith, F.F. (1986), *Inner Bridges: A Guide to Energy Movement and Body Structure*, Atlanta, GA: Humanics Ltd.

Smith, F.F. (2005), *The Alchemy of Touch: Moving Towards Mastery*, Taos, NM: Complementary Medicine Press.

Smith, M. (2007), *Sensory History*, Oxford: Berg Publishers.

Sontag, S. (1977), *Illness as Metaphor*, Harmondsworth: Penguin.

Sontag, S. (1988), *Illness as Metaphor and AIDS and its Metaphors*, New York: Doubleday.

Soskice, J.M. (1996), 'Sight and Vision in Medieval Christian Thought', in T. Brennan and M. Jay (eds), *Vision in Context: Historical and Contemporary Perspectives on Sight*, New York: Routledge, pp. 29–43.

Spintge, R. (1996), 'Physiology, Mathematics, Music, and Medicine: Definitions and Concepts for Research', in R.R. Pratt and R. Spintge (eds), *MusicMedicine: Volume 2*, Selected papers from the International Society for Music in Medicine V, St Louis, MO: International Society for Music in Medicine, pp. 3–13.

Srinivasananda, Swami (2003), *Meditations for Inner Freedom*, compact disc, Simon & Schuster.

Stacey, J. (1997), *Teratologies: A Cultural Study of Cancer*, London: Routledge.

Stacey, J. (2000), 'The Global Within', in S. Franklin, C. Lury and J. Stacey (eds), *Global Nature, Global Culture*, London: Sage, pp. 97–145.

Stacey, M. (1986), 'Concepts of Health and Illness and the Division of Labour in Health Care', in C. Currer and M. Stacey (eds), *Concepts of Health, Illness and Healing*, Leamington Spa: Berg, pp. 9–26.

Stafford, B.M. (1991), *Body Criticism: Imaging the Unseen in Enlightenment Art and Medicine*, Cambridge, MA: MIT Press.

Stallybrass, P. and White, A. (1986), *The Politics and Poetics of Transgression*, Ithaca, NY: Cornell University Press.

Star, S.L. (1991), 'The Politics of Left and Right: Sex Differences in Hemispheric Brain Asymmetry', in S. Gunew (ed.), *A Reader in Feminist Knowledge*, London: Routledge, pp. 237–48.

Steingart, M. (2006), 'You Can Achieve Anything You Imagine ...', viewed 20 July 2010, http://www.yourdailymotivation.com/motivational-message-5.htm

Stoller, P. (2004), *Stranger in the Village of the Sick: A Memoir of Cancer, Sorcery, and Healing*, Boston, MA: Beacon Press.

Sullivan, L.E. (1997), 'Enchanting Powers: An Introduction', in *Enchanting Powers: Music in the World's Religions*, Cambridge, MA: Harvard University Press, pp. 1–11.

Sutcliffe, S.J. (2006), 'Practising New Age Soteriologies in the Rational Order', in L. Hume and K. McPhillips (eds), *Popular Spiritualities: The Politics of Contemporary Enchantment*, Aldershot: Ashgate, pp. 159–74.

Sutherland, J-A., Poloma, M.M. and Pendleton, B.F. (2003) 'Religion, Spirituality and Alternative Health Practices: The Baby Boomer and Cold War Cohorts', *Journal of Religion and Health*, 42(4): 315–38.

Synnott, A. (1993), *The Body Social: Symbolism, Self and Society*, London: Routledge.

Taylor, J. Bolte (2006), *My Stroke of Insight: A Brain Scientist's Personal Journey*, New York: Viking/Penguin.

Thomas, K. (2005), 'Magical Healing: The King's Touch', in C. Classen (ed.), *The Book of Touch*, Oxford: Berg Publishers, pp. 354–62.

Tokalon, C. (n.d.), 'Playshops & Sound Journeys', Sound Body Sound Mind website, viewed 24 Aug. 2007, www.soundman.co.za/workshops.html

Tompkins, P. and Bird, C. (1974), *The Secret Life of Plants*, Harmondsworth: Penguin.

Toning for Peace (n.d.), viewed 21 April 2010, http://www.toningforpeace.org/

Tortora, G.J. and Grabowski, S.R. (1993), *Principles of Anatomy and Physiology*, 7th edn, New York: HarperCollinsCollege Publications.

Turnbull, C., Grimmer-Somers, K., Kumar, S., May, E., Law. D. and Ashworth, E. (2009), 'Allied, Scientific and Complementary Health Professionals: A New Model for Australian Allied Health', *Australian Health Review*, 33(1): 27–37.

Turner, B.S. (1992), *Regulating Bodies: Essays in Medical Sociology*, London: Routledge.

Turner, B.S. (1996), *The Body and Society*, 2nd edn, London: Sage Publications.

Tyler, H.M. (2000), 'The Music Therapy Profession in Modern Britain', in P. Horden (ed.), *Music as Medicine: The History of Music Therapy Since Antiquity*, Aldershot: Ashgate, pp. 375–93.

Van Dijck, J. (2005), *The Transparent Body: A Cultural Analysis of Medical Imaging*, Seattle, WA: University of Washington Press.

Vasseleu, C. (1996), 'Illuminating Passion: Irigaray's Transfiguration of Night', in T. Brennan and M. Jay (eds), *Vision in Context: Historical and Contemporary Perspectives on Sight*, New York: Routledge, pp. 129–37.

Vasseleu, C. (1998), *Textures of Light: Vision and Touch in Irigaray, Levinas, and Merleau-Ponty*, London: Routledge.

Voss, A. (2000), 'Marsilio Ficino, The Second Orpheus', in P. Horden (ed.), *Music as Medicine: The History of Music Therapy Since Antiquity*, Aldershot: Ashgate, pp. 154–72.

Weir, M. (2003), 'Obligation to Advise of Options for Treatment: Medical Doctors and Complementary and Alternative Medicine Practitioners', *Journal of Law and Medicine*, 10: 296–307.

Weiten, W. (2010), *Psychology: Themes and Variations*, 8th edn, Belmont, CA: Wadsworth.

White, A. (2000), 'Integration … Beyond Placebo?' Editorial, *Complementary Therapies in Medicine*, 8(4): 225.

Wilde, A. (2006), *Allied Health: Australia*, Ultimo: Career FAQs Pty Ltd.

Willard, B.E. (2005), 'Feminist Interventions in Biomedical Discourse: An Analysis of the Rhetoric of Integrative Medicine', *Women's Studies in Communication*, 28(1): 115–48.

Williams, A. (1998), 'Therapeutic Landscapes in Holistic Medicine', *Social Science and Medicine*, 46(9): 1193–203.

Willis, E. and White, K. (2004), 'Evidence-Based Medicine and CAM', in P. Tovey, G. Easthope and J. Adams (eds), *The Mainstreaming of Complementary and Alternative Medicine: Studies in Social Context*, London: Routledge, pp. 49–63.

Wilson, E.A. (2004), 'Gut Feminism', *differences: A Journal of Feminist Cultural Studies*, 15(3): 66–94.

Young, K. (2002), 'The Memory of the Flesh: The Family Body in Somatic Psychology', *Body & Society*, 8(3): 25–47.

Ziebland, S., Chapple, A., Dumelow, C., Evans, J., Prinjha, S. and Rozmovits, L. (2004), 'Information in Practice: How the Internet Affects Patients' Experience of Cancer: A Qualitative Study', *British Medical Journal*, 328, 6 March: 564.

Zipkis, L. (2006), *Beyond the Binary: Wilhelm Reich: Somatic Theories of Embodiment*, Honours thesis, Department of Gender and Cultural Studies, University of Sydney, Australia.

Zola, I. (1972), 'Medicine as an Institution of Social Control', *Sociological Review*, 20: 487–54.

INDEX

acupuncture 7–8, 26
  medical acupuncture 15–16, 222n12
  see also Traditional Chinese Medicine
ageing 39, 223n29
allied health 9–10, 221n6
alternative therapies *see* Complementary and
  Alternative Medicine
anatomy 61, 65, 78, 82
animality 3, 112, 114, 141, 223n29
anxiety 9, 33, 37, 41, 62, 81, 85
Aristotle 57, 112, 117, 142
aromatherapy 4, 15, 51–2 139, 215
Augustine 88, 142
AUM *see* OM
auras 26, 60, 196, 197–8
  Kirlian photography 6
Ayurveda 38–9, 49, 52, 72, 129, 147–8, 151,
  163, 223n36, 229n3

Benor, Daniel 187, 193, 194, 199
biomedicine
  acceptance outside the West 8, 13
  convergence with CAM 16, 39, 42, 52, 64,
    66, 218
    see also integrative medicine
  dissatisfaction with 23, 32–4
  names for 12, 221n3
  relations with alternative medicine 7,
    12–20, 37–8
  successes of 2, 18, 19, 33, 213
  see also anatomy; evidence-based medicine;
    medical pluralism; medicalization;
    palliative care; vision – medical gaze
body
  as communicative 52, 78–9, 138–9, 151–2,
    168–9, 171, 185, 186

  see also touch – as a medium of
    communication
  as 'fluid', 152–4, 167
  interpretation of 4, 71, 75–80, 83–5, 138,
    139, 147, 170, 176–84
  rhythmicity of 116–17, 120, 125, 153–4
bodywork 147–84
Borg-Olivier, Simon 19, 134, 135, 219
Bowen technique 8–9, 22
brain, the 81, 85, 107, 117, 119, 138, 170,
  175
  hemispheres of 205–8
  see also neuroplasticity
Brennan, Barbara 19, 31, 229n3
Byrne, Rhonda 102

Cage, John 111
chakras 26, 101, 116, 133, 151, 186, 193,
  222n18
chanting 8, 19, 116, 123, 125, 133–5
chi 26, 147, 149, 169, 170
  chi body 136, 138
  see also energy
chiropractic 7, 10, 21, 23
choice 8–9, 33, 37, 41, 213
Chopra, Deepak 26–7, 38–9, 223n28, 229n3
clairvoyance 45, 73, 198
  ethics of 92–7
  feminization of 88, 90, 186
  medical clairvoyance 4, 15, 185–212
  vision and 47, 87–96, 197–9
Classen, Constance 4, 50, 57
colonialism 63, 98
Complementary and Alternative Medicine
  (CAM)
  accreditation of practitioners 15

as cultural practice 2–3, 16, 21–2, 214
attractions of 4, 32, 34, 215–18 passim
contradictions of 4–5, 41–2
core principles of 22–31
definitions of 6
diversity within 11, 20, 214
domestication of 11, 13–15
feminization of 3, 8, 9, 18, 49, 186, 217
legitimization of 9–10, 13, 16, 210–11
medical effectiveness of 3, 19, 71–2, 89,
    149, 187–8, 213–14
opposition to 17, 18, 24–5, 31, 74
practitioner-client relations 22–3, 34, 36,
    72, 136, 160, 162–9, 196
patterns of usage 2, 8, 9, 11–12, 186, 217,
    229n1
privilege associated with 2, 11–12, 36, 41,
    109–10, 149, 217–18, 222n8
professional ethics see ethics
professionalization of 11, 13–15, 52, 86,
    161–2
relations to biomedicine 6–11, 187, 190,
    204–5
resistance to biomedicine 217
social factors behind rise of 32–42
studies of 42–4
taxonomies of 20–1, 192
terms for 6–12
see also allied health; evidence-based
    medicine; integrative medicine; and
    separate listings for particular therapies
complementarity 6, 8, 9, 206–8
consumerism 4–8 passim, 21, 31, 35–7
    aestheticisation of everyday life 36
    body maintenance and 41–2
    commodification of traditional techniques
        12, 35, 44, 95, 97, 173, 221n3
    hedonism and 4, 35, 41–2, 213, 215, 216
control 31, 32, 38–41, 64, 70, 106, 108
craniosacral therapy (CST), 148, 151–9
    passim 172
    see also Milne, Hugh
Cultural Studies 3, 4, 5, 42–6, 48, 78, 129,
    218–19, 220

Damasio, Antonio 209
depression 81, 85
Derrida, Jacques 114

Descartes, René 144, 169, 202, 209
diagnosis 4, 7, 18, 23, 60, 68–97, 150, 195–6,
    205, 222n16
    intuitive 194, 209–10
dreams 59, 88, 113, 177, 179
dualism 9, 30, 33, 166–7, 191, 208, 218

'East', the 4, 21, 44, 221n3
emotions 30, 33–5 passim, 141, 167, 189–90
    emotional body 26, 205
    emotional release 15, 23, 26, 80–1, 91–2,
        158–9, 177
    music and 118, 123, 130–1
    relation to reason 208–9
    role in illness 28–30, 80–1
    stored in the body 78–9, 86, 147, 151
empowerment 8, 33, 37, 40–1, 43, 70, 72, 98,
    105, 106, 190
energy 26–7, 102, 186, 194
    see also chi; prana; subtle body; vibrations
energy medicine 65, 194–5, 210–11
    see also reiki; spiritual healing
epigenetics 107, 175, 176, 195
ethics 67, 77, 102, 105, 216
    of intersubjectivity 27–8, 122, 124, 132,
        215
    professional 52–3, 71–3, 75, 79–80, 86,
        154, 158, 177–81 passim, 200, 204
    research 89, 149, 173, 189–90, 219
    somatic 213, 220
    see also clairvoyance – ethics of
evidence-based medicine 10, 11, 14, 18, 175,
    210, 218
eyes see iridology; vision

fascia 147, 148, 156, 170–1
    see also myofascial release
feminism 6, 56, 58, 63, 68, 108, 143, 187,
    217, 219
    the body and 46–7
    the brain and 205–8
Ficino, Marsilio 125, 127
Foucault, Michel 24, 42, 46, 61–2, 67, 77, 80,
    103, 189
    biopolitics 213
    Foucauldian approaches 42, 66, 72, 76, 87,
        180
    see also Rose, Nikolas

freedom 38, 41, 58, 59, 106
Freud, Sigmund 28, 29, 55, 79, 80–2, 112, 136, 143, 178, 227n20

Gawain, Shakti 27, 102, 105
Gender Studies 3, 42
    see also feminism
globalization 6, 13, 44, 46

hands, the 146–7, 171–2, 178
harmony 206, 207
    see also sound – harmony and
Hay, Louise L., 29, 30, 38, 80, 83
healing 24
    absent 166, 172, 181–2, 193, 194, 195
    mutuality of 166
    self-healing 22–3, 98, 148–9
    vs. cure 23, 106, 138, 158, 169, 210
holism 4, 7, 15, 23–7, 34, 65, 78, 82, 85, 133, 135, 148, 151–2, 197, 206, 222n17
homeopathy 6, 22, 65, 140, 221n4
Howes, David 4, 36, 47, 50
Hypnobirthing 107–8
hypnotherapy 22, 100, 109–10

Illich, Ivan 24
illness 33, 216
    metaphor and 43–4
        see also Sontag, Susan
    metaphysical theories of 29–31, 80–1, 105–6, 181, 196–7
    pedagogic concept of 31, 39
    psychosocial factors and 25, 28
    responsibility for 37, 39–40, 43, 105
    social conceptions of 30, 197
incommensurability 5, 14, 16, 48–9, 133, 188–90, 204
individualism 2, 4, 5, 28, 38, 167, 216–17
information 63–4, 65, 67, 70, 169, 171, 186, 195–8
    see also body – interpretation of; touch – as a medium of communication
integrative medicine 8, 17–18, 53, 109, 209–10, 211, 218–19
intercorporeality 3, 162–82, 201
interpretation see body – interpretation of
intersubjectivity 3, 107, 165, 201–2, 215
    see also intercorporeality

intuition 27, 43, 45, 77, 90, 96, 149, 185–212
    as a gift 185,
    as transcending other senses 51, 202–3
    bodily dimensions of 178
    gendering of 3, 27, 186
    relation to reason 3, 191, 201, 203, 206–9
    training of 97–8, 139, 172, 185, 191, 202
    see also clairvoyance – medical; diagnosis – intuitive
iridology 4, 23, 69–75, 202–3
Irigaray, Luce 58, 59
IVF 9, 40
Iyengar, B.K.S. 133, 222n18

Jung, Carl 104, 109, 112, 225n21

Kant, Immanuel 172, 178, 220
Keleman, Stanley 82–6, 153

Lacan, Jacques 132, 133, 144
Leadbeater, Charles Webster 90, 97, 198
life force 22
    see also vitalism
light 56, 99–100

McLuhan, Marshall 12, 225n1
Marx, Karl 215
massage 12, 18, 75, 149, 160, 161, 163
    different styles of 21, 23, 151, 152, 157–9, 161, 164–5
    eroticism and 160–2
    intimacy of 34, 160–1, 163
    pleasures of 36, 40, 51
Mateos, René 19, 109–10
materiality
    of the body 65, 66, 186, 214
    of sound 133–40
    of the senses 218–19
    of thought 176
medical imaging techniques 62–4, 224n2
    see also X-ray
medical intuition see clairvoyance – medical
medical pluralism 1, 2, 3, 13, 33, 159, 188
medicalization 24, 213
meditation 26, 57, 60, 68, 77, 99, 100, 107, 119, 138, 155, 180
    see also visualization – creative

memory 4
  bodily 170–1, 214
  encoded in sound 136, 138–9, 170
  music and 119, 120–1, 123, 131
Menuhin, Yehudi 117, 122, 125
Merleau-Ponty, Maurice 58, 59, 132, 146,
  165, 168, 169, 215–16, 228n17
metaphysics *see* illness – metaphysical theories
  of; presence; religion – US metaphysical
Milne, Hugh 77, 101, 151–5 passim, 158,
  166,
modernity 35, 55, 61, 90, 112–15, 189
music
  as visceral 115, 117, 128
  dangers of 123, 127–31
  divinity and 122, 131–2
  effects on cells 129–31
  effects on plants 130
  emotions and *see* emotions – music and
  healing power of 115–16, 118–19, 122
  memory and *see* memory – music and
  New Age 122
  rap 128, 131
  singing 131–2
  sociality and 121–4
music therapy 116, 118–20, 123–4
myofascial release (MFR) 75, 83, 148, 151,
  152, 166
Myss, Caroline 19, 209–10, 211

nature
  as God's mediator 113, 114
  as musical 126
  'Easternised' 21
  ideologies of 4, 6, 7, 23–4, 44
naturopathy 12, 15, 52, 140, 197
neoliberalism 5, 8, 37–41, 64, 66, 70, 95,
  103, 216–17
neuroplasticity 77, 175
New Age 4, 17, 20, 27, 38, 49, 84, 95, 97–8,
  99, 123, 180
  apoliticism of 28, 43
  artistic merits of 221n1
  beliefs 26, 29–31, 38, 180, 203, 206, 214
  critiques of 42–3
  individualism of 27–8, 35, 43, 102, 103,
  216–17
  links with alternative medicine 6, 31, 34

manifestation techniques 102–5
  rise of 34–5
  use of science 26–7, 195
  workshops 71, 83, 107
  see also illness – metaphysical theories of
noise 111, 113, 120–1, 128–9
Novalis 117, 120, 125, 142

OM 116, 126–7, 133–4, 226–7n18
Ong, Walter 50, 112, 137, 225n1
Orientalism 5
osteopathy 7, 15, 75, 153
  see also craniosacral therapy; Milne, Hugh

palliative care 24, 28
perception, subtle 101, 154–7, 176
  see also intuition
phenomenology 90, 144, 165, 175
  see also Merleau-Ponty, Maurice; Sartre,
  Jean-Paul
physical therapy (PT), *see* physiotherapy
physiotherapy 151
placebo 16, 130
Plato 55, 56, 101, 125, 142, 206, 229n4
pleasure 4, 39, 51, 69, 71, 86, 147, 216–18
  see also consumerism – hedonism; senses,
  the – pleasure of
post-structuralism 2, 24, 47, 88, 114, 133,
  149, 220
psychoneuroimmunology (PNI), 25, 175,
  195
power 38, 40–1, 51, 57, 66–8, 78, 98, 113,
  143, 146, 155, 157–9, 160, 179–80
  biomedical 16, 17, 61–4
  practitioner's 70–6, 83–7, 92–6, 105, 169,
  176–7, 190–1, 196
  see also empowerment; neoliberalism;
  surveillance; vision – and power
prana 26, 100, 138, 147, 149, 151, 169
prayer 20, 28, 114, 193, 194, 211, 229n2
presence 114–15, 122, 179, 181, 225n1
  see also metaphysics
psychoanalysis *see* Freud, Sigmund; Reich,
  Wilhelm
Psychophonetics 135–40
psychotherapy 6, 24, 100
  somatic psychotherapy 81, 85, 151
  see also Keleman, Stanley; Reich, Wilhelm

rationality 35, 36, 55, 70, 113, 182, 191
    see also intuition; reason
    scientific 17, 28, 57, 88, 90, 194, 205
reason 90, 173, 174, 175, 182–3, 189, 202,
    218
    death of 17, 88–9, 176, 211–12
    gender and 88, 175, 203
reciprocity 132, 146, 149, 165–6, 168, 172,
    216, 227n3
    see also intercorporeality
Reich, Wilhelm 81–2, 83, 85, 151, 153, 170
reiki 4, 12, 22, 34, 65, 148–9, 169–84, 211
    academic accounts of 176
    author's experiences with 45, 48–9, 51, 149,
        163–4, 172–84, 212, 227–8n6
religion 46
    Christianity 22, 97, 103, 113–14
    music and 131–2
    US metaphysical 28, 29, 31, 103
responsibility 64, 95, 96–7, 213
    see also illness – responsibility for;
        neoliberalism
Rolfing 75, 148, 158, 228n12
Rose, Nikolas 4, 6, 24, 43, 64, 66, 213, 216,
    220
Rubik, Beverly 65, 67, 210, 217

Sartre, Jean-Paul 55, 58
scepticism 16, 42, 46, 113, 177, 183, 189,
    220
Sedgwick, Eve Kosofsky 43, 47, 182, 229n22
Schulz, Mona Lisa 19, 29, 196, 206–9, 219
senses, the 4, 35–6
    gendering of 50, 57, 88, 141
    intersensoriality 51, 145–6, 155–6, 165,
        178–9, 215
    pleasures of 50–1, 52, 142, 160–2
        see also consumerism
    see also sensory studies; smell; synaesthesia;
        taste; touch; vision
sensory studies 4, 50–1, 59
Serres, Michel 144, 145–6, 165, 182–3
Shealy, Norman 19, 209–10, 211
silence 111–15, 127
skin 30, 144–6, 164, 171
smell 51–2, 199–200
Smith, Fritz Frederick 19, 79, 148, 150
Sontag, Susan 29, 43–4

sound
    danger and 127–31
    divinity and 133–5
    harmony and 124–7
    materiality of see materiality – of sound
    sociality and 121–4, 132–3
    temporality and 120–1
sound therapies 8, 116–18, 133
spiritual healing 12, 65, 185–212
spirituality
    Cultural Studies and 46
    discourse of 194–5
    rise of 22, 35
    the body and 4, 35, 106–7
    see also New Age
Stacey, Jackie 4, 21, 38, 39, 42, 44, 63–4,
    80–1, 106, 176, 181, 195
Steiner, Rudolf 135–6, 170
subtle body 119, 147, 151, 159, 194–5, 214
    definition of 26–7, 48
    illness and 30
    knowledge and 176, 191
    lack of distinction between mind and
        matter 29, 66, 166–7
    Psychophonetics and 138–40
    Theosophy and 126, 135–6
surveillance 24, 37, 38, 42, 61, 66, 87, 112
    surveillance medicine 66–7
synaesthesia 122, 156, 215–16
    see also intersensoriality

Tagar, Yehuda 135–40, 170, 214
taste 52
Theosophy 90, 97, 126, 135–6
toning 116, 124
touch
    as a medium of communication 171–84
    as a medium of connection 143, 146,
        157
    dangers of 142, 160–1, 167–8
    eroticism and 161–2
    gender and 141, 158–9, 160–1
    healing power of 150
    intimacy of 76, 141, 161–2
    moral coding of 142, 162
    pleasures of 142, 162–3
    power and 143, 146, 162
    primacy of 141, 143–4, 162–3

role in development 142–5, 157
see also hands; skin
Touch for Health 34, 149
Traditional Chinese Medicine (TCM), 12, 26,
49, 52, 71, 223n35
truth 141–2, 171–2, 177

vibration 116, 119
effect on the body 117, 119, 126, 127,
129–30, 133–5, 138
of the body 119–20, 136, 138–9
see also body, the – as rhythmic
vision
as a tool of reason 55
dominance of 55, 57, 112–14
eyes 60, 69, 73
in Western philosophy 55, 59
male gaze 56, 57
medical gaze 61–4
power and 55, 58–9, 63, 66, 69
relationship to touch 58, 77–8
suspicion of 55–6, 59, 67
therapeutic uses of 99–110
truth and 55, 57, 69
visual techniques 59, 60, 63, 87
see also clairvoyance – vision and;
visualization

visualization 77, 136, 140, 155, 164, 193
creative visualization 59, 60, 99–110
vitalism 15, 23, 172
see also life force
voice, the 112–15
as carrier of meaning 137–7
as guarantor of presence 114, 132
in psychoanalysis 136
speech sounds 136–8
therapeutic power of 121

X-ray 63, 90
see also medical imaging techniques

yoga 77, 97, 99–102, 133
mantras 133–5, 226n13, 226n17
pranayama 100
self-control and 38, 106–7
see also prana
Tratak 101
yoga nidra 100, 104, 160
see also Borg-Olivier, Simon; *chakras*;
chanting; Iyengar, B.K.S.; meditation;
OM

Zero Balancing 79, 148, 154, 164
Zola, Irving 24